The Action of Bioactive Compounds on Human Health or Disease

The Action of Bioactive Compounds on Human Health or Disease

Guest Editor

Jacqueline Isaura Alvarez-Leite

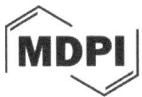

Basel • Beijing • Wuhan • Barcelona • Belgrade • Novi Sad • Cluj • Manchester

Guest Editor
Jacqueline Isaura
Alvarez-Leite
Departamento de Bioquímica
e Imunologia
Universidade Federal de
Minas Gerais
Belo Horizonte
Brazil

Editorial Office
MDPI AG
Grosspeteranlage 5
4052 Basel, Switzerland

This is a reprint of the Special Issue, published open access by the journal *Nutrients* (ISSN 2072-6643), freely accessible at: https://www.mdpi.com/journal/nutrients/special_issues/P0DJ98GP3X.

For citation purposes, cite each article independently as indicated on the article page online and as indicated below:

Lastname, A.A.; Lastname, B.B. Article Title. *Journal Name* **Year**, *Volume Number*, Page Range.

ISBN 978-3-7258-3989-6 (Hbk)
ISBN 978-3-7258-3990-2 (PDF)
https://doi.org/10.3390/books978-3-7258-3990-2

© 2025 by the authors. Articles in this book are Open Access and distributed under the Creative Commons Attribution (CC BY) license. The book as a whole is distributed by MDPI under the terms and conditions of the Creative Commons Attribution-NonCommercial-NoDerivs (CC BY-NC-ND) license (https://creativecommons.org/licenses/by-nc-nd/4.0/).

Contents

About the Editor vii

Preface ix

Jacqueline I. Alvarez-Leite
The Role of Bioactive Compounds in Human Health and Disease
Reprinted from: *Nutrients* **2025**, *17*, 1170, https://doi.org/10.3390/nu17071170 1

Nicola Cecchi, Roberta Romanelli, Flavia Ricevuti, Maria Grazia Carbone, Michele Dinardo, Elisabetta Cesarano, et al.
Bioactives in Oral Nutritional Supplementation: A Pediatric Point of View
Reprinted from: *Nutrients* **2024**, *16*, 2067, https://doi.org/10.3390/nu16132067 6

Montserrat Torres-Vanda and Ruth Gutiérrez-Aguilar
Mexican Plants Involved in Glucose Homeostasis and Body Weight Control: Systematic Review
Reprinted from: *Nutrients* **2023**, *15*, 2070, https://doi.org/10.3390/nu15092070 36

Karenia Lorenzo, Garoa Santocildes, Joan Ramon Torrella, José Magalhães, Teresa Pagès, Ginés Viscor, et al.
Bioactivity of Macronutrients from *Chlorella* in Physical Exercise
Reprinted from: *Nutrients* **2023**, *15*, 2168, https://doi.org/10.3390/nu15092168 61

Bincheng Han, Jinhai Luo and Baojun Xu
Insights into the Chemical Compositions and Health Promoting Effects of Wild Edible Mushroom *Chroogomphus rutilus*
Reprinted from: *Nutrients* **2023**, *15*, 4030, https://doi.org/10.3390/nu15184030 78

Agnieszka Kopystecka, Ilona Kozioł, Dominika Radomska, Krzysztof Bielawski, Anna Bielawska and Monika Wujec
Vaccinium uliginosum and *Vaccinium myrtillus*—Two Species—One Used as a Functional Food
Reprinted from: *Nutrients* **2023**, *15*, 4119, https://doi.org/10.3390/nu15194119 96

Janayne L. Silva, Elandia A. Santos and Jacqueline I. Alvarez-Leite
Are We Ready to Recommend Capsaicin for Disorders Other Than Neuropathic Pain?
Reprinted from: *Nutrients* **2023**, *15*, 4469, https://doi.org/10.3390/nu15204469 123

Mohd Farhan and Asim Rizvi
The Pharmacological Properties of Red Grape Polyphenol Resveratrol: Clinical Trials and Obstacles in Drug Development
Reprinted from: *Nutrients* **2023**, *15*, 4486, https://doi.org/10.3390/nu15204486 140

Marisabel Mecca, Marzia Sichetti, Martina Giuseffi, Eugenia Giglio, Claudia Sabato, Francesca Sanseverino and Graziella Marino
Synergic Role of Dietary Bioactive Compounds in Breast Cancer Chemoprevention and Combination Therapies
Reprinted from: *Nutrients* **2024**, *16*, 1883, https://doi.org/10.3390/nu16121883 164

Mariana Grancieri, Mirelle Lomar Viana, Daniela Furtado de Oliveira, Maria das Graças Vaz Tostes, Mariana Drummond Costa Ignacchiti, André Gustavo Vasconcelos Costa and Neuza Maria Brunoro Costa
Yacon (*Smallanthus sonchifolius*) Flour Reduces Inflammation and Had No Effects on Oxidative Stress and Endotoxemia in Wistar Rats with Induced Colorectal Carcinogenesis
Reprinted from: *Nutrients* **2023**, *15*, 3281, https://doi.org/10.3390/nu15143281 190

Seulmin Hong, Seonkyeong Park, Jangho Lee, Soohyun Park, Jaeho Park and Yugeon Lee
Anti-Obesity Effects of *Pleurotus ferulae* Water Extract on 3T3-L1 Adipocytes and High-Fat-Diet-Induced Obese Mice
Reprinted from: *Nutrients* **2024**, *16*, 4139, https://doi.org/10.3390/nu16234139 . . . . **206**

About the Editor

Jacqueline Isaura Alvarez-Leite

Dr. Alvarez-Leite is a physician specialized in Nutritional Medicine, with a Ph.D. in Biochemistry and Immunology from the Federal University of Minas Gerais (UFMG). She completed her doctoral internship at INRA-France and technical internship at NIH-USA, along with postdoctoral research at Harvard Medical School. She is a Full Professor at UFMG, leading the Laboratory of Atherosclerosis and Nutritional Biochemistry (LABIN-UFMG) and coordinating the Nutritional and Nutritional Therapy Team for Extreme Obesity (ETNNO/UFMG). Her research focuses on Nutritional Biochemistry, particularly antioxidants, obesity, atherosclerosis, and inflammatory bowel diseases.

Preface

We present the reprint "Bioactive Compounds in Health and Disease". Designed for researchers and healthcare professionals, this reprint emphasizes the antioxidant, anti-inflammatory, and antimicrobial properties of bioactive compounds found in foods and herbs. Our goal is to provide valuable and innovative insights into their mechanisms of action and therapeutic potential in health and disease.

Jacqueline Isaura Alvarez-Leite
Guest Editor

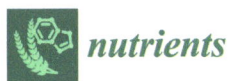

Editorial

The Role of Bioactive Compounds in Human Health and Disease

Jacqueline I. Alvarez-Leite

Departamento of Biochemistry and Immubology, Federal University of Minas Gerais, Belo Horizonte 31270-901, MG, Brazil; jalvarezleite@gmail.com

1. Introduction

Bioactive compounds, natural chemicals found in foods, herbs, and other natural sources, have attracted significant attention for their potential to influence health and fight disease. Unlike macro- and micronutrients necessary for metabolism and human nutrition, bioactive compounds offer benefits that can improve overall well-being and prevent or mitigate various health conditions.

Bioactive compounds have several biological activities. They exert effects such as antioxidants, anti-inflammatories, antimicrobials, and immunomodulator agents [1]. These properties have made these compounds a focus of interest in health and disease prevention [2]. Polyphenols, found in fruits and vegetables, act as antioxidants with therapeutic or adjuvant potential in therapies for diseases such as obesity, diabetes, cardiovascular disease, and cancer, among others [3]. Compounds such as resveratrol, found in grapes and red wine, have shown promising anticancer properties by inhibiting the growth and proliferation of cancer cells [4,5]. Bioactive peptides derived from proteins can modulate blood pressure and glucose metabolism, offering benefits for controlling hypertension and diabetes [6,7]. In addition, numerous phytochemicals in spices and herbs have been identified as possessing anti-obesity and lipid-lowering effects, contributing to weight management and metabolic health [7,8].

This Special Issue of *Nutrients* delves into the multifaceted effects of bioactive compounds, showcasing groundbreaking research and analysis that explores their potential in combating various health challenges. Below is an overview of the articles contained in this Special Issue.

1.1. Anti-Obesity Potential of Pleurotus ferulae

Hong et al. (contribution 1) investigate the anti-obesity effects of *Pleurotus ferulae*, a mushroom used mainly in Asian cuisine. The authors showed that *P. ferulae* extracts reduced weight gain and adiposity in obese mice fed high-fat diets. *P. ferulae* extract also reduced serum lipid, improved profiles, and impaired adipocyte differentiation, suggesting its potential to prevent and control obesity.

1.2. Pediatric Perspective on Bioactive Compounds

Bioactive compounds are not well studied in pediatric populations. In this regard, Cecchi et al. (contribution 2) presented a systematic narrative review that evaluated the literature concerning bioactive compounds present in supplements from a pediatric standpoint. They focused on types, sources, bioavailability, physiological effects, and clinical implications. Several bioactives reinforce the immune system, reducing the incidence and severity of infections in children. They could also support optimal growth trajectories and cognitive function. By functioning as prebiotics, these compounds could improve digestion, enhance nutrient absorption, and improve overall gastrointestinal health. However, clinical trials are necessary to establish the safety and efficacy of bioactives in pediatric populations. Ensuring the quality, purity, and consistency of bioactive-enriched supplements is crucial. While current evidence is promising, more research is needed to confirm their long-term benefits and potential risks.

1.3. Resveratrol: Pharmacological Properties and Challenges

Farhan and Rizvi (contribution 3) present a summary of recent research on the pharmacological properties of resveratrol, known mainly for its potent antioxidant activity. Resveratrol has shown anticancer capabilities by blocking all stages of carcinogenesis. It can also benefit other non-communicable diseases such as diabetes and cardiovascular disease. Clinical and experimental studies suggest that moderate resveratrol supplementation could benefit health. However, there is a long pathway before total knowledge of its action mechanism and bioavailability is achieved, so further research is required before indicating it as a therapy for the prevention of disease.

1.4. Capsaicin and Non-Communicable Diseases

Silva et al. (contribution 4) present a comprehensive examination of capsaicin, the spicy component of chili peppers, in the treatment of non-communicable diseases such as obesity, diabetes, and dyslipidemia. Recent studies highlight the benefits of capsaicin, including improved antioxidant status and gut health. Although research on the use of capsaicinoids and capsinoids as adjuvants for treating obesity, diabetes, dyslipidemia, and cancer is growing, extensive studies remain limited. Capsaicin is shown to improve antioxidant and anti-inflammatory status, induce thermogenesis, and reduce white adipose tissue while also affecting food intake and intestinal health. Despite promising clinical results, most studies are limited to under 12 weeks, and additional investigations are needed to determine optimal dosage, treatment duration, and long-term safety. The impact of capsaicin on gut microbiota and its role in cancer prevention is still in the early stages, requiring further exploration to clarify whether capsaicin is protective or promoting in cancer cases.

1.5. Health-Promoting Effects of Chroogomphus rutilus

Han, Luo, and Xu (contribution 5) revised the chemical compositions and health-promoting effects of *Chroogomphus rutilus*, a wild edible mushroom. Rich in vitamins, proteins, minerals, polysaccharides, and phenolics, C. rutilus exhibits antioxidant, antitumor, immunomodulatory, antifatigue, hypoglycemic, gastroprotective, hypolipidic, and neuronal protective properties that could be beneficial as an adjuvant in the treatment of several diseases. However, the mechanism driving such actions has been poorly studied. Studies addressing *C. rutilus* actions are still restricted to cellular or animal experiments. Further clinical research and practice are needed to verify its safety and efficacy and to promote its use in clinical practice. Despite the remarkable pharmacological effects of *C. rutilus* in vitro and in vivo, there is a lack of information on its safe use, therapeutic index, and risk–benefit ratio in humans. These data will be essential for the development of new pharmaceutical preparations based on the active principles of *C. rutilus*.

1.6. Health Benefits of Anthocyanin-Rich Vaccinium Species

Kopystecka et al. (contribution 6) explore the health benefits of anthocyanin-rich *Vaccinium uliginosum* and *Vaccinium myrtillus*, known as bilberry. These berries exhibit antioxidant, anti-inflammatory, anti-cancer, and apoptosis-reducing activities. The authors believe that they could be helpful as dietary supplements for preventing cancer diseases and cataracts or as a part of sunscreen preparations. Clinical studies confirm their anti-inflammatory, anticancer, and apoptosis-reducing activities, making them valuable additions to a healthy diet. Although studies suggest the prevention and possible treatment of cancer with *V. uliginosum* blueberries, their benefits are still unconfirmed and more clinical research is needed.

1.7. Yacon Flour and Colorectal Cancer

Grancieri et al.'s original study (contribution 7) investigated the effects of yacon flour on inflammation and colorectal cancer in an animal model. They showed that yacon flour reduces inflammation in mice with induced colorectal cancer, indicating its potential as a dietary intervention. The treatment with yacon flour increased fecal secretory immunoglobulin A levels and decreased lipopolysaccharides, tumor necrosis factor-alpha, and interleukin-12. Although yacon flow ingestion did not influence oxidative stress, it reduced inflammation by increasing fecal secretory immunoglobulin A levels and decreasing lipopolysaccharides, tumor necrosis factor-alpha, and interleukin-12. These results make yacon flour a promising food for reducing the damage caused by colorectal cancer. Nonetheless, clinical studies are necessary to confirm its action and safety in those patients.

1.8. Chlorella Macronutrient Bioactivity

Lorenzo et al. (contribution 8) review the bioactivity of the macronutrients of Chlorella, a marine microalga rich in protein and containing all the essential amino acids. The macronutrients in Chlorella have been shown to improve exercise performance and reduce fatigue, attributed to its antioxidant, anti-inflammatory, and metabolic activities. The authors claim that Chlorella proteins increase intramuscular free amino acids and their utilization, sparing glycogen and improving the fatty acid β-oxidation capacity. The cell wall of Chlorella possesses carbohydrates that help maintain a gut microbiota balance and diversity. The authors also state that alpha-linolenic and linolenic fatty acids can contribute to physical performance by favorably modifying the fluidity of cell membranes. This makes Chlorella a promising dietary supplement for exercise-related nutrition. However, as it occurs with several bioactive compounds, more scientific and metabolic studies are necessary to confirm its benefits for humans.

1.9. Mexican Medicinal Plants in Glucose Homeostasis and Weight Management

Torres-Vanda and Gutiérrez-Aguilar (contribution 9), in their systematic review, explore the use of Mexican medicinal plants such as *Momordica charantia* L., *Cucurbita ficifolia bouché*, *Coriandrum sativum* L., *Persea americana* Mill., and *Bidens pilosa* in managing glucose homeostasis and controlling body weight. It has been observed that aqueous and organic extracts from these plants can have hypoglycemic effects by increasing insulin secretion and sensitivity, improving pancreatic β cell function and glucose tolerance, and regulating body weight. It is assumed that these effects are due to the different compounds, such as saponins, phenolic compounds, antioxidants, tannins, triterpenes, avocation B, cytoglobin, etc. Besides the analysis of the action mechanism of each of these plant-derived compounds, there are few studies of their toxicologic potential. In this way, it is still not possible to recommend doses for their hypoglycemic and body weight control effect. Therefore, it is necessary to study the different extracts using in vivo and in vitro models to validate their implications for glucose homeostasis and body weight control.

1.10. Bioactive Compounds and Breast Cancer

Breast cancer remains a major cause of death worldwide. This review (contribution 10) highlights the potential effects of polyunsaturated fatty acids and other bioactive compounds in terms of inhibiting molecular and signaling pathways associated with breast cancer. This review offers valuable insights into how these dietary components may provide natural strategies for the prevention of breast cancer and treatment. The authors conclude that Bromelain, ω-3 PUFAs, sulforaphane, and indole-3-carbinol are promising adjuvants for traditional treatment and chemoprevention for breast cancer due to the low risk of side effects and toxicity. However, using dietary compounds and phytochemicals as part of standard treatment for BC requires further investigation.

2. Conclusions

In summary, bioactive compounds play a key role in improving health and fighting diseases, mainly due to their anti-inflammatory and antioxidant properties. Their ability to modulate physiological processes and target specific disease pathways makes them a focal point in nutritional and medical research. As our understanding of these compounds deepens, their applications in preventive health care and therapeutic interventions continue to expand, offering promising avenues for improving human health and well-being.

Conflicts of Interest: The author declares no conflict of interest.

List of Contributions

1. Hong, S.; Park, S.; Lee, J.; Park, J.; Lee, Y. Anti-Obesity Effects of *Pleurotus ferulae* Water Extract on 3T3-L1 Adipocytes and High-Fat-Diet-Induced Obese Mice. *Nutrients* **2024**, *16*, 4139.
2. Cecchi, N.; Romanelli, R.; Ricevuti, F.; Carbone, M.G.; Dinardo, M.; Cesarano, E.; De Michele, A.; Messere, G.; Morra, S.; Scognamiglio, A.; et al. Bioactives in Oral Nutritional Supplementation: A Pediatric Point of View. *Nutrients* **2024**, *16*, 2067.
3. Farhan, M.; Rizvi, A. The Pharmacological Properties of Red Grape Polyphenol Resveratrol: Clinical Trials and Obstacles in Drug Development. *Nutrients* **2023**, *15*, 4486.
4. Silva, J.L.; Santos, E.A.; Alvarez-Leite, J.I. Are We Ready to Recommend Capsaicin for Disorders Other Than Neuropathic Pain? *Nutrients* **2023**, *15*, 4469.
5. Han, B.; Luo, J.; Xu, B. Insights into the Chemical Compositions and Health Promoting Effects of Wild Edible Mushroom *Chroogomphus rutilus*. *Nutrients* **2023**, *15*, 4030.
6. Kopystecka, A.; Kozioł, I.; Radomska, D.; Bielawski, K.; Bielawska, A.; Wujec, M. *Vaccinium uliginosum* and *Vaccinium myrtillus*—Two Species—One Used as a Functional Food. *Nutrients* **2023**, *15*, 4119.
7. Grancieri, M.; Viana, M.L.; de Oliveira, D.F.; Vaz Tostes, M.d.G.; Costa Ignacchiti, M.D.; Costa, A.G.V.; Brunoro Costa, N.M. Yacon (*Smallanthus sonchifolius*) Flour Reduces Inflammation and Had No Effects on Oxidative Stress and Endotoxemia in Wistar Rats with Induced Colorectal Carcinogenesis. *Nutrients* **2023**, *15*, 3281.
8. Lorenzo, K.; Santocildes, G.; Torrella, J.R.; Magalhães, J.; Pagès, T.; Viscor, G.; Torres, J.L.; Ramos-Romero, S. Bioactivity of Macronutrients from *Chlorella* in Physical Exercise. *Nutrients* **2023**, *15*, 2168.
9. Torres-Vanda, M.; Gutiérrez-Aguilar, R. Mexican Plants Involved in Glucose Homeostasis and Body Weight Control: Systematic Review. *Nutrients*. **2023**, *15*, 2070.
10. Mecca, M.; Sichetti, M.; Giuseffi, M.; Giglio, E.; Sabato, C.; Sanseverino, F.; Marino, G. Synergic Role of Dietary Bioactive Compounds in Breast Cancer Chemoprevention and Combination Therapies. *Nutrients* **2024**, *16*, 1883.

References

1. Babbar, R.; Kaur, A.; Vanya; Arora, R.; Gupta, J.K.; Wal, P.; Tripathi, A.K.; Koparde, A.A.; Goyal, P.; Ramniwas, S.; et al. Impact of Bioactive Compounds in the Management of Various Inflammatory Diseases. *Curr. Pharm. Des.* **2024**, *30*, 1880–1893. [CrossRef] [PubMed]

2. Direito, R.; Barbalho, S.M.; Sepodes, B.; Figueira, M.E. Plant-Derived Bioactive Compounds: Exploring Neuroprotective, Metabolic, and Hepatoprotective Effects for Health Promotion and Disease Prevention. *Pharmaceutics* **2024**, *16*, 577. [CrossRef] [PubMed]
3. Mamun, M.A.A.; Rakib, A.; Mandal, M.; Kumar, S.; Singla, B.; Singh, U.P. Polyphenols: Role in Modulating Immune Function and Obesity. *Biomolecules* **2024**, *14*, 221. [CrossRef] [PubMed]
4. Brown, K.; Theofanous, D.; Britton, R.G.; Aburido, G.; Pepper, C.; Sri Undru, S.; Howells, L. Resveratrol for the Management of Human Health: How Far Have We Come? A Systematic Review of Resveratrol Clinical Trials to Highlight Gaps and Opportunities. *Int. J. Mol. Sci.* **2024**, *25*, 747. [CrossRef] [PubMed]
5. Wu, S.X.; Xiong, R.G.; Huang, S.Y.; Zhou, D.D.; Saimaiti, A.; Zhao, C.N.; Shang, A.; Zhang, Y.-J.; Gan, R.-Y.; Li, H.-B. Effects and mechanisms of resveratrol for prevention and management of cancers: An updated review. *Crit. Rev. Food Sci. Nutr.* **2023**, *63*, 12422–12440. [CrossRef] [PubMed]
6. Purohit, K.; Reddy, N.; Sunna, A. Exploring the Potential of Bioactive Peptides: From Natural Sources to Therapeutics. *Int. J. Mol. Sci.* **2024**, *25*, 1391. [CrossRef] [PubMed]
7. Joshua Ashaolu, T.; Joshua Olatunji, O.; Can Karaca, A.; Lee, C.C.; Mahdi Jafari, S. Anti-obesity and anti-diabetic bioactive peptides: A comprehensive review of their sources, properties, and techno-functional challenges. *Food Res. Int.* **2024**, *187*, 114427. [CrossRef] [PubMed]
8. Hidalgo-Lozada, G.M.; Villarruel-López, A.; Nuño, K.; García-García, A.; Sánchez-Nuño, Y.A.; Ramos-García, C.O. Clinically Effective Molecules of Natural Origin for Obesity Prevention or Treatment. *Int. J. Mol. Sci.* **2024**, *25*, 2671. [CrossRef] [PubMed]

Disclaimer/Publisher's Note: The statements, opinions and data contained in all publications are solely those of the individual author(s) and contributor(s) and not of MDPI and/or the editor(s). MDPI and/or the editor(s) disclaim responsibility for any injury to people or property resulting from any ideas, methods, instructions or products referred to in the content.

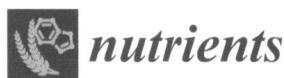

Systematic Review

Bioactives in Oral Nutritional Supplementation: A Pediatric Point of View

Nicola Cecchi [1], Roberta Romanelli [1], Flavia Ricevuti [1,*], Maria Grazia Carbone [1], Michele Dinardo [1], Elisabetta Cesarano [1], Alfredo De Michele [1], Giovanni Messere [1], Salvatore Morra [1], Armando Scognamiglio [1] and Maria Immacolata Spagnuolo [2]

[1] Clinical Nutrition Unit, A.O.R.N. Santobono-Pausilipon Children's Hospital, 80129 Naples, Italy; n.cecchi@santobonopausilipon.it (N.C.); robe.romanelli@gmail.com (R.R.)
[2] Department of Pediatrics, University Federico II of Naples, Via Sergio Pansini 5, 80131 Naples, Italy; mariaimmacolata.spagnuolo@unina.it
* Correspondence: fricevuti@gmail.com; Tel.: +39-3921857397

Abstract: Background: Oral nutritional supplements (ONSs) are crucial for supporting the nutritional needs of pediatric populations, particularly those with medical conditions or dietary deficiencies. Bioactive compounds within ONSs play a pivotal role in enhancing health outcomes by exerting various physiological effects beyond basic nutrition. However, the comprehensive understanding of these bioactives in pediatric ONSs remains elusive. Objective: This systematic narrative review aims to critically evaluate the existing literature concerning bioactive compounds present in oral nutritional supplements from a pediatric standpoint, focusing on their types, sources, bioavailability, physiological effects, and clinical implications. Methods: A systematic search was conducted across the major academic databases, including PubMed, Scopus, and Web of Science, employing predefined search terms related to oral nutritional supplements, bioactives, and pediatrics. Studies published between 2013 and 2024 were considered eligible for inclusion. Data extraction and synthesis were performed according to the PRISMA guidelines. Results: The initial search yielded 558 of articles, of which 72 met the inclusion criteria. The included studies encompassed a diverse range of bioactive compounds present in pediatric ONS formulations, including, but not limited to, vitamins, minerals, amino acids, prebiotics, probiotics, and phytonutrients. These bioactives were sourced from various natural and synthetic origins and were found to exert beneficial effects on growth, development, immune function, gastrointestinal health, cognitive function, and overall well-being in pediatric populations. However, variations in bioavailability, dosing, and clinical efficacy were noted across different compounds and formulations. Conclusions: Bioactive compounds in oral nutritional supplements offer promising avenues for addressing the unique nutritional requirements and health challenges faced by pediatric populations. However, further research is warranted to elucidate the optimal composition, dosage, and clinical applications of these bioactives in pediatric ONS formulations. A deeper understanding of these bioactive compounds and their interplay with pediatric health may pave the way for personalized and effective nutritional interventions in pediatric clinical practice.

Keywords: pediatric; oral nutritional supplements; enteral nutrition; immunonutrition; fibers; inflammatory; immunity; clinical nutrition; bioactive compounds

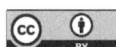

1. Introduction

Oral nutritional supplements (ONSs) are part of the nutritional products for medical nutrition therapy, designed to address specific health conditions and improve overall health and well-being. These products are used under the guidance of healthcare professionals and can include a range of specialized foods, supplements, and enteral or parenteral nutrition solutions. Enteral nutrition (EN) products designed to deliver both macronutrients and/or micronutrients encompass various forms of nutritional support involving the utilization of "Nutritional Products for Medical Nutrition Therapy" as defined by the 2017 European Society for Clinical Nutrition and Metabolism (ESPEN) guidelines [1] on the definitions and terminology of clinical nutrition.

These supplements find extensive application in health settings, particularly for individuals facing challenges in meeting their nutritional needs solely through their oral dietary intake [2].

ONSs are designed to complement the diet of individuals who can eat orally but need extra nutrition: provide balanced nutrition, high protein content for muscle maintenance, and high calories for weight gain or maintain.

ONSs might be recommended for a brief duration during acute illness or for individuals managing long-term chronic conditions and are frequently prescribed or recommended for those at risk of malnutrition. The purpose of ONSs is to supplement nutritional intake, and accompanying guidance on enhancing oral intake should be offered concurrently. Evidence from studies involving adults indicates that the use of ONSs is linked to a decreased length of stay (LOS) [3], lower inpatient episode costs [4], reduced complication rates [5], alleviation of depressive symptoms, lower readmission rates, and enhanced recovery of lean body mass. In pediatrics, nutritional support is crucial for the optimal growth and development of children, and ONSs play a pivotal role in addressing nutritional deficiencies and promoting overall well-being. Furthermore, ONSs, looking at them from the side of children, do not instill that fear of the classic pharmacological/therapeutic treatment of drugs.

ONSs come in diverse formats, such as convenient ready-to-drink beverages (available in milk or juice varieties), powders ideal for meal integration, and delectable dessert-style puddings. Certain products offer a high-fiber variant designed to support optimal bowel function. Additionally, there are products with a denser consistency specifically crafted for individuals dealing with dysphagia. For patients who can fulfill their protein needs but struggle to meet their energy requirements, fat emulsion shots can offer a concentrated source of energy. Table 1 [6] shows the classifications of oral nutritional supplements, clinical indications, and potential advantages linked to the use of these products.

Table 1. Summary of characteristics of oral nutritional supplements and recommendations for use.

Formula Type	Summary of Characteristics	Recommendations for Use
Polymeric	Comprise macronutrients such as unhydrolyzed proteins, fats, and carbohydrates. Varies in concentration within the range of 1–2 kcal/mL. Include essential vitamins and minerals. Might be tailored for specific diseases and/or incorporate prebiotics and probiotics.	Designed for patients without severe malabsorptive disorders.
Fiber-containing	The inclusion of fiber is meant to enhance the well-being of the gastrointestinal tract by regulating the frequency and/or consistency of stool through the maintenance of a healthy GI flora. The fiber content generally falls below the recommended total daily fiber intake. These products may include prebiotics in the form of fructooligosaccharides, oligofructose, or inulin. May incorporate probiotics.	Suggested for patients experiencing diarrhea and/or to support or sustain the gut microbiota.

Table 1. Cont.

Formula Type	Summary of Characteristics	Recommendations for Use
Whole food/blenderized	Whole foods blended to create a texture suitable for enteral consumption, enabling patients to obtain nutritional qualities not present in typical enteral formulas, such as phytochemicals.	Only deemed suitable for application in medically stable patients with a healed feeding tube site and no indications of infection. Should be administered as bolus feeds to uphold safe food practices. Involvement of a dietitian is crucial in formulating the feeding composition to ensure sufficient nutrient delivery.
Diabetes/glucose intolerance	Designed to alleviate hyperglycemia by incorporating a macronutrient composition of 40% carbohydrates, 40% fats, and 20% protein. The presence of fats and soluble fibers in the diet may impede gastric emptying, thereby averting an increase in blood glucose levels.	Current research does not strongly support the use of enteral formulas specifically designed for individuals with diabetes mellitus (DM). Instead, emphasis should be placed on avoiding overfeeding.
Renal	Fluid restricted. Designed with reduced levels of electrolytes, particularly potassium and phosphorus, to avoid excessive supply in patients with renal insufficiency. Protein content may vary.	The initial choice for patients with renal insufficiency should be a standard enteral formula. If there are notable electrolyte imbalances or they arise, contemplation of a renal formula is warranted until electrolyte levels stabilize.
Hepatic	Formulated with reduced protein content featuring a higher proportion of branched-chain amino acids and lower aromatic amino acids to mitigate the risk of hepatic encephalopathy. The lower protein content, however, may lead to insufficient protein delivery. Designed with restrictions on fluid and sodium to lessen the impact of ascites.	As the initial approach, the standard enteral nutrition (EN) formula is recommended for patients with hepatic encephalopathy. Reserve only for individuals with encephalopathy where conventional treatment with luminal-acting antibiotics and lactulose fails to improve the condition.
Elemental/semielemental	Macronutrients are hydrolyzed to maximize absorption.	The objective is to limit enteral delivery to 60–70% of the target energy requirements while ensuring sufficient protein intake. Designed for individuals with malabsorptive disorders; not recommended for regular use.
Pulmonary/fish oil	In efforts to reduce carbon dioxide production, these formulas contain >50% total calories from fat, with lower carbohydrate (<30%) and similar protein content (16–18%). Typically, they also contain ω-3 fatty acids derived from fish oil to increase the delivery of the anti-inflammatory properties of EPA/DHA.	Implement measures to avoid excessive enteral nutrition (EN) delivery, aiming to minimize complications linked to overfeeding. Exercise caution when considering the use of pulmonary formulas in septic and critically ill patients.
Immunonutrition/ immunomodulating	Contain pharmacologically active substances, such as arginine, glutamine, ω-3 fatty acids, γ linolenic acid, nucleotides, and/or antioxidants in efforts to modulate immune function.	Providing immune-modulating substances as part of enteral nutrition (EN) may offer potential benefits for patients undergoing elective surgery. However, the existing research is insufficient to endorse the routine use of immune-modulating formulas for critically ill patients.

In recent years, researchers have investigated the potential benefits of incorporating bioactive molecules into ONS formulations to address specific nutritional needs in children, so the aim of this paper is to discuss the various aspects of ONSs in pediatric nutrition, emphasizing oral supplements enriched with specific functional molecules with specific physiological activities that extend beyond their nutritional value. These molecules exhibit various bioactivities, including antioxidant, anti-inflammatory, and immunomodulatory properties. Understanding the mechanisms of action of these molecules is crucial for elucidating their potential benefits in pediatric nutrition. This review aims to explore the potential advantages of incorporating biocompounds into ONSs for pediatric use.

2. Materials and Methods

This systematic review followed the PRISMA (Preferred Reporting Items for Systematic Reviews and Meta-Analyses) guidelines to ensure comprehensive and transparent reporting of the methods and findings. A PRISMA flow diagram was used to depict the study selection process (Figure 1).

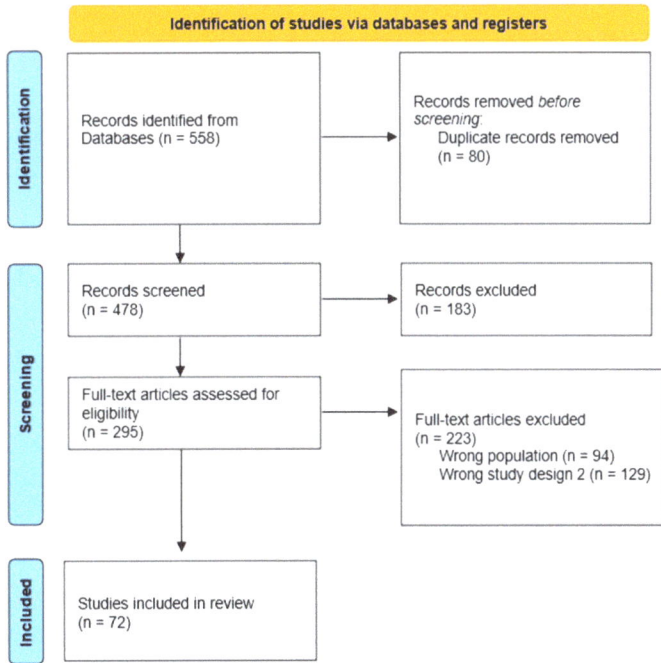

Figure 1. PRISMA flow chart. An overview of the employed systematic search strategy.

In most cases, systematic reviews culminate in either a statistical (quantitative) or narrative (qualitative) summary of findings. Given the nature of the research questions and designs involved in this review, a narrative review approach was employed to synthesize the data. Narrative reviews are particularly useful for exploring studies that investigate the effects of interventions, the factors influencing the implementation of interventions, the needs and preferences of specific population groups, and the causes of particular social and health problems.

2.1. Data Sources and Study Selection

Comprehensive searches were performed across three major academic databases: PubMed, Scopus, and Web of Science. The search strategy utilized a combination of keywords and Medical Subject Headings (MeSH) terms, including "oral nutritional supplements", "bioactives", "pediatrics", "children", "nutritional support", and "health outcomes". Boolean operators (AND and OR) were employed to refine the search queries. The search was restricted to studies published from January 2013 to April 2024. The inclusion criteria encompassed studies published in English, involving pediatric populations aged 0–18 years, investigating bioactive components within oral nutritional supplements, and reporting outcomes related to efficacy, safety, or both. The exclusion criteria comprised studies not relevant to the pediatric population, non-English publications, and those lacking full-text availability. Two independent reviewers screened in blind titles, abstracts, and full texts of identified studies for eligibility, with disagreements resolved through discussion or consultation with a third reviewer.

2.2. Data Extraction

Data were independently extracted by two reviewers (RR and FR) using a standardized form using software for systematic reviews [7]. The extracted information included study characteristics (author, year, country, and study design), population details (age and sample size), types of bioactive compounds, sources of bioactives (natural or synthetic), the outcomes measured, and key findings related to the effects of bioactives on the specified outcomes.

2.3. Results

The initial search identified 558 articles, of which 72 met the inclusion criteria. These studies examined a wide range of bioactive compounds present in pediatric ONS formulations, including vitamins, minerals, amino acids, prebiotics, probiotics, and phytonutrients. These bioactives, sourced from both natural and synthetic origins, demonstrated beneficial effects on growth, development, immune function, gastrointestinal health, cognitive function, and overall well-being in pediatric populations. However, there were noted variations in bioavailability, dosing, and clinical efficacy across different compounds and formulations.

3. Dietary Fibers as Bioactive Compounds in Oral Nutritional Supplements

Dietary fibers encompass a diverse array of substances crucial for gut health and a healthy microbiome, but not all oral nutritional supplements contain fiber. Why? Many children with digestive diseases or conditions (e.g., strictures or recurrent small bowel obstructions) need to avoid fiber in the short- or long-term. Oral nutritional supplements with added fiber can be a valuable tool in promoting the overall health of children, especially those facing nutritional challenges. The American Gastroenterology Association (AGA) and the European Society of Pediatric Gastroenterology, Hepatology, and Nutrition (ESPGHAN) recently published different evidence-based recommendations.

This paragraph reviews the physiological effects of dietary fiber, the impact of fiber on gastrointestinal health, and the potential synergies between fiber and essential nutrients in ONSs in the pediatric population. Additionally, we discuss the challenges and opportunities associated with formulating ONSs with added fiber, along with emerging research directions in this evolving field. By delving into the scientific and clinical aspects of ONSs with added fiber, this paper aims to contribute to the growing body of knowledge surrounding nutritional and dietary supplementation.

The importance of the dietary fiber children consume is just as significant as the quantity they intake. The majority of oral nutritional supplements, including those with added fiber, are still considered to be low-fiber and below the recommended amount per day. Fiber is crucial for preserving the structure and function of the gut microbiome, promoting overall host health [8]. The latest agreement suggests that dietary fiber consists of carbohydrate polymers that undergo neither digestion nor absorption in the human intestine. Instead, they proceed to the large bowel, where the colonic microbiota partially or completely ferment them.

Dietary fibers and whole grains consist of a unique blend of bioactive components, incorporating plant non-starch polysaccharides like cellulose, pectin, gums, hemicelluloses, and β-glucans, as well as vitamins, minerals, phytochemicals, and antioxidants. Natural fibers refer specifically to dietary fibers naturally occurring in the cell wall or inner layer of diverse edible plants, fruits, vegetables, cereals, nuts, pulses, and seaweed. Furthermore, fibers can be derived from plants or food and undergo modifications through different processing techniques [9]. The physicochemical properties of various dietary fibers, including solubility, viscosity, and fermentability, exhibit significant variations based on their origin and processing. These factors play a crucial role in determining the functional characteristics and clinical efficacy of dietary fibers. Even with advancements in comprehending these connections, numerous clinical inquiries persist, such as determining the optimal dosage, type, and source of fiber essential for effectively managing clinical symptoms and preventing gastrointestinal disorders [10]. Despite endeavors to promote healthy eating habits, certain factors, such as picky eating, medical conditions, or lifestyle constraints, may impede some children from meeting their nutritional needs. In such instances, oral nutritional supplements (ONSs) serve as a valuable tool to bridge nutritional gaps. The incorporation of fiber into ONSs for children is particularly noteworthy due to its contributions to digestive health, satiety, and disease prevention.

In studies evaluating the effects of fibers in children, no serious adverse events have been reported. Since fibers are resistant to digestion and are not absorbed in the human small intestine, partial or complete fermentation occurs in the large intestine, leading to flatulence, diarrhea, abdominal distention, and discomfort. These effects vary based on the quantity and type of fibers, other food components, the gut microbiota, and individual response and sensitivity [11–14].

3.1. Prebiotic Fibers in Oral Nutritional Supplementations for Children

Non-digestible fermentable carbohydrates, or fermentable or "prebiotic" fibers, are a heterogeneous group of polysaccharides and oligosaccharides constituting dietary fiber. These compounds, therefore, could be defined as "nourishment for the intestinal microbiota", which can be modulated and regulated, thus promoting microbial diversity, which in turn affects the regulation of energy metabolism, intestinal homeostasis, and the production of metabolites that actively participate in immune responses. Currently, the literature extensively documents only resistant oligosaccharides, such as fructans and galactans, as accepted prebiotics. Other fibers are regarded as potential prebiotics or possess prebiotic potential, while some seem to lack a discernible prebiotic effect on humans [15]. Among the fermentable fibers, galacto-oligosaccharides (or GOSs, present in breast milk and yogurts) and fructo-oligosaccharides (or FOSs, present in *Liliaceae*, bananas, rye, and wheat) are especially well known, with a prebiotic role mainly on the colon microbiota [16]. These functional food components, as shown, may be naturally present in plant-based foods or produced synthetically through the enzymatic conversion of sugars [17]. Functional oligosaccharides, including galacto-oligosaccharides (GOSs), fructo-oligosaccharides (FOSs), xylo-oligosaccharides, isomaltose, and human milk oligosaccharides, reach the colon and act with unique physiological functions: preventing intestinal obstruction or diarrhea, regulating intestinal flora, or promoting the proliferation of bifidobacteria, positive effect on lipid metabolism, stimulating mineral absorption, and immunomodulatory properties [11,18] (Table 2).

Table 2. Summary of characteristics of prebiotics and recommendations for use [11,18].

Prebiotic	Health Benefits
FOS	Enhances gut health by fostering the proliferation and function of beneficial gut bacteria; aids in regulating blood sugar levels by delaying carbohydrate digestion; potentially lowers the risk of specific cancers; may contribute to better bone health through enhanced calcium absorption; and could diminish the risk of heart disease by lowering cholesterol levels and inflammation.
GOS	Enhances gut health by stimulating the growth and function of beneficial gut bacteria; alleviates the risk of constipation and related digestive problems by promoting regular bowel movements; boosts the immune system through heightened production of beneficial bacteria; lowers the likelihood of infections and inflammatory bowel conditions; and may aid in weight management by enhancing satiety and reducing calorie consumption.

Why are some oral nutritional supplements added with functional oligosaccharides/prebiotic fibers such as GOSs, FOSs, or a mixture? See Figure 2 [19,20].

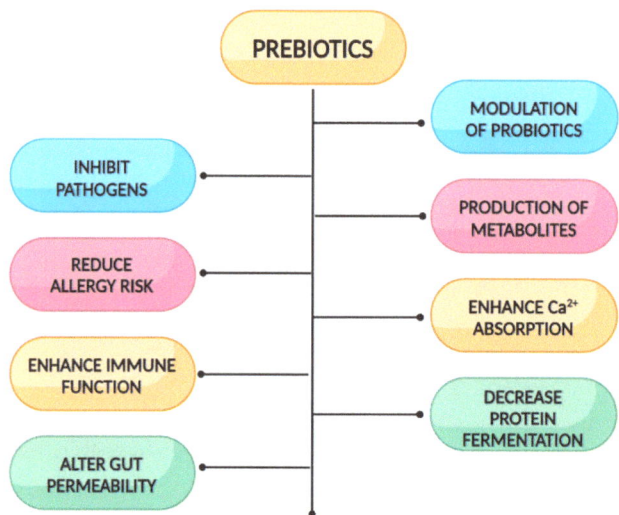

Figure 2. The effects of prebiotics on pediatric health outcomes. Prebiotics contribute to various health benefits by inhibiting pathogens, reducing allergy risk, enhancing immune function, and altering gut permeability. They also modulate probiotics, produce beneficial metabolites, enhance calcium absorption, and decrease protein fermentation. These multifaceted effects highlight the importance of prebiotics in oral nutritional supplements for pediatric populations.

3.1.1. Fructo-Oligosaccharides (FOSs)

Fructo-oligosaccharides and inulin (fructans) are made up of fructose chains of variable lengths with a terminal glucose molecule. Fructose units are joined by β $(1\rightarrow2)$ bonds while glucose units are connected by α $(1\rightarrow1)$ bonds, similar to that present in sucrose. From a chemical point of view, FOSs and inulin differ in their degree of polymerization (DP): from 3 to 10 for FOSs, up to 60 for inulin (polymer). Fructo-oligosaccharides (FOSs) remain structurally unchanged as they bypass hydrolysis by small intestinal glycosidases and reach the cecum. In the intestinal environment, they undergo metabolism by the gut microflora, resulting in the production of short-chain carboxylic acids, L-lactate, CO(2), hydrogen, and other metabolites. FOSs possess several intriguing characteristics, including mild sweetness, zero calorie content, non-cariogenic properties, and recognition as soluble dietary fiber. Additionally, FOSs offer significant physiological benefits, such as reduced carcinogenicity, a prebiotic impact, enhanced mineral absorption, and lowered levels of serum cholesterol, triacylglycerols, and phospholipids [21].

Although consensus on the optimal type and quantity of fiber for children remains elusive, evidence suggests that dietary fibers play a crucial role in maintaining healthy gastrointestinal functions and preventing childhood constipation. Constipation, a prevalent condition affecting 3–29% of children globally, often begins in infancy and persists in 35–52% of cases for years [22]. The ESPGHAN/NAPGHAN guidelines advocate for a standard dietary fiber intake for children with functional constipation, although data on the most advantageous fiber type or source for these children are scarce, and recommendations are lacking [23]. Recently, a prospective study tested a mixture of polydextrose (4.17 g) and FOSs (0.45 g) in a daily dose of food supplement in 77 children. The number of children with less than three bowel movements per week dropped from 59.7% to 11.7%, hard stools (Bristol type 1 and 2) decreased from 68.8% to 7.8%, pain during defecation decreased from 79.2% to 10.4%, fear of defecation decreased from 68.8% to 3.9%, and the number of children with abdominal pain symptoms reduced from 84.2% to 2.6% at the end of the study. Significantly, there was no comparison conducted with a control group [24].

Microbiome-targeted treatments, such as fiber and prebiotics, hold promise for rebalancing the gut microbiome and improving both gut health and clinical outcomes for the host. Indeed, research on adult patients with inflammatory bowel disease (IBD) shows that fiber and prebiotics can positively influence the microbiome and ameliorate disease progression. However, as of now, there have been no studies assessing the therapeutic efficacy of fiber and prebiotics in pediatric IBD patients [25].

3.1.2. Biological Effects of Galacto-Oligosaccharides (GOSs)

This paper tries to also explore the association of galacto-oligosaccharides with oral nutritional supplements, aiming to understand their potential health-promoting properties. These investigations explore the impact of such supplements on various aspects of health, including intestinal barrier function, lactose intolerance, constipation relief, and potentially other health-related outcomes. Researchers have aimed to understand the potential advantages and mechanisms of action associated with GOSs in oral nutritional supplements. GOSs have been shown to enhance the production of health-related short-chain fatty acids (SCFAs), stimulate the growth and differentiation of colonic epithelial cells, improve energy transduction in colonocytes, and influence lipid and carbohydrate metabolism. GOSs serve essential functions in milk and are a widely employed prebiotic substance [11]. The presence of GOSs in the diet has been associated with various beneficial biological activities. Research conducted by He et al. in 2021 indicated that the supplementation of GOSs to a high-fat diet effectively stimulates the growth of bifidobacteria. Bifidobacteria, known for their ability to produce lactic acid, contribute to the acidification of the intestinal environment [26]. This acidification helps in restraining the growth of pathogenic bacteria and enhances the mucosal barrier's function. Infants who received prebiotic supplements had softer stools compared to those receiving standard formula, with stool consistency resembling that of breastfed infants.

Numerous studies in both animals and humans have indicated the positive impact of GOSs on bone composition and structure. Several mechanisms have been proposed: firstly, bacterial fermentation of acidic metabolites in the colon lowers the local pH in the intestine, leading to an increased luminal concentration of calcium ions and enhanced passive calcium absorption; secondly, short-chain fatty acids (SCFAs) alter the charge of calcium, stimulate calcium channels, and promote increased calcium absorption [27].

GOSs perform a crucial function in alleviating lactose intolerance and preventing constipation (Figure 3 [28]). Oligosaccharides found in human milk contribute to the development of beneficial intestinal microbiota in infants, particularly *Bifidobacterium* and *Lactobacillus* [29]. While human milk oligosaccharides are limited and primarily found in the colostrum of various mammals, making the cost of HMOs high, GOSs derived from lactose exhibits notable prebiotic properties and share a structural resemblance to HMOs. Comprising two to seven galactose units with a glucose molecule at the terminus, GOSs are a cost-effective alternative [28]. Oral nutritional supplements enriched with GOSs present a promising avenue for promoting health and addressing specific gastrointestinal issues. This review consolidates existing knowledge, highlighting the potential benefits of incorporating GOSs into oral nutritional supplements and suggesting avenues for future research.

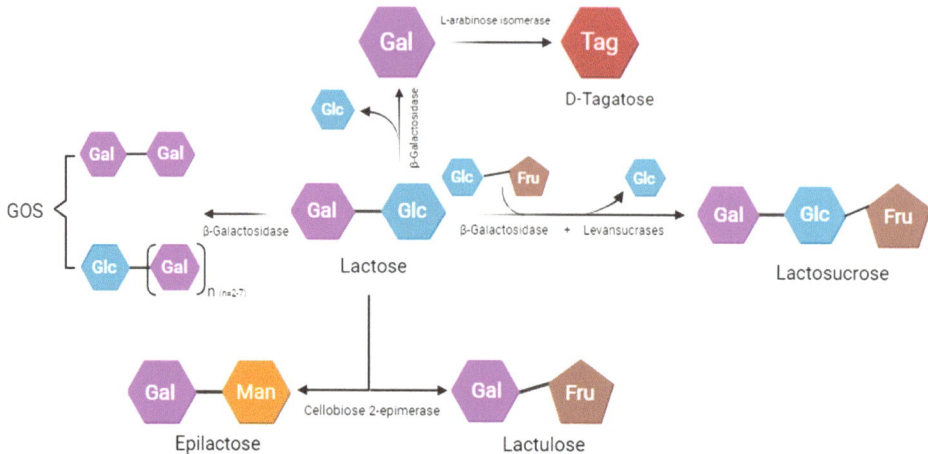

Figure 3. An overview of the enzymatic production of functional lactose derivatives.

4. Oral Nutritional Supplements Enriched with Transforming Growth Factor-Beta 2 (TGF-Beta)

Nutritional support plays an important role in the treatment of inflammatory bowel diseases (IBDs). Oral nutritional supplements enriched with specific bioactive peptides seem to have a direct effect on the intestinal mucosa by suppressing the inflammatory process [30]. Moreover, supplementary enteral nutrition after primary therapy and after remission is induced may be associated with the prolongation of remission and promotion of linear growth in patients with IBD [31], particularly in Crohn's disease (CD), a chronic, relapsing transmural inflammation characterized by skip intestinal lesions anywhere in the GI tract [32]. The leading biocompound that appears to play important roles in the inflammatory processes exhibited in IBD is the transforming growth factor (TGF)-β superfamily (thirty-three genes that encode for homodimeric or heterodimeric secreted cytokines) [33], which includes TGF-β (TGF-β1, TGF-β2, and TGF-β3) and related proteins (activins, growth and differentiation factors (GDFs), the bone morphogenetic proteins (BMPs), the müllerian inhibiting substance (MIS), and the nodal). TGF-β is a multifunctional cytokine expressed by many types of cells [34], such as epithelial cells, fibroblasts, and immune cells, particularly leukocytes and macrophages, with various immunomodulatory roles especially relevant to the GI tract. This cytokine contributes to the regulation of several key cellular functions, including cell proliferation, differentiation, migration, apoptosis, and extracellular matrix production [35]. TGF-β ligands bind to pairs of transmembrane receptors known as receptor types I and II [36]. The resulting TGF-β receptor complex triggers intracellular signaling via both the Smad-dependent canonical and the Smad-independent non-canonical pathways. SMAD proteins are the major effector molecules in the TGF-β signaling pathway, through phosphorylation at specific Ser residues in their C-terminal regions. These SMAD proteins, called "receptor-regulated SMADs" (R-SMADs), associate with the common mediator SMAD4 protein, form trimeric complexes, and are then shuttled to the nucleus. These complexes can directly bind on specific DNA sequences that have been characterized as being SMAD-binding elements (SBEs) and cooperate with DNA-binding transcription factors and chromatin modifiers to regulate the expression of TGF-β-responsive genes (Figure 4a,b) [37].

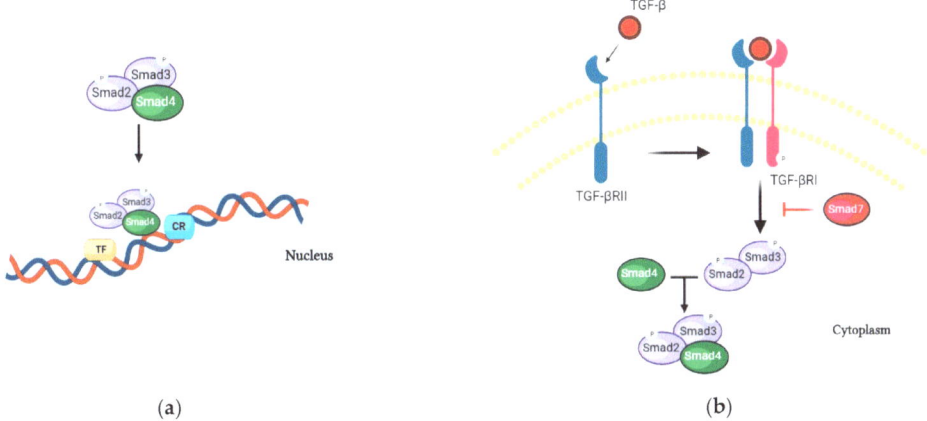

Figure 4. (**a**). TGF-β intracellular signaling through the Smad-dependent canonical pathway. TGF-β binds to transmembrane type I and type II receptors. Receptor-regulated SMADs associate with the common mediator SMAD4 protein and form trimeric complexes. (**b**). The SMAD complex is shuttled to the nucleus, where it binds to specific DNA sequences and cooperates with DNA-binding transcription factors and chromatin modifiers to regulate the expression of TGF-β-responsive genes.

SMADs are capable of regulating gene expression at the post-transcriptional level as well, impacting mRNA splicing, stability, and translation through interactions with RNA-binding proteins (RBPs) and non-coding RNAs (ncRNAs) [38]. Among the various recognized mechanisms, TGF-β seems to be a key modulator of innate and adaptive immunity, acting as a general enforcer of immune tolerance and a suppressor of inflammation. For this reason, TGF-β has been considered, in particular, for the treatment of IBD, administered directly or through formulas added with TGF-β content. Some studies have shown that the consumption of a formula enriched with TGF-β is associated with a reduction in the expression of cytokines in the intestinal mucosa with a concomitant improvement in histologic parameters in children and teenagers [39]. TGF-β regulates multiple immune processes of T-cells. A major function of TGF-β signaling in T-cells is to regulate and balance the differentiation of naive T-cells into specific effector subsets, in particular, to suppress T-cell proliferation and activation through Treg differentiation. TGF-β inhibits, through the induction of Foxp3 (a master regulator of Tregs), the maturation of naive CD4+ T-cells into TH1 and TH2 T helper cells and of naive CD8+ T-cells into cytotoxic T lymphocytes (CTLs), promoting instead their differentiation to the Treg stage [40], a specialized subpopulation of T-cells that act to suppress the immune response, is able to inhibit T-cell proliferation and cytokine production, and plays a critical role in preventing autoimmunity.

TGF-β also inhibits the function of dendritic cells (DCs), responsible for the antigen presentation to CD4+ T-cells and CD8+ T-cells [41] and suppresses natural killer (NK) cells and their production of interferon-γ (IFN-γ) (Figure 5) [42].

TGF-β also plays an integral role in the process of healing of the intestinal mucosa and in the development of fibrosis and strictures [43] through regulation of fibroblast activity, the main producers of connective tissue matrix which play a key role in tissue repair. TGF-β potently induces the recruitment, proliferation, and activation of fibroblasts that produce collagens, fibronectin, and other components required for extracellular matrix (ECM) assembly, as well as integrins that mediate cell adhesion to the ECM [44] (see Table 3).

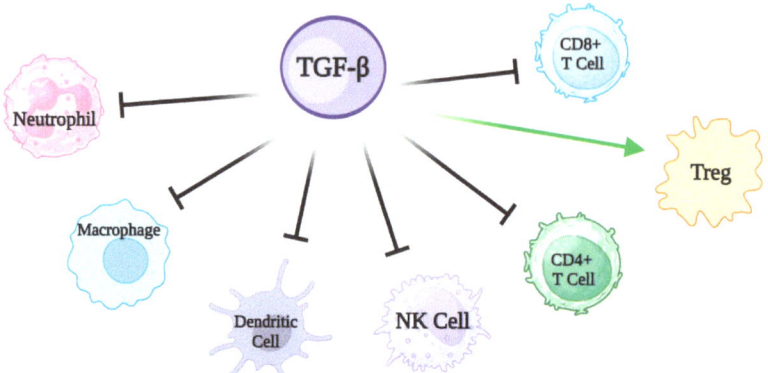

Figure 5. TGF-β's effects on different cells of the immune system. TGF-β suppresses all kinds of cells of the immune system, such as CD8(+) and CD4(+) T-cells, NK cells, dendritic cells, macrophages, and neutrophils. In addition, TGF-β induces Treg cells.

Table 3. The role of TGF-β present in ONSs.

	Disease	Functions
ONSs Supplemented with TGF-β	IBD	Immunomodulatory roles especially relevant to the GI tract.
		Healing of the intestinal mucosa and in the development of fibrosis and stenosis through the regulation of fibroblast activity.

In studies conducted on nutritional supports enriched with TGF-β, was found an improvement on mucosal healing and remission induction. Furthermore, it was demonstrated that C-Reactive Protein levels, sedimentation rates, reductions in PCDAI, and albumin levels showed significant improvement in these patients [45,46]. In the light of these data, oral nutritional supplements enriched with TGF-β, given in addition to medical treatments without restricting normal diets, avoided the potential side effects of steroids in CD patients, remained in remission for longer durations, and contributed to improving anthropometrics data.

In studies investigating oral nutritional supplements enhanced with TGF-beta (transforming growth factor-beta), no serious side effects were reported among the patients. The minor side effects that were occasionally observed, such as abdominal pain and abdominal distention, were infrequent and typically resolved quickly [47].

5. Immunonutrition and Oral Nutritional Supplements

Immunonutrition (IN) is characterized as the utilization of particular nutritional substrates, referred to as "immunonutrients", which possess the capability to modulate specific mechanisms involved in various immune and inflammatory pathways. Numerous nutrients could fit into this description, and among these, the most defined are Omega 3 polyunsaturated fatty acids, arginine, branched-chain amino acids, trace metals (e.g., zinc, copper, and iron), vitamin D, and nucleotides [48]. These immunonutrients primarily target mucosal barrier function, cellular defense, and either local or systemic inflammation [49]. Recent research works have indicated that combinations of immunonutrients, incorporating omega-3 fatty acids, glutamine, arginine, and nucleotides, may be advantageous for certain patient populations. This is usually associated with a decrease in both hospital length of stay and infection rates. Nevertheless, there was no observed reduction in mortality. Moreover, various immunonutrients like proteins, vitamins, trace metals, and enzymes possess antioxidant properties, mitigating tissue damage and lowering the risk of carcinogenesis [50]. Therefore, the proposition of utilizing oral nutritional supplements enriched with certain immunonutrients is suggested as a nutritional treatment approach. This method could serve as an option to meet nutritional needs and regulate the immune response in patients with particular pathologies, cancer, or those preparing for surgery. However, evidence-based recommendations for the use of these formulations in pediatric clinical practice are scarce and confined to specific populations. This discussion focuses on the characteristic changes in innate and acquired immunity that occur during critical illness, as well as the mechanisms through which immune nutrients can beneficially influence the immune response (Table 4).

Table 4. Bioactive nature of the components and their roles within oral nutrition supplements targeted at enhancing physiological functions in pediatric populations.

Oral Nutrition Supplements	Characteristics	Where Is It?	Functions
Arginine	Conditionally essential amino acid in situations such as developmental stages and certain pathological conditions (infection or inflammation, or under conditions of impaired renal and/or intestinal metabolic functions), where endogenous production is insufficient.	Seafood, watermelon juice, nuts, seeds, algae, meats, rice protein concentrate, and soy protein isolate.	- Plays a role in immunoregulation. - Precursor of proteins, nitric oxide, proline, creatine, agmatine, and polyamine. - Induces the secretion of hormones such as insulin, glucagon, growth hormone, and prolactin.
Omega-3	Are polyunsaturated fatty acids (PUFAs) characterized by a double bond at the n-3 position. These PUFAs include eicosapentaenoic acid (EPA), alpha-linolenic acid (ALA), and docosahexaenoic acid (DHA). Alpha-linolenic acid is essential (ALA).	EPA and DHA are mainly found in the marine ecosystem, fish and seafood, but also in leafy vegetables and nuts, which are famous for their high n-3 FA content, making them the main source of ALA. Leafy vegetables and nuts are also famous for their high n-3 FA content, making them the main source of ALA.	- Affects the structure and function of biological membranes, such as elasticity, membrane organization, and ion permeability. - Reduces the production of inflammatory cytokines TNFα and IL-6.
Nucleotides	Consist of a sugar molecule (ribose in RNA or deoxyribose in DNA), a phosphate group, and a nitrogen-containing base. The bases found in DNA are adenine (A), cytosine (C), guanine (G), and thymine (T), while RNA substitutes uracil (U) for thymine. Both DNA and RNA molecules are polymers composed of extended chains of nucleotides.	Nucleotides are obtained in the diet and are also synthesized from common nutrients by the liver. Naturally found in all foods of both animal and plant origin (healthy individuals typically consume 1–2 g of nucleotides daily through their diet), or through endogenous synthesis, which serves as the primary source of nucleotides.	- Play a fundamental role in organismal physiology, serving as the fundamental units of nucleic acids and repositories of chemical energy. - Carriers of activated metabolites for biosynthesis, structural components of coenzymes, and regulators of metabolism.

5.1. Arginine

L-arginine is categorized as a conditionally essential amino acid. In fact, there are instances, such as developmental stages and certain pathological conditions (infection or inflammation, or under conditions in which renal and/or intestinal metabolic functions are impaired), where the endogenous production is insufficient. Consequently, a dietary intake becomes necessary in these situations [51]. Arginine freely available in the body is sourced from the diet (it is abundant in seafood, watermelon juice, nuts, seeds, algae, meats, rice protein concentrate, and soy protein isolate [52]), de novo synthesis, and protein turnover. While the synthesis of arginine from citrulline is possible in various cell types [53], a significant portion of endogenous synthesis takes place through a cooperative process involving the epithelial cells of the small intestine and the proximal tubule cells of the kidney [54], a pathway known as the "Intestinal-Renal Axis" of arginine synthesis. In fact, the gut is the main source of citrulline for the synthesis of L-arginine. Enterocytes in the small intestine express carbamyl phosphate synthetase I and ornithine transcarbamylase. This expression allows for the synthesis of citrulline from glutamine, proline, or ornithine. Citrulline is absorbed by the proximal tubules of the kidney and undergoes efficient conversion to arginine through the sequential action of argininosuccinate synthetase and argininosuccinate lyase (ASL) (Figure 6) [54].

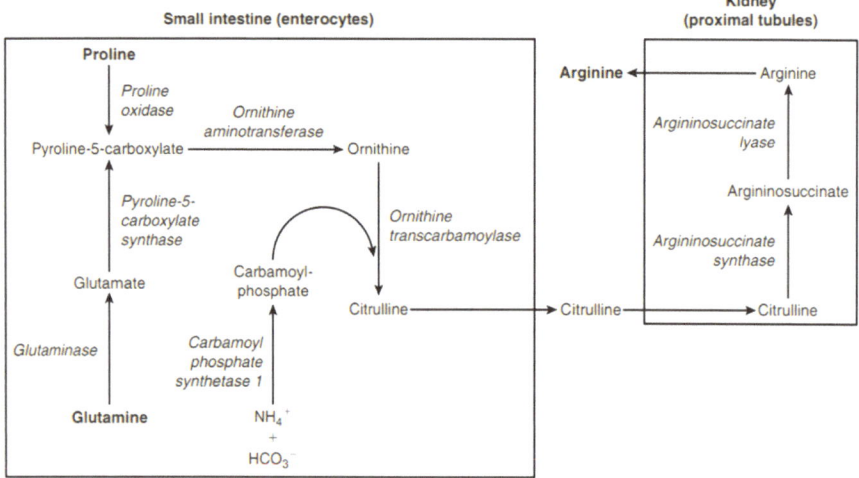

Figure 6. Intestinal–renal axis for the endogenous synthesis of arginine in adult animals.

Within the liver, possessing a fully functional urea cycle, arginine is synthesized from ornithine, carbamoyl phosphate, and the amino group sourced from aspartate. However, the hepatic urea cycle does not yield a net production of arginine, as the synthesis of arginine within the cycle precisely matches its breakdown. Consequently, the liver does not serve as a net source of arginine.

Arginine serves as the precursor for several crucial substances within the organism, including proteins, nitric oxide, proline, creatine, agmatine, and polyamine. Additionally, it can trigger the secretion of hormones such as insulin, glucagon, growth hormone, and prolactin. Furthermore, it plays a role in immunoregulation [55]. Numerous enzymes are involved in the degradation of arginine, including arginase, three variants of nitric oxide synthase (NOS), arginine decarboxylase (ADC), and arginine:glycine amidinotransferase (AGAT) [56]. The three NOS isoenzymes (I/nNOS; II/iNOS; and III/eNOS) [57] exhibit variations in structural properties, distribution, regulation, and the production of nitric oxide quantities. Each of the three NOS enzymes utilizes L-arginine as a substrate, leading to a reaction where N-hydroxy-L-arginine (L-NOHA) serves as an intermediate, releasing both nitric oxide (NO) and L-citrulline [58]. NOS I and NOS III operate in a Ca^{2+}-dependent and constitutively expressed manner, while NOS II functions independently of Ca^{2+} and is abundantly expressed in response to immunological challenges [56]. NOS relies on various cofactors, such as flavin adeninedinucleotide (FAD), flavin mononucleotide (FMN), heme, and tetrahydrobiopterin (BH4), which is crucial and acts as the rate-limiting factor [59]. NO governs multiple signaling pathways across various tissues, playing diverse physiological roles. Its most recognized and established functions are associated with the immune, cardiovascular, and neuronal systems. Notably, NO is generated by various immune cells, primarily macrophages, serving as a crucial regulator of immunity and inflammation [60]. Within the cardiovascular system, NO derived from the endothelium acts as a potent vasodilator, playing a pivotal role in determining vascular tone and blood pressure [61]. Finally, in the nervous system, NO originating from neurons is recognized for its role in regulating neural development and influencing diverse brain functions, including cognition and response to stress [62]. New findings indicate that NO plays a significant role in governing the homeostasis of both the fetus and neonate [63].

Similar to the production of NO, arginine plays a unique role as the exclusive amino acid supplying the amidino group for creatine synthesis. In this process, arginine acts as a donor for transferring the amidino group to a glycine backbone. The catalysis of this reaction is carried out by L-arginine glycine amidinotransferase (AGAT), resulting in the generation of ornithine and guanidinoacetic acid. Creatine plays a major role in energy metabolism in skeletal muscle and neuronal cells [64]. Instead, arginase is a classical enzyme in the urea cycle that facilitates the hydrolysis of L-arginine into urea and L-ornithine. There are two distinct forms of mammalian arginase: type I and type II, each governed by separate genes. Type I arginase is a cytosolic enzyme prominently present in the liver. It plays a crucial role as a key element in the transport, storage, and excretion of nitrogen, serving as an essential factor in ammonia detoxification through the urea cycle. This function aids in averting metabolic disruptions caused by heightened levels of tissue ammonia [65]. Type II arginase is a mitochondrial enzyme characterized by modest expression levels in various tissues, such as the small intestine, kidney, brain, endothelium, mammary gland, and macrophages [66]. It plays an important role in regulating the synthesis of NO, proline, and polyamines [67]. Polyamines, such as putrescine, spermine, and spermidine, play roles in membrane transport as well as in cell growth, cell proliferation, and cell differentiation [68]. Additionally, arginine triggers the release of growth hormones and insulin in mammals, including preterm infants, thereby playing a crucial role in overseeing protein, lipid, and carbohydrate metabolism [69].

The significance of arginine in metabolic pathways leading to protein synthesis and the elimination of nitrogenous waste, along with its involvement in cell signaling, proliferation, differentiation, and stimulation of the immune system, is firmly established. What still needs clarification is whether dietary arginine can be supplemented at pharmacological levels to influence metabolic outcomes. In fact, maintaining an adequate supply of arginine has been closely linked to enhancing immune responses. Beyond its role as a building block for protein synthesis, arginine functions as a substrate for various metabolic pathways that significantly impact the biology of immune cells, particularly macrophages, dendritic cells, and T-cells. For instance, the administration of additional arginine exhibits positive effects on the immune system, specifically influencing thymus-dependent and T-cell-dependent immune responses. Initial animal experiments illustrated the thymotropic effects of arginine, evident in increased thymic weight, elevated thymic lymphocyte content, and heightened reactivity of thymic lymphocytes [65]. In various experimental models, additional immunomodulatory effects of arginine have been observed. Arginine supplementation has been shown to alleviate the diminished delayed-type hypersensitivity response typically associated with extreme youth age [70]. In 2001, Waugh and colleagues conducted a preliminary phase II clinical trial involving five pediatric participants (aged 10–18 years) diagnosed with sickle cell disease. Their trial revealed that administering oral L-citrulline at doses ranging from 0.09 to 0.13 g/kg twice daily over a four-week period led to a 65% increase in plasma arginine concentrations, resulting in the normalization of leukocyte and neutrophil counts [71].

In a double-blind, randomized, placebo-controlled trial investigating enteral arginine supplementation in burned children, Veronica B. Marin et al. aimed to address the existing gap in data for pediatric burn patients [72]. Their study compared the effects of supplemental dietary arginine with an isocaloric and isonitrogenous placebo diet, seeking to elucidate the specific roles of arginine in immune and metabolic responses in children affected by burns. Twenty-eight children who met the criteria were randomly divided into two groups: one receiving an arginine-supplemented diet (AG; $n = 14$) and the other receiving an isocaloric isonitrogenous diet (CG; control, $n = 14$) for a duration of 14 days. This study found that a diet exclusively supplemented with arginine enhances mitogen-stimulated lymphocyte proliferation in burned children. The immunological advantage noted in the AG group was linked to heightened arginine disposal and metabolism. This was evidenced by elevated ornithine levels resulting from the pharmacokinetic properties of arginine, including increased turnover and oxidation, restricted synthesis, and irreversible conversion to ornithine. Following the noted immunostimulatory effects of arginine, there has been a growing interest in dietary arginine supplementation, aiming to formulate what are referred to as immune-enhancing diets [73]. Nutrition formulas enriched with arginine have demonstrated benefits in both animal and human trials. However, there is limited evidence suggesting that arginine alone is accountable for these positive effects, as the immune-enhancing diets also included other pharmacologically active components [74].

Reports of side effects from arginine administration are primarily derived from animal studies or in vitro studies, which indicate that these side effects are minimal and generally transient. Theoretically, an overdose of arginine could lead to hypotension due to its vasodilatory effects [75].

5.2. Omega 3

Omega-3 (n-3) are polyunsaturated fatty acids (PUFAs) characterized by a double bond at the n-3 position. These PUFAs include eicosapentaenoic acid (EPA), alpha-linolenic acid (ALA), and docosahexaenoic acid (DHA). Mammals lack the ability to produce the essential alpha-linolenic acid (ALA). Nevertheless, they have the capacity to synthesize EPA and DHA from alpha-linolenic acid, albeit at a conversion rate of less than 5% for EPA and 1% for DHA. As a result, mammals rely on acquiring these fatty acids from their diet. EPA and DHA predominantly come from the marine ecosystem, with fish and seafood serving as the primary reservoir of n-3 PUFAs [76]. Additionally, leafy vegetables and nuts are renowned for their elevated content of n-3 FAs, establishing themselves as the principal source of ALA [77].

Numerous studies have identified the potential health advantages associated with the intake of n-3 PUFAs, such as changes in the physical characteristics of the membrane (referred to as "fluidity") [78], impacts on cellular signaling pathways [79], or changes in the production pattern of lipid mediators [80].

Publications from the early 1990s on human infants indicated that preterm infants, when fed a formula enriched with n-3 LCPUFA, primarily in the form of DHA, exhibited enhanced retinal sensitivity and visual acuity in comparison to preterm infants fed the standard unsupplemented formulas of that time [81,82]. Research has also brought attention to the potential impact of extremely long-chain omega-3 fatty acids on mental development, enhancing childhood learning and behavior [83]. For instance, research has shown a direct correlation between elevated levels of DHA in the mother's plasma, especially in breast milk, and enhanced growth and development of the brain and visual system in children [84]. However, these areas of potential action are still subjects of controversy and demand more substantial scientific support. On this matter, there is a hypothesis suggesting that n-3 PUFAs play a role in influencing the structure and function of biological membranes, such as elasticity, membrane organization, and ion permeability. Consequently, these fatty acids may potentially aid in brain glucose uptake, neurotransmission, and neuronal function [85].

Many studies have examined the various mechanisms through which omega-3 fatty acids exert their beneficial actions on the body. In one study, researchers demonstrated that DHA induced PPARγ (peroxisome proliferator-activated receptor gamma) and several established target genes of PPARγ in dendritic cells. These outcomes were associated with a reduction in the production of the inflammatory cytokines TNFα and IL-6 following endotoxin stimulation. Consequently, by activating PPARs, n-3 PUFAs can govern metabolism and various cellular and tissue responses, such as adipocyte differentiation and inflammation [86,87]. Moreover, EPA and DHA exhibit the capability to hinder the production of various inflammatory proteins, including COX-2, inducible NO synthase, TNFα, IL-1, IL-6, IL-8, and IL-12 in cultured endothelial cells [88], monocytes [89], macrophages [90], and dendritic cells [91]. These inhibitory effects of n-3 PUFAs appear to be associated with reduced IkB phosphorylation and diminished activation of NFκB [92], a crucial transcription factor that triggers the expression of genes encoding diverse proteins linked to inflammation and necessitates the activation achieved through phosphorylation of its inhibitory subunit, IkB. Additionally, n-3 PUFAs reduce the accessibility of arachidonic acid for eicosanoid synthesis, impeding its metabolism. This reduction in eicosanoid production from arachidonic acid can impact the actions regulated by these mediators [93].

Interventional trials with n-3 PUFAs have not reported any serious therapy-related side effects. Compared to the placebo, n-3 PUFAs show similar rates of adverse reactions during short-term use, primarily including nausea and other gastrointestinal symptoms [94].

5.3. Nucleotides

Nucleotides (NTs) play a crucial role in nearly all biological processes within the body, serving as essential components of nucleic acids, namely DNA and RNA. NTs are composed of heterocyclic nitrogenous bases, which can be either pyrimidine or purine. Nucleotides can be acquired either through the presence of nucleoproteins (proteins linked to a nucleic acid) naturally found in all foods of both animal and plant origin (healthy individuals typically consume 1–2 g of nucleotides daily through their diet [95]) or through endogenous synthesis, which serves as the primary source of nucleotides [96]. Due to the substantial presence of NTs in breast milk, they are regarded as conditionally essential nutrients for infants. These biocompounds hold significant physiological significance in supporting immune function, lipid metabolism, and growth. Primarily, they act as precursors to nucleic acids—monomeric units found in DNA and RNA, pivotal in storing and transferring genetic information, facilitating cell division, and enabling protein synthesis [97]. Moreover, nucleotides and their derivatives play various roles in energy metabolism (adenosine triphosphate—ATP), enzymatic regulation, and signal transduction and serve as structural components of coenzymes such as NAD, coenzyme A, and NADP+ [98]. Recent research on the impact of NTs on the immune system suggests their potential as immunomodulators. In vitro and animal model studies indicate that nucleotides stimulate the differentiation and proliferation of lymphocytes. Consequently, stages of lymphocyte activation and function also affect nucleotide metabolism to some extent, leading to increase de novo synthesis and salvage in stimulated lymphocytes [99]. Furthermore, the absence of nucleotides led to substantial reductions in host immune responses, resulting in the downregulation of T-cell function and antigen stimulation [100]. Supplementing the diet with nucleotides improves disease resistance, potentially ascribed to increased peritoneal macrophage phagocytosis, heightened NK cell activity, augmented secretion of T-cell-dependent antibodies, elevated production of interleukin-2, and increased levels of bone marrow cells and neutrophils in peripheral blood. Moreover, NT supplementation has the potential to enhance growth, immunity, and stress tolerance, modify intestinal structure, and strengthen the body's defenses against viral, bacterial, and parasitic infections. Nucleotides have also exhibited robust anti-inflammatory properties. Specifically, in vitro studies involving macrophages, or the endothelium have demonstrated that extracellular adenosine can effectively downregulate the potent inflammatory cytokine, tumor necrosis factor alpha (TNF-α) [101]. As crucial elements in immunonutrition, nucleotides showcase diverse physiological activities. These include improving the prognosis of individuals undergoing physiological stress, reducing levels of DNA damage, extending lifespan, serving as anti-fatigue agents, and accelerating carbon turnover in the fundic stomach. Research has suggested that dietary nucleotides play a vital role in intestinal development, liver and immune function, and the rapid growth of cells under physiological stress [102].

To investigate the impact of nucleotides on immune function and sepsis in infants, two clinical studies were undertaken involving healthy term young children. These infants were either breastfed (HM group) or fed with one of two infant formulas—one supplemented with nucleotides (NFM group) and the other not supplemented (FM group). Physical growth, hematological indices, and plasma biochemistry profiles were not significantly different among the three groups. Natural killer cell activity and interleukin-2 activity were significantly higher at 2 months of age in the NFM group compared to the FM group. However, no significant difference was found at 4 months of age [103]. Additional research exploring the potential advantageous impact of dietary nucleotides, in particular clinical scenarios among high-risk neonates, is recommended. These scenarios encompass extreme prematurity, small for gestational age (SGA), gut injuries such as necrotizing enterocolitis (NEC), and extended periods of restricted enteral or parenteral nutrient intake.

6. Potential Bioactive Candidates Added to ONSs

Bioactive peptides exhibit diverse biological actions influenced by factors such as amino acid class, net charge, secondary structures, sequence, and molecular mass. Numerous studies have identified the bioactivities of peptides, associating them with enhanced overall health and reduced risk of specific chronic diseases, including cancer, diabetes, and heart diseases (Figure 7) [104].

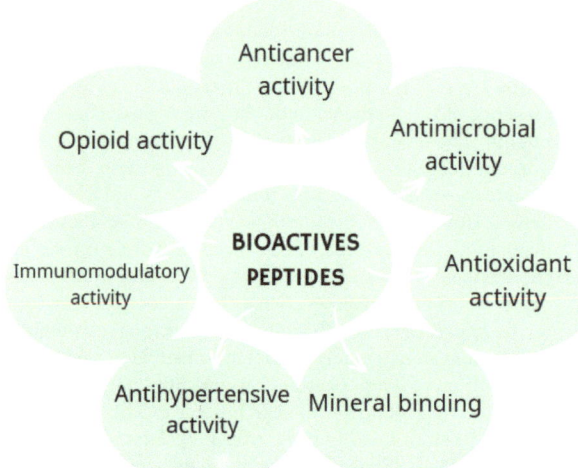

Figure 7. Therapeutic potential of bioactives peptides.

6.1. Glutamine

Glutamine is the most abundant and versatile amino acid in the body, constituting greater than 50% of the total free amino acid pool [105], with a concentration of between 0.6 and 0.7 mmol/L. This molecule takes on the role of a conditionally essential amino acid in situations where there is a deficiency, such as in sepsis [106], traumas [107], cancer [108], infections [109], surgeries [110], or prolonged intense physical exercise [111]. In a study examining glutamine levels in critically ill children, it was observed that they experienced significant early glutamine depletion (glutamine 0.31 mmol/L) compared to convalescent levels (0.40 mmol/L). The glutamine levels during the acute phase of illness were 52% below the lower limit of the normal reference range, while in the convalescent samples, levels were 26% below, suggesting depletion rather than an ongoing consequence of fluid shifts [112]. Nevertheless, the utilization of glutamine in children is not clearly defined, and there is a lack of sufficient data regarding the advantages of glutamine as a pharmacological agent in pediatric critical illness. Anyway, a reduction in plasma glutamine availability has been noted to contribute to compromised immune function in various clinical conditions. Specifically, glutamine depletion diminishes lymphocyte proliferation, hinders the expression of surface activation proteins, reduces cytokine production, and triggers apoptosis in these cells [113]. Present in nearly every cell, glutamine serves as a substrate for various biosynthetic pathways essential for cellular integrity and function, including nucleotide synthesis (purines, pyrimidines, and amino sugars), nicotinamide adenine dinucleotide phosphate (NADPH), antioxidants, and more [114]. The concentration and availability of glutamine in the entire body hinge on the equilibrium between its synthesis and/or release and its uptake by human organs and tissues.

The two main intracellular enzymes involved in glutamine metabolism are glutamine synthetase (GS), found in the cytosol, which initiates the reaction that synthesizes glutamine from ammonium ions (NH^{4+}) and glutamate, involving the consumption of ATP, and phosphate-dependent glutaminase (GLS), mainly found within the mitochondria, which is accountable for the hydrolysis of glutamine, transforming it back into glutamate and NH^{4+} (Figure 8).

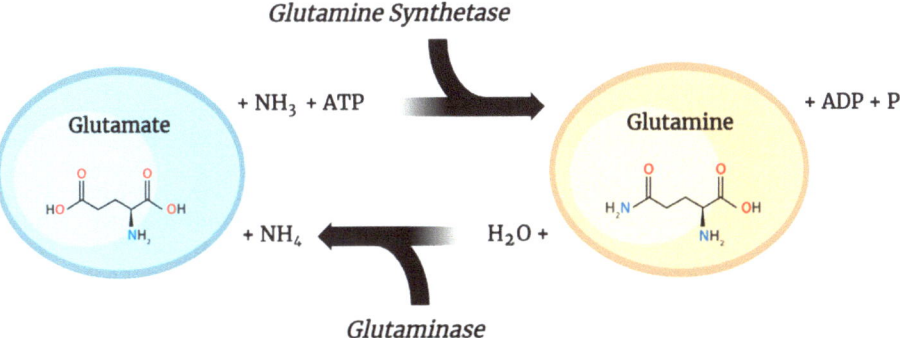

Figure 8. Glutamine metabolism.

Mitochondrial glutamate is transformed into alpha-ketoglutarate (α-KG) through the action of glutamate dehydrogenase 1 (GLUD1 or GDH1) or various mitochondrial aminotransferases. α-KG can be exported from the mitochondria to the cytosol through SLC25A11, where it engages in fatty acid biosynthesis and NADH generation, or can then participate in the tricarboxylic acid (TCA) cycle, supporting either the oxidative phosphorylation (OXPHOS) pathway or the reductive carboxylation pathway [115,116]. The primary contributors of glutamine, with notable activity in tissue-specific glutamine synthesis (GS), include the lungs, liver, brain, adipose tissue, and skeletal muscles. Conversely, through the actions of enzymes like GLS that degrade glutamine, the amino acid can undergo degradation at varying rates. Tissues such as the intestinal mucosa, renal tubules, and, particularly, leukocytes are prominent consumers of glutamine [117]. In fact, glutamine serves as a vital energy source for leukocytes, enough to be considered "fuel for the immune system" [118]. Lymphocytes and macrophages have high rates of glutamine utilization, especially during inflammatory states such as sepsis and injury. In a study, Newsholme and Parry-Billings [119] established a strong correlation between the phagocytosis rate in murine macrophages and the concentrations of glutamine. Furthermore, in vitro studies have shown that glutamine supplementation in vitro optimizes macrophage functions [118]. On the other hand, a reduction in plasma glutamine availability has been documented as a factor contributing to compromised immune function in various clinical scenarios. Specifically, the depletion of glutamine diminishes the proliferation of lymphocytes, hinders the expression of surface activation proteins, reduces cytokine production, and triggers apoptosis in these cells [113]. The role of glutamine extends to its significant antioxidant capabilities, particularly crucial in the context of critical and severe illnesses. In fact, glutamine acts as a precursor for the formation of glutathione (GSH) through the conversion of glutamate. In rat-based in vivo experiments, it has been shown that administering glutamine before ischemia/reperfusion injury or surgical procedures can boost GSH concentrations [120], enhancing cellular resilience against damage and mitigating oxidative stress [118]. Another noteworthy aspect is the function of glutamine as the favored energy source for intestinal epithelial cells [121]. Remarkably, glutamine stands out as the most plentiful free amino acid found in milk. This observation implies that glutamine could play a role in supporting intestinal health and development during the lactation period [122]. It is well known that the small intestinal epithelium undergoes frequent renewal, experiencing regeneration approximately every 2–5 days, a continuously high level of cell proliferation required to maintain homeostasis [123]. Glutamine exerts its influence on various signaling pathways (Figure 9) [121] responsible for regulating the cell cycle and proliferation, such as epidermal growth factor (EGF), transforming growth factor, mitogen-activated protein kinases (MAPKs), and insulin-like growth factor 1 (IGF-1) [124,125]. Various sources of evidence have suggested that glutamine also regulates the expression of tight junction proteins (occludin, the claudin-family proteins, junction adhesion molecules (JAMs), zonula occludens (ZO-1, ZO-2, and ZO-3), which create a physical barrier that seals neighboring epithelial cells, establishing a separation between epithelial and endothelial cells [126]. The reduction of glutamine is correlated with a decrease in the tight junction protein claudin-1, resulting in the breakdown of barrier function [127]. This breakdown is often associated with the initiation of various gastrointestinal diseases, which are frequently linked to the initial disruption of tight junctions. Other significant factors contributing to the development of intestinal conditions like ulcerative colitis, Crohn's disease, and colorectal cancer include inflammatory processes [128]. Multiple lines of evidence indicate that glutamine demonstrates anti-inflammatory properties by modulating various inflammatory signaling pathways, including those involving nuclear factor κB (NF-κB) (an essential controller of immune responses with implications in the pathogenesis of various inflammatory diseases) and signal transducer and activator of transcription (STAT) [129]. STAT proteins serve as transcription factors regulating the immune system, cellular proliferation, and development [130]. Glutamine plays a role in inhibiting STAT activation and suppressing the expression of inflammatory cytokines, such as IL-6 and IL-8, in intestinal tissues.

There is also a strong association between intestinal inflammatory disorders and increased apoptosis of intestinal epithelial cells. Glutamine has been demonstrated to exhibit anti-apoptotic properties in the intestine through various mechanisms: (1) by maintaining normal cellular redox status as a precursor for GSH [131]; (2) by regulation of caspase activation, a group of protease enzymes that holds significant roles in triggering apoptosis [132]; and (3) enhancing the expression of heat shock proteins (HSPs) (i.e., HSP10, HSP40, HSP60, HSP70, HSP90 and HSP100), proteins with chaperone function, preventing the aggregation of newly synthesized polypeptide chains during folding or by clearing improperly folded and unfolded proteins [133], through glutamine-mediated increase the heat shock factors (HSF1) expression, activator of HSPs [134].

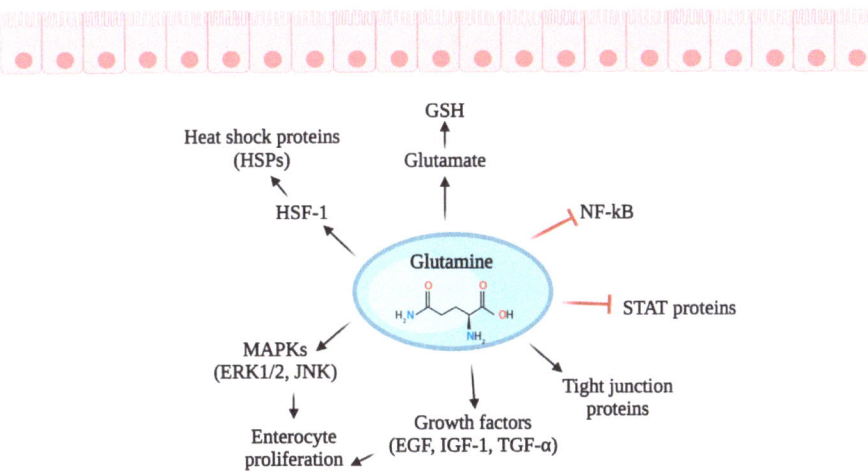

Figure 9. Glutamine's functions.

In conclusion, the dietary presence of glutamine has been demonstrated to play a crucial role in maintaining the integrity of the intestinal mucosal barrier. This is achieved through the regulation of gene and protein expression related to cell proliferation, differentiation, apoptosis, protein turnover, anti-oxidative properties, and immune responses. For this reason, a new ONS added with glutamine should be evaluated in the future, involving in vivo studies to enhance our understanding of the molecular mechanisms underlying the impact of glutamine on gut barrier function and to contribute to the development of personalized glutamine regimens for the therapeutic management of various diseases.

6.2. Lactoferrin

Lactoferrin is a non-heme iron-binding glycoprotein found in exocrine biological fluids like breast milk, tears, bronchial secretions, and gastrointestinal fluids, playing a crucial role in both human and bovine milk [135]. Lactoferrin, possessing antimicrobial and immune-modulating properties, is released from activated neutrophil granules, leading to increased concentrations in plasma and feces during infection and inflammation due to neutrophil recruitment. Human lactoferrin (hLf) shares structural and functional similarities with bovine lactoferrin (bLf). Although lactoferrin concentrations are notably higher in human milk compared to bovine milk, bLf can be efficiently extracted from bovine milk in substantial amounts. Bovine lactoferrin is progressively utilized as a nutritional supplement across various patient populations and conditions and is generally considered safe and well-tolerated.

Specifically, given that bLf receptors are present in the intestinal mucosa and lymphatic tissue cells of the intestine, the preservation of bLf's structural integrity is crucial for binding to these receptors [136]. Nevertheless, studies have demonstrated that bLf can directly stimulate the growth and proliferation of enterocytes, depending on its concentration [137]. Consequently, the absorption of lactoferrin in the intestine may vary during different life stages. During early life, infants who are breastfed or fed with infant formula fortified with bLf will experience a high concentration of lactoferrin in the intestinal lumen. This is attributed to minimal proteolytic degradation and heightened cell proliferation.

The mucosal development stimulated by lactoferrin can lead to an increase in mucosal surface area, thereby improving the absorption not only of iron but also of other nutrients. As the infant matures, protein digestion becomes more efficient, resulting in a significant decrease in lactoferrin concentration and an increase in differentiation.

To ensure the orally administered protein reaches the intestine without undergoing degradation in the stomach, protective measures must be implemented. Various approaches have been employed in formulating bLf oral delivery systems to enhance its oral bioavailability. Some of the commonly utilized methods to safeguard bLf during the oral and gastric passage include iron saturation, microencapsulation, PEGylation, and absorption enhancers [138].

The evidence supporting the impact of lactoferrin supplementation on inflammation, immune function, and respiratory tract infections (RTIs) in humans has demonstrated the crucial role in host defense by performing a range of physiological functions, encompassing antiviral, antimicrobial, antioxidant, and immunomodulatory activities. The protective functions of lactoferrin can rely on its capacity to bind iron or operate independently of it [139]. Probably, as Kruzel et al. [140] reviewed, through iron sequestration, LTF regulates the natural equilibrium of reactive oxygen species (ROS) production and their elimination rate, thereby providing a natural defense against direct oxidative cell damage. A compelling hypothesis suggests that by managing oxidative stress, LTF influences the responsiveness of the innate immune system, leading to changes in the production of immune regulatory mediators crucial for shaping the development of adaptive immune function. Numerous studies have indeed demonstrated the significant modulatory effects of LTF on the adaptive immune system.

In recent times, it has been that lactoferrin may play a role in safeguarding against common viral infections by boosting type I interferon (IFN) production, enhancing NK cell activity, and promoting type 1 T-helper (Th1) cell cytokine responses [141]. Numerous in vitro studies have indicated that lactoferrin treatment hinders virus growth, cellular entry, and the cytopathic effect after exposure to prevalent respiratory viruses, such as respiratory syncytial virus [142] and influenza virus [143]. Furthermore, colostrum, rich in lactoferrin at approximately 7 g/L, has demonstrated protective effects against RTIs in both adults and children [144]. Recent preliminary evidence using pseudo-viruses has suggested that Lf may provide protection against emerging viruses like severe acute respiratory syndrome coronavirus 2 (SARS-CoV-2), which was responsible for the COVID-19 pandemic [145].

Many points of evidence from several randomized clinical trials support the role of bLf in reducing systemic inflammation, specifically IL-6, due to various mechanisms. The regulation of iron homeostasis by bLf is emerging as the most pertinent aspect in the context of the presented evidence; in particular, IL-6 downregulates ferroportin, the transporter responsible for moving iron from tissues to the systemic circulation, while IL-6 upregulates hepcidin, which inhibits iron transport [146].

As the RCT from Widjaja et al. [147] showed, the lactoferrin in oral nutritional supplements affects IL-6 and IL-10 levels in children experiencing failure to thrive and infections over a 90-day intervention, functions as a regulator of innate immunity and serves as a defense mechanism owing to its antimicrobial properties.

Lactoferrin possesses both bacteriostatic and bactericidal effects while also being capable of stimulating the immune response in an organism. This helps mitigate tissue damage resulting from an excessive pro-inflammatory response, often seen in chronic infections. Consequently, it has the potential to decrease the occurrence of acute gastrointestinal symptoms and shorten the duration of respiratory symptoms in children under 12 months old, whether stemming from viral or bacterial infections.

In a 2020 randomized, double-blind, placebo-controlled trial, researchers investigated the effects of lactoferrin (LF)-fortified formula on acute gastrointestinal and respiratory symptoms in children [148]. As result, the occurrence of acute gastrointestinal symptoms was notably lower in the LF group (22 out of 53 (41.5%)) compared to the placebo group (30 out of 48 (62.5%), $p = 0.046$). Additionally, the overall duration of acute respiratory symptoms was significantly reduced in the LF group (9.0 days) compared to the placebo group (15.0 days, $p = 0.030$).

It is becoming evident that LTF plays a pivotal role in shaping and fully activating adaptive host immune responses. At the molecular level, homeostasis is governed by a complex network involving the neuroendocrine and immune systems, where LTF assumes a central role, primarily owing to its capacity to bind ferric ions.

In a randomized controlled trial, no safety issues were observed. Liver enzyme levels were monitored, and no anomalies were found. Overall, there were no adverse effects associated with lactoferrin [149].

6.3. Butyrate

Butyrate, a four-carbon short-chain fatty acid, derives principally from the fermentation of undigested carbohydrates, particularly resistant starch and dietary fiber, and, to a lesser degree, dietary and endogenous proteins [150], by the gut microbiota. The gut microbiota generates around 500–600 mmol of short-chain fatty acids (SCFAs), with butyrate estimated to contribute to 20% of the overall SCFA production [151]. SCFAs are absorbed in both the small and large intestines through similar mechanisms, which involve the diffusion of the undissociated form and the active transport of the dissociated form facilitated by SCFA transporters [152,153]. The ionized form of butyrate is actively transported across the apical surface of intestinal epithelial cells via H+-monocarboxylate transporter-1 (MCT1) [154]. The absorbed butyrate is metabolized in the intestinal epithelial cells, liver cells, and other tissues and cells [155]. Within the epithelial cells, butyrate undergoes conversion into acetyl-CoA and enters the tricarboxylic acid (TCA) cycle within the mitochondria to generate ATP, serving as an energy source for colon epithelial cells.

In addition to its energy function for colonocytes, butyrate has garnered significant attention due to its wide-ranging benefits, such as playing a crucial role as a mediator in anti-inflammatory and antitumorigenic activities [156]. Butyrate functions by either inhibiting histone deacetylase (HDAC) or signaling through various G protein-coupled receptors (GPCRs). Its recent attention stems from its advantageous impacts on intestinal homeostasis and energy metabolism. With its anti-inflammatory attributes, butyrate improves intestinal barrier function and mucosal immunity [157].

Butyrate interacts with G protein-coupled receptors such as GPR41, GPR43, and GPR109A, which are found on the surface of intestinal epithelial cells, adipocytes, and immune cells. The activation of GPR41 by butyrate regulates body energy expenditure and upholds metabolic balance [158]; meanwhile, GPR109A (HCAR2) triggers signaling that activates the inflammasome pathway in colonic macrophages and dendritic cells. This activation leads to the differentiation of regulatory T-cells and T-cells producing IL-10, functioning as an anti-inflammatory and anticancer agent in the colon [159].

Butyrate can function as a modulator of the chemotaxis and adhesion of immune cells [160]. It has the ability to influence the migration of neutrophils to inflammatory sites mediated by intestinal epithelial cells and engages various signaling pathways in both gut immune cells and epithelial cells to restore impaired colonic barrier function and maintain gut homeostasis. The heightened reassembly of tight junctions (TJs) and the restoration of transepithelial electrical resistance (TER) were attributed to the activation of AMP-activated protein kinase (AMPK) induced by butyrate [161]. Additionally, butyrate stimulates the production or release of chemokines in neutrophils, dendritic cells (DCs), and endothelial cells, thereby regulating the recruitment of leukocytes [162]. In addition to its effects on cells, these microbial metabolites inhibit HDAC (histone deacetylase) activities both in vitro and in vivo [163,164]. However, the mechanism behind this remains unclear. Butyrate's effects, primarily mediated through HDAC inhibition, encompass the inhibition of cell proliferation, induction of cell differentiation or apoptosis, and modulation of gene expression [165], acting as an antitumor agent. In addition to this role, butyrate also contributes to anti-inflammatory effects, partially through HDAC inhibition. Multiple human and animal studies have indicated that butyrate downregulates proinflammatory cytokines such as IFN-γ, TNF-α, IL-1β, IL-6, and IL-8 while simultaneously upregulating IL-10 and TGF-β.

Postbiotics show considerable promise as supplements for human health. Specifically, their beneficial impact on microbiota development, intestinal maturation, and various immunomodulatory effects make them particularly intriguing for children, as childhood represents a critical window of opportunity for long-term health. Butyrate shows promise as a valuable intervention for improving the health of newborns and premature infants, potentially preventing serious conditions like necrotizing enterocolitis [166] and late-onset sepsis by enhancing the integrity of the intestinal barrier through promoting the production of the characteristic mucins of the intestinal epithelium (MUC2). Moreover, obesity is increasingly prevalent among children globally, and butyrate could offer a promising supplement in combating this widespread epidemic. In a randomized clinical trial by Coppola et al., researchers discovered that supplementation with butyrate reduced HOMA-IR and fasting insulin levels in children with obesity. Additionally, the analysis of the gut microbiota supported butyrate's role in glucose metabolism, with children showing a more favorable response if they had a higher abundance of butyrate-producing bacteria at the beginning of the study [167].

In summary, appropriate concentrations of butyrate aid in preserving intestinal barrier function and modulating the immune response within the gut. Both clinical trials and animal studies have demonstrated that butyrate has the potential to alleviate mucosal inflammation and enhance barrier function. Hence, formulations of butyrate and butyrogenic compounds could offer alternative therapeutic strategies for various diseases.

In pediatric patients, butyrate administration has been associated with some adverse effects. Specifically, transient mild nausea and headaches have been observed as side effects [167].

7. Conclusions

Products known as oral nutritional supplements (ONSs) are FSMPs (Food for Special Medical Purposes) intended for the prevention or management of caloric-protein malnutrition. They are available in liquid, creamy, or powder form for individuals who can still feed themselves naturally. ONSs are currently available in a wide range of nutritional variants with either standard or disease-specific formulations, as per the document prepared by the European Society of Clinical Nutrition and Metabolism (ESPEN).

Overall, the systematic review revealed evidence supporting the significant role of ONSs in pediatric nutrition. Many studies reported significant improvements in patient outcomes, particularly in clinical nutrition, which provides therapeutic benefits.

The evidence suggests that integrating ONSs with routine medical care can enhance treatment outcomes for children with specific clinical conditions whose dietary management cannot be achieved through natural food modifications alone.

However, the heterogeneity of the studies limits the generalizability of the results. The importance of thorough nutritional assessments, early detection of malnutrition, and addressing nutritional deficiencies is underscored to prevent complications such as muscle weakness, immune deficits, increased infection susceptibility, microbiota–immune system dysregulation, and severe growth and developmental delays. According to the European Society for Paediatric Gastroenterology, Hepatology, and Nutrition (ESPGHAN), "insufficient oral intake" is defined as failing to meet 60–80% of nutritional needs for more than 10 consecutive days in children over one year of age, necessitating timely supplementation.

For children aged one year and older, ONSs are recommended to counteract protein-calorie malnutrition when oral feeding is inadequate. In children with fragile or impaired digestive systems, easily digestible supplements are preferred to prevent and manage malnutrition. This review broadens the definition of "malnutrition" to include selective deficits of bioactive molecules.

This review also explores the growing interest in incorporating bioactive compounds into ONSs, tailored to meet the specific nutritional needs of children. These bioactive compounds exhibit a range of benefits, including antioxidant, anti-inflammatory, and immunomodulatory properties. Understanding the mechanisms of these compounds is crucial for leveraging their potential in pediatric nutrition.

Key conclusions from this systematic narrative review include:

Enhanced nutritional profiles: bioactives contribute to the overall nutritional value of oral supplements, ensuring that children receive a balanced intake of essential nutrients. This is particularly crucial for children with specific dietary restrictions or health conditions that impair nutrient absorption. Healthcare providers should consider personalized nutrition plans that incorporate specific bioactives based on individual patient needs. For example, children with a history of gastrointestinal issues may benefit more from probiotics and prebiotics, while those with bone health concerns may require increased vitamin D supplementation.

Immune support: Several bioactives have been shown to bolster the immune system, reducing the incidence and severity of infections in children.

Growth and development: Omega-3 fatty acids and other essential nutrients play a critical role in the cognitive and physical development of children. Bioactive-enriched supplements can support optimal growth trajectories and cognitive function.

Gut health: Probiotics and prebiotics are instrumental in maintaining a healthy gut microbiota, which is linked to improved digestion, enhanced nutrient absorption, and overall gastrointestinal health.

Disease prevention and management: Bioactives have therapeutic potential in managing chronic pediatric conditions such as obesity, diabetes, and gastrointestinal disorders. They offer a non-pharmacological approach to disease management, which is particularly advantageous in pediatric care.

Safety and efficacy: This review highlights the importance of rigorous clinical trials to establish the safety and efficacy of bioactives in pediatric populations. While current evidence is promising, more research is needed to confirm their long-term benefits and potential risks. In summary, oral nutritional supplements containing bioactives are generally well-tolerated. While minor and transient side effects may occur, serious adverse effects are rare. Nevertheless, monitoring and proper dosing are essential to minimize potential risks.

Personalized nutrition: The inclusion of bioactives in supplements allows for a more tailored approach to pediatric nutrition, addressing individual health needs and dietary gaps. This personalized strategy can lead to better health outcomes and enhanced quality of life for children.

Regulatory and quality control: Ensuring the quality, purity, and consistency of bioactive-enriched supplements is crucial. Regulatory frameworks need to adapt to the growing use of bioactives to guarantee safety and efficacy standards are met.

However, further research and clinical validation are needed to fully establish the efficacy and safety of biocompound-enriched ONSs in pediatric populations. Additionally, practical considerations such as taste, texture, and palatability must be addressed to ensure acceptance and compliance among young patients.

Future advancements in this field will require collaboration among healthcare professionals, researchers, and industry partners. Through combined efforts and resources, continued innovation and refinement of ONS formulations can more effectively meet the nutritional needs of children globally.

Author Contributions: F.R. and R.R. contributed equally to this work. N.C., R.R., F.R. and M.I.S. contributed to the conception, writing, review, and editing of the study. All authors contributed to the manuscript revision. All authors have read and agreed to the published version of the manuscript.

Funding: This research received no external funding.

Data Availability Statement: Not applicable.

Acknowledgments: All of the figures in this article have been created with BioRender.com; the content is not changed and is properly referenced.

Conflicts of Interest: The authors declare no conflicts of interest.

References

1. Cederholm, T.; Barazzoni, R.; Austin, P.; Ballmer, P.; Biolo, G.; Bischoff, S.C.; Compher, C.; Correia, I.; Higashiguchi, T.; Holst, M.; et al. ESPEN guidelines on definitions and terminology of clinical nutrition. *Clin. Nutr.* **2017**, *36*, 49–64. [CrossRef]
2. Susan, M. Hill, Oral nutritional supplementation: A user's guide. *Paediatr. Child Health* **2017**, *27*, 378–382. [CrossRef]
3. Philipson, T.J.; Snider, J.T.; Lakdawalla, D.N.; Stryckman, B.; Goldman, D.P. Impact of oral nutritional supplementation on hospital outcomes. *Am. J. Manag. Care* **2013**, *19*, 121–128. [CrossRef]
4. Lim, S.L.; Ong, K.C.B.; Chan, Y.H.; Loke, W.C.; Ferguson, M.; Daniels, L. Malnutrition and its impact on cost of hospitalization, length of stay, readmission and 3-year mortality. *Clin. Nutr.* **2012**, *31*, 345–350. [CrossRef]
5. Schoonhoven, L.; Grobbee, D.E.; Donders, A.R.T.; Algra, A.; Grypdonck, M.H.; Bousema, M.T.; Schrijvers, A.J.P.; Buskens, E. Prediction of pressure ulcer development in hospitalized patients: A tool for risk assessment. *Qual. Saf. Health Care* **2006**, *15*, 65–70. [CrossRef]
6. Brown, B.; Roehl, K.; Betz, M. Enteral nutrition formula selection: Current evidence and implications for practice. *Nutr. Clin. Pract.* **2015**, *30*, 72–85. [CrossRef]
7. Ouzzani, M.; Hammady, H.; Fedorowicz, Z.; Elmagarmid, A. Rayyan—A web and mobile app for systematic reviews. *Syst. Rev.* **2016**, *5*, 210. [CrossRef]
8. Hojsak, I.; Benninga, M.A.; Hauser, B.; Kansu, A.; Kelly, V.B.; Stephen, A.M.; Lopez, A.M.; Slavin, J.; Tuohy, K. Benefits of dietary fibre for children in health and disease. *Arch. Dis. Child.* **2022**, *107*, 973–979. [CrossRef]
9. Stephen, A.M.; Champ, M.M.; Cloran, S.J.; Fleith, M.; van Lieshout, L.; Mejborn, H.; Burley, V.J. Dietary fibre in Europe: Current state of knowledge on definitions, sources, recommendations, intakes and relationships to health. *Nutr. Res. Rev.* **2017**, *30*, 149–190. [CrossRef]
10. Gill, S.K.; Rossi, M.; Bajka, B.; Whelan, K. Dietary fibre in gastrointestinal health and disease. *Nat. Rev. Gastroenterol. Hepatol.* **2021**, *18*, 101–116. [CrossRef]
11. Mei, Z.; Yuan, J.; Li, D. Biological activity of galacto-oligosaccharides: A review. *Front. Microbiol.* **2022**, *13*, 993052. [CrossRef]
12. François, I.E.; Lescroart, O.; Veraverbeke, W.S.; Marzorati, M.; Possemiers, S.; Hamer, H.; Windey, K.; Welling, G.W.; Delcour, J.A.; Courtin, C.M.; et al. Effects of wheat bran extract containing arabinoxylan oligosaccharides on gastrointestinal parameters in healthy preadolescent children. *J. Pediatr. Gastroenterol. Nutr.* **2014**, *58*, 647–653. [CrossRef] [PubMed]
13. Tabbers, M.M.; DiLorenzo, C.; Berger, Y.M.; Faure, C.; Langendam, W.M.; Nurko, S.; Staiano, A.; Vandenplas, Y.; Benninga, A.M. Evaluation and treatment of functional constipation in infants and children: Evidence-based recommendations from ESPGHAN and NASPGHAN. *J. Pediatr. Gastroenterol. Nutr.* **2014**, *58*, 258–274. [CrossRef]
14. Axelrod, C.H.; Saps, M. The Role of Fiber in the Treatment of Functional Gastrointestinal Disorders in Children. *Nutrients* **2018**, *10*, 1650. [CrossRef]
15. Rezende, E.S.V.; Lima, G.C.; Naves, M.M.V. Dietary fibers as beneficial microbiota modulators: A proposal classification by prebiotic categories. *Nutrition* **2021**, *89*, 111217. [CrossRef]
16. Xu, B.; Cao, J.; Fu, J.; Li, Z.; Jin, M.; Wang, X.; Wang, Y. The effects of nondigestible fermentable carbohydrates on adults with overweight or obesity: A meta-analysis of randomized controlled trials. *Nutr. Rev.* **2022**, *80*, 165–177. [CrossRef]
17. Whisner, C.M.; Castillo, L.F. Prebiotics, Bone and Mineral Metabolism. *Calcif. Tissue Int.* **2018**, *102*, 443–479. [CrossRef]
18. Salvatore, S.; Battigaglia, M.S.; Murone, E.; Dozio, E.; Pensabene, L.; Agosti, M. Dietary Fibers in Healthy Children and in Pediatric Gastrointestinal Disorders: A Practical Guide. *Nutrients* **2023**, *15*, 2208. [CrossRef]
19. Coppa, G.V.; Bruni, S.; Morelli, L.; Soldi, S.; Gabrielli, O. The first prebiotics in humans: Human milk oligosaccharides. *J. Clin. Gastroenterol.* **2004**, *38* (Suppl. S6), S80–S83. [CrossRef]
20. Divyashri, G.; Sadanandan, B.; Chidambara Murthy, K.N.; Shetty, K.; Mamta, K. Neuroprotective Potential of Non-Digestible Oligosaccharides: An Overview of Experimental Evidence. *Front. Pharmacol.* **2021**, *12*, 712531. [CrossRef]
21. Sabater-Molina, M.; Larqué, E.; Torrella, F.; Zamora, S. Dietary fructooligosaccharides and potential benefits on health. *J. Physiol. Biochem.* **2009**, *65*, 315–328. [CrossRef] [PubMed]
22. Connor, F.; Salvatore, S.; D'Auria, E.; Baldassarre, M.E.; Acunzo, M.; Di Bella, G.; Farella, I.; Sestito, S.; Pensabene, L. Cows' Milk Allergy-Associated Constipation: When to Look for It? A Narrative Review. *Nutrients* **2022**, *14*, 1317. [CrossRef] [PubMed]
23. Wegh, C.A.M.; Baaleman, D.F.; Tabbers, M.M.; Smidt, H.; Benninga, M.A. Nonpharmacologic Treatment for Children with Functional Constipation: A Systematic Review and Meta-analysis. *J. Pediatr.* **2022**, *240*, 136–149.e5. [CrossRef] [PubMed]
24. Toporovski, M.S.; de Morais, M.B.; Abuhab, A.; Crippa, J.M.A. Effect of Polydextrose/Fructooligosaccharide Mixture on Constipation Symptoms in Children Aged 4 to 8 Years. *Nutrients* **2021**, *13*, 1634. [CrossRef] [PubMed]
25. Healey, G.R.; Celiberto, L.S.; Lee, S.M.; Jacobson, K. Fiber and Prebiotic Interventions in Pediatric Inflammatory Bowel Disease: What Role Does the Gut Microbiome Play? *Nutrients* **2020**, *12*, 3204. [CrossRef] [PubMed]
26. He, N.; Wang, Y.; Zhou, Z.; Liu, N.; Jung, S.; Lee, M.S.; Li, S. Preventive Prebiotic Effect of α-Galacto-Oligosaccharide against Dextran Sodium Sulfate-Induced Colitis Gut Microbiota Dysbiosis in Mice. *J. Agric. Food Chem.* **2021**, *69*, 9597–9607. [CrossRef]
27. Weaver, C.M.; Martin, B.R.; Nakatsu, C.H.; Armstrong, A.P.; Clavijo, A.; McCabe, L.D.; McCabe, G.P.; Duignan, S.; Schoterman, M.H.C.; van den Heuvel, E.G.H.M. Galactooligosaccharides improve mineral absorption bone properties in growing rats through gut fermentation. *J. Agric. Food Chem.* **2011**, *59*, 6501–6510. [CrossRef] [PubMed]
28. Xiao, Y.; Chen, Q.; Guang, C.; Zhang, W.; Mu, W. An overview on biological production of functional lactose derivatives. *Appl. Microbiol. Biotechnol.* **2019**, *103*, 3683–3691. [CrossRef]

29. Sims, I.M.; Tannock, G.W. Galacto- and Fructo-oligosaccharides Utilized for Growth by Cocultures of Bifidobacterial Species Characteristic of the Infant Gut. *Appl. Environ. Microbiol.* **2020**, *86*, e00214-20. [CrossRef]
30. O'Sullivan, M.; O'Morain, C. Nutritional therapy in inflammatory bowel disease. *Curr. Treat. Options Gastroenterol.* **2004**, *7*, 191–198. [CrossRef]
31. Verma, S.; Kirkwood, B.; Brown, S.; Giaffer, M.H. Oral nutritional supplementation is effective in the maintenance of remission in Crohn's disease. *Dig. Liver Dis.* **2000**, *32*, 769–774. [CrossRef] [PubMed]
32. Roda, G.; Ng, S.C.; Kotze, P.G.; Argollo, M.; Panaccione, R.; Spinelli, A.; Kaser, A.; Peyrin-Biroulet, L.; Danese, S. Crohn's disease. *Nat. Rev. Dis. Primers* **2020**, *6*, 22. [CrossRef] [PubMed]
33. Derynck, R.; Budi, E.H. Specificity, versatility, and control of TGF-β family signaling. *Sci. Signal.* **2019**, *12*, eaav5183. [CrossRef] [PubMed]
34. Morikawa, M.; Derynck, R.; Miyazono, K. TGF-β and the TGF-β family: Context-dependent roles in cell and tissue physiology. *Cold Spring Harb. Perspect. Biol.* **2016**, *8*, a021873. [CrossRef] [PubMed]
35. Massagué, J.; Blain, S.W.; Lo, R.S. TGFβ signaling in growth control, cancer, and heritable disorders. *Cell* **2000**, *103*, 295–309. [CrossRef] [PubMed]
36. Shi, Y.; Massagué, J. Mechanisms of TGF-beta signaling from cell membrane to the nucleus. *Cell* **2003**, *113*, 685–700. [CrossRef] [PubMed]
37. Massagué, J.; Sheppard, D. TGF-β signaling in health and disease. *Cell* **2023**, *186*, 4007–4037. [CrossRef]
38. Davis, B.N.; Hilyard, A.C.; Lagna, G.; Hata, A. SMAD proteins control DROSHA-mediated microRNA maturation. *Nature* **2008**, *454*, 56–61. [CrossRef]
39. Triantafillidis, J.K.; Stamataki, A.; Gikas, A.; Malgarinos, G. Maintenance treatment of Crohn's disease with a polymeric feed rich in TGF-β. *Ann. Gastroenterol.* **2010**, *23*, 113–118.
40. Strainic, M.; Shevach, E.; An, F.; Lin, F.; Medof, M.E. Absence of signaling into CD4+ cells via C3aR and C5aR enables autoinductive TGF-β1 signaling and induction of Foxp3+ regulatory T cells. *Nat. Immunol.* **2013**, *14*, 162–171. [CrossRef]
41. Brown, C.C.; Rudensky, A.Y. Spatiotemporal regulation of peripheral T cell tolerance. *Science* **2023**, *380*, 472–478. [CrossRef] [PubMed]
42. Nixon, B.G.; Gao, S.; Wang, X.; Li, M.O. TGFb control of immune responses in cancer: A holistic immuno-oncology perspective. *Nat. Rev. Immunol.* **2023**, *23*, 346–362. [CrossRef] [PubMed]
43. Burke, J.P.; Mulsow, J.J.; O'Keane, C.; Docherty, N.G.; Watson, R.W.G.; O'connell, P.R. Fibrogenesis in Crohn's disease. *Am. J. Gastroenterol.* **2007**, *102*, 439–448. [CrossRef] [PubMed]
44. Buechler, M.B.; Pradhan, R.N.; Krishnamurty, A.T.; Cox, C.; Calviello, A.K.; Wang, A.W.; Yang, Y.A.; Tam, L.; Caothien, R.; Roose-Girma, M.; et al. Cross-tissue organization of the fibroblast lineage. *Nature* **2021**, *593*, 575–579. [CrossRef] [PubMed]
45. Heuschkel, R.B.; Menache, C.C.; Megerian, J.T.; Baird, A.E. Enteral nutrition and corticosteroids in the treatment of acute Crohn's disease in children. *J. Pediatr. Gastroenterol. Nutr.* **2000**, *31*, 8–15. [PubMed]
46. Levine, A.; Wine, E.; Assa, A.; Boneh, R.S.; Shaoul, R.; Kori, M.; Cohen, S.; Peleg, S.; Shamaly, H.; On, A.; et al. Crohn's disease exclusion diet plus partial enteral nutrition induces sustained remission in a randomized controlled trial. *Gastroenterology* **2019**, *157*, 440–450. [CrossRef]
47. Agin, M.; Yucel, A.; Gumus, M.; Yuksekkaya, H.A.; Tumgor, G. The Effect of Enteral Nutrition Support Rich in TGF-β in the Treatment of Inflammatory Bowel Disease in Childhood. *Medicina* **2019**, *55*, 620. [CrossRef] [PubMed]
48. Vetvicka, V.; Vetvickova, J. Concept of Immuno-Nutrition. *J. Nutr. Food Sci.* **2016**, *6*, 1000500. [CrossRef]
49. Calder, P.C. Immunonutrition may have beneficial effects in surgical patients. *BMJ* **2003**, *327*, 117–118. [CrossRef]
50. Grimble, R. Basics in clinical nutrition: Immunonutrition—Nutrients which influence immunity: Effect and mechanism of action. *E-SPEN Eur. E-J. Clin. Nutr. Metab.* **2009**, *4*, e10–e13. [CrossRef]
51. Luiking, Y.C.; Ten Have, G.A.; Wolfe, R.R.; Deutz, N.E. Arginine de novo and nitric oxide production in disease states. *Am. J. Physiol. Endocrinol. Metab.* **2012**, *303*, E1177–E1189. [CrossRef] [PubMed]
52. Hou, Z.P.; Yin, Y.L.; Huang, R.L.; Li, T.; Hou, R.; Liu, Y.; Wu, X.; Liu, Z.; Wang, W.; Xiong, H.; et al. Rice protein concentrate partially replaces dried whey in the diet for early-weaned piglets and improves their growth performance. *J. Sci. Food Agric.* **2008**, *88*, 1187–1193. [CrossRef]
53. Morris, S.M., Jr. Arginine synthesis. In *Cellular and Molecular Biology of Nitric Oxide*; Laskin, J.D., Laskin, D.L., Eds.; Marcel Dekker, Inc.: New York, NY, USA, 1999; pp. 57–85.
54. Brosnan, M.E.; Brosnan, J.T. Renal arginine metabolism. *J. Nutr.* **2004**, *134*, 2791S–2795S. [CrossRef] [PubMed]
55. Szefel, J.; Danielak, A.; Kruszewski, W.J. Metabolic pathways of L-arginine and therapeutic consequences in tumors. *Adv. Med. Sci.* **2019**, *64*, 104–110. [CrossRef] [PubMed]
56. Wu, G.; Bazer, F.W.; Davis, T.A.; Kim, S.W.; Li, P.; Rhoads, J.M.; Satterfield, M.C.; Smith, S.B.; Spencer, T.E. Arginine metabolism and nutrition in growth, health and disease. *Amino Acids* **2009**, *37*, 153–168. [CrossRef]
57. Förstermann, U.; Kleinert, H. Nitric oxide synthase: Expression and expressional control of the three isoforms. *Naunyn-Schmiedeberg's Arch. Pharmacol.* **1995**, *352*, 351–364. [CrossRef] [PubMed]
58. Li, H.; Poulos, T.L. Structure-function studies on nitric oxide synthases. *J. Inorg. Biochem.* **2005**, *99*, 293–305. [CrossRef]
59. Crabtree, M.J.; Channon, K.M. Synthesis and recycling of tetrahydrobi-opterin in endothelial function and vascular disease. *Nitric Oxide* **2011**, *25*, 81–88. [CrossRef]

60. Predonzani, A.; Calì, B.; Agnellini, A.H.; Molon, B. Spotlights on immunological effects of reactive nitrogen species: When inflammation says nitric oxide. *World J. Exp. Med.* **2015**, *5*, 64–76. [CrossRef]
61. Zhao, Y.; Vanhoutte, P.M.; Leung, S.W. Vascular nitric oxide: Beyond eNOS. *J. Pharmacol. Sci.* **2015**, *129*, 83–94. [CrossRef]
62. Prast, H.; Philippu, A. Nitric oxide as modulator of neuronal function. *Prog. Neurobiol.* **2001**, *64*, 51–68. [CrossRef] [PubMed]
63. Fakler, C.R.; Kaftan, H.A.; Nelin, L.D. Two cases suggesting a role for the L-arginine nitric oxide pathway in neonatal blood pressure regulation. *Acta Paediatr.* **1995**, *84*, 460–462. [CrossRef] [PubMed]
64. Wu, G.; Morris, S.M., Jr. Arginine metabolism: Nitric oxide and beyond. *Biochem. J.* **1998**, *336*, 1–17. [CrossRef] [PubMed]
65. Tong, B.C.; Barbul, A. Cellular and physiological effects of arginine. *Mini Rev. Med. Chem.* **2004**, *4*, 823–832. [CrossRef]
66. Flynn, N.E.; Meininger, C.J.; Haynes, T.E.; Wu, G. The metabolic basis of arginine nutrition and pharmacotherapy. *Biomed. Pharmacother.* **2002**, *56*, 427. [CrossRef]
67. Orlando, G.F.; Wolf, G.; Engelmann, M. Role of neuronal nitric oxide synthase in the regulation of the neuroendocrine stress response in rodents: Insights from mutant mice. *Amino Acids* **2008**, *35*, 17–27. [CrossRef]
68. Langkamp-Henken, B.; Johnson, L.R.; Viar, M.J.; Geller, A.M.; Kotb, M. Differential effect on polyamine metabolism in mitogen- and superantigen-activated human T-cells. *Biochim. Biophys. Acta* **1998**, *425*, 337–347. [CrossRef]
69. Reitano, G.; Grasso, S.; Distefano, G.; Messina, A. The serum insulin and growth hormone response to arginine and to arginine with glucose in the premature infant. *J. Clin. Endocrinol.* **1971**, *33*, 924–928. [CrossRef]
70. Lewis, B.; Langkamp-Henken, B.J. Arginine enhances in vivo immune responses in young, adult and aged mice. *J. Nutr.* **2000**, *130*, 1827–1830. [CrossRef]
71. Waugh, W.H.; Daeschner, C.W., 3rd; Files, B.A.; McConnell, M.E.; Strandjord, S.E. Oral citrulline as arginine precursor may be beneficial in sickle cell disease: Early phase two results. *J. Natl. Med. Assoc.* **2001**, *93*, 363–371.
72. Marin, V.B.; Rodriguez-Osiac, L.; Schlessinger, L.; Villegas, J.; Lopez, M.; Castillo-Duran, C. Controlled study of enteral arginine supplementation in burned children: Impact on immunologic and metabolic status. *Nutrition* **2006**, *22*, 705–712. [CrossRef]
73. Martí I Líndez, A.A.; Reith, W. Arginine-dependent immune responses. *Cell. Mol. Life Sci.* **2021**, *78*, 5303–5324. [CrossRef]
74. Pérez-Cano, F.J.; Franch, À.; Castellote, C.; Castell, M. The suckling rat as a model for immunonutrition studies in early life. *Clin. Dev. Immunol.* **2012**, *2012*, 537310. [CrossRef]
75. Rashid, J.; Kumar, S.S.; Job, K.M.; Liu, X.; Fike, C.D.; Sherwin, C.M. Therapeutic Potential of Citrulline as an Arginine Supplement: A Clinical Pharmacology Review. *Pediatr. Drugs* **2020**, *22*, 279–293. [CrossRef]
76. Tocher, D.R.; Betancor, M.B.; Sprague, M.; Olsen, R.E.; Napier, J.A. Omega-3 long-chain polyunsaturated fatty acids, EPA and DHA: Bridging the gap between supply and demand. *Nutrients* **2019**, *11*, 89. [CrossRef]
77. Bishop, K.S.; Erdrich, S.; Karunasinghe, N.; Han, D.Y.; Zhu, S.; Jesuthasan, A.; Ferguson, L.R. An investigation into the association between DNA damage and dietary fatty acid in men with prostate cancer. *Nutrients* **2015**, *7*, 405–422. [CrossRef]
78. Calder, P.C.; Yaqoob, P. Lipid rafts—Composition, characterization and controversies. *J. Nutr.* **2007**, *137*, 545–547. [CrossRef]
79. Miles, E.A.; Calder, P.C. Modulation of immune function by dietary fatty acids. *Proc. Nutr. Soc.* **1998**, *57*, 277–292. [CrossRef]
80. Calder, P.C. The relationship between the fatty acid composition of immune cells and their function. *Prost. Leuk. Essent. Fatty Acids* **2008**, *79*, 101–108. [CrossRef]
81. Uauy, R.D.; Birch, D.G.; Birch, E.E.; Tyson, J.E.; Hoffman, D.R. Effect of dietary n-3 fatty acids on retinal function of very low birthweight neonates. *Pediatr. Res.* **1990**, *28*, 485–492. [CrossRef]
82. Carlson, S.E.; Werkman, S.H.; Rhodes, P.G.; Tolley, E. Visualacuity development in healthy preterm infants: Effect of marine-oil supplementation. *Am. J. Clin. Nutr.* **1993**, *58*, 35–42. [CrossRef]
83. Richardson, A.J. Clinical trials of fatty acid treatment in ADHD, dyslexia, dyspraxia and the autistic spectrum. *Prost. Leuk. Essent. Fatty Acids* **2004**, *70*, 383–390. [CrossRef]
84. Sanders, T.A.; Naismith, D.J. A comparison of the influence of breast-feeding and bottle-feeding on the fatty acid composition of the erythrocytes. *Br. J. Nutr.* **1979**, *41*, 619–623. [CrossRef]
85. Luchtman, D.W.; Song, C. Cognitive enhancement by omega-3 fatty acids from child-hood to old age: Findings from animal and clinical studies. *Neuropharmacology* **2013**, *64*, 550–565. [CrossRef]
86. Kong, W.; Yen, J.H.; Vassiliou, E.; Adhikary, S.; Toscano, M.G.; Ganea, D. Docosahexaenoic acid prevents dendritic cell maturation and in vitro and in vivo expression of the IL-12 cytokine family. *Lipids Health Dis.* **2010**, *9*, 12. [CrossRef]
87. Zapata-Gonzalez, F.; Rueda, F.; Petriz, J.; Domingo, P.; Villarroya, F.; DiazDelfin, J.; de Madariaga, M.A.; Domingo, J.C. Human dendritic cell activities are modulated by the omega-3 fatty acid, docosahexaenoic acid, mainly through PPAR(gamma): RXR heterodimers: Comparison with other polyunsaturated fatty acids. *J. Leukoc. Biol.* **2008**, *84*, 1172–1182. [CrossRef]
88. De Caterina, R.; Libby, P. Control of endothelial leukocyte adhesion molecules by fatty acids. *Lipids* **1996**, *31*, S57–S63. [CrossRef]
89. Babcock, T.A.; Novak, T.; Ong, E.; Jho, D.H.; Helton, W.S.; Espat, N.J. Modulation of lipopolysaccharide-stimulated macrophage tumor necrosis factor-α production by v-3 fatty acid is associated with differential cyclooxygenase-2 protein expression and is independent of interleukin-10. *J. Surg. Res.* **2002**, *107*, 135–139.
90. Lee, J.Y.; Sohn, K.H.; Rhee, S.H.; Hwang, D. Saturated fatty acids, but not unsaturated fatty acids, induce the expression of cyclooxygenase-2 mediated through Toll-like receptor 4. *J. Biol. Chem.* **2001**, *276*, 16683–16689. [CrossRef]
91. Draper, E.; Reynolds, C.M.; Canavan, M.; Mills, K.H.; Loscher, C.E.; Roche, H.M. Omega-3 fatty acids attenuate dendritic cell function via NF-kB independent of PPARg. *J. Nutr. Biochem.* **2011**, *22*, 784–790. [CrossRef]

92. Novak, T.E.; Babcock, T.A.; Jho, D.H.; Helton, W.S.; Espat, N.J. NF-kappa B inhibition by omega-3 fatty acids modulates LPS-stimulated macrophage TNF-alpha transcription. *Am. J. Physiol. Lung Cell Mol. Physiol.* **2003**, *284*, L84–L89. [CrossRef]
93. Calder, P.C. N-3 polyunsaturated fatty acids, inflammation, and inflammatory diseases. *Am. J. Clin. Nutr.* **2006**, *83*, S1505–S1519. [CrossRef]
94. Podpeskar, A.; Crazzolara, R.; Kropshofer, G.; Hetzer, B.; Meister, B.; Müller, T.; Salvador, C. Omega-3 Fatty Acids and Their Role in Pediatric Cancer. *Nutrients* **2021**, *13*, 1800. [CrossRef]
95. Suchner, U.; Kuhn, K.S.; Furst, P. The scientific basis of immunonutrition. *Proc. Nutr. Soc.* **2000**, *59*, 553–563. [CrossRef]
96. Schloerb, P.R. Immune-enhancing diets: Products, components, and their rationales. *JPEN J. Parenter. Enter. Nutr.* **2001**, *25*, S3–S7. [CrossRef]
97. Hess, J.R.; Greenberg, N.A. The role of nucleotides in the immune and gastrointestinal systems: Potential clinical applications. *Nutr. Clin. Pract.* **2012**, *27*, 281–294. [CrossRef]
98. Steinberg, G.R.; Kemp, B.E. AMPK in health and disease. *Physiol. Rev.* **2009**, *89*, 1025–1078. [CrossRef]
99. Rudolph, F.B.; Kulkarni, A.D.; Fanslow, W.C.; Pizzini, R.P.; Kumar, S.; Van Buren, C.T. Role of RNA as a dietary source of pyrimidines and purines in immune function. *Nutrition* **1990**, *6*, 45–52.
100. Jyonouchi, H.; Lei, Z.-S.; Tomita, Y.; Yokoyama, H. Nucleotide-free diet impairs T-helper cell functions in antibody production in response to T-dependent antigens in normal C57BL/6 mice. *J. Nutr.* **1994**, *124*, 475–484. [CrossRef]
101. Hasko, G. Adenosine inhibits IL-12 and TNF-α production via adenosine A2a receptor-dependent and independent mechanisms. *FASEB J.* **2000**, *14*, 2065–2074. [CrossRef]
102. Ding, T.; Song, G.; Liu, X.; Xu, M.; Li, Y. Nucleotides as optimal candidates for essential nutrients in living organisms: A review. *J. Funct. Foods* **2021**, *82*, 104498. [CrossRef]
103. Carver, J.D.; Pimentel, B.; Cox, W.I.; Barness, L.A. Dietary nucleotide effects upon immune function in infants. *Pediatrics* **1991**, *88*, 359–363. [CrossRef]
104. Zaky, A.A.; Simal-Gandara, J.; Eun, J.-B.; Shim, J.-H.; Abd El-Aty, A.M. Bioactivities, Applications, Safety, and Health Benefits of Bioactive Peptides from Food and By-Products: A Review. *Front. Nutr.* **2022**, *8*, 815640. [CrossRef]
105. Mizock, B. Immunonutrition and critical illness: An update. *Nutrition* **2010**, *26*, 701–707. [CrossRef]
106. Cruzat, V.F.; Pantaleao, L.C.; Donato, J., Jr.; de Bittencourt, P.I.H., Jr.; Tirapegui, J. Oral supplementations with free and dipeptide forms of l-glutamine in endotoxemic mice: Effects on muscle glutamine-glutathione axis and heat shock proteins. *J. Nutr. Biochem.* **2014**, *25*, 345–352. [CrossRef]
107. Rodas, P.C.; Rooyackers, O.; Hebert, C.; Norberg, A.; Wernerman, J. Glutamine and glutathione at icu admission in relation to outcome. *Clin. Sci.* **2012**, *122*, 591–597. [CrossRef]
108. Altman, B.J.; Stine, Z.E.; Dang, C.V. From Krebs to clinic: Glutamine metabolism to cancer therapy. *Nat. Rev. Cancer* **2016**, *16*, 619–634. [CrossRef]
109. Rogero, M.M.; Borges, M.C.; Pires, I.S.D.; Borelli, P.; Tirapegui, J. Ffect of glutamine supplementation and in vivo infection with mycobacterium bovis (bacillus calmette-guerin) in the function of peritoneal macrophages in early weaned mice. *Ann. Nutr. Metab.* **2007**, *51*, 173–174.
110. Flaring, U.B.; Rooyackers, O.E.; Wernerman, J.; Hammarqvist, F. Glutamine attenuates post-traumatic glutathione depletion in human muscle. *Clin. Sci.* **2003**, *104*, 275–282. [CrossRef]
111. Leite, J.S.; Raizel, R.; Hypolito, T.M.; Rosa, T.D.; Cruzat, V.F.; Tirapegui, J. L-glutamine and l-alanine supplementation increase glutamine-glutathione axis and muscle hsp-27 in rats trained using a progressive high-intensity resistance exercise. *Appl. Physiol. Nutr. Metab.* **2016**, *41*, 842–849. [CrossRef]
112. Marino, L.V.; Pathan, N.; Meyer, R.; Wright, V.; Habibi, P. Glutamine depletion and heat shock protein 70 (HSP70) in children with meningococcal disease. *Clin. Nutr.* **2014**, *33*, 915–921. [CrossRef] [PubMed]
113. Roth, E. Nonnutritive effects of glutamine. *J. Nutr.* **2008**, *138*, 2025S–2031S. [CrossRef] [PubMed]
114. Curi, R.; Newsholme, P.; Marzuca-Nassr, G.N.; Takahashi, H.K.; Hirabara, S.M.; Cruzat, V.; Krause, M.; de Bittencourt, P.I.H., Jr. Regulatory principles in metabolism-then and now. *Biochem. J.* **2016**, *473*, 1845–1857. [CrossRef] [PubMed]
115. Mullen, A.R.; Hu, Z.; Shi, X.; Jiang, L.; Boroughs, L.K.; Kovacs, Z.; Boriack, R.; Rakheja, D.; Sullivan, L.B.; Linehan, W.M.; et al. Oxidation of alpha-ketoglutarate is required for reductive carboxylation in cancer cells with mitochondrial defects. *Cell Rep.* **2014**, *7*, 1679–1690. [CrossRef] [PubMed]
116. Yang, L.F.; Venneti, S.; Nagrath, D. Glutaminolysis: A hallmark of cancer metabolism. *Annu. Rev. Biomed. Eng.* **2017**, *19*, 163–194. [CrossRef]
117. Newsholme, P.; Diniz, V.L.S.; Dodd, G.T.; Cruzat, V. Glutamine metabolism and optimal immune and CNS function. *Proc. Nutr. Soci.* **2023**, *82*, 22–31. [CrossRef] [PubMed]
118. Cruzat, V.; Macedo Rogero, M.; Noel Keane, K.; Curi, R.; Newsholme, P. Glutamine: Metabolism and Immune Function, Supplementation and Clinical Translation. *Nutrients* **2018**, *10*, 1564. [CrossRef] [PubMed]
119. Newsholme, E.A.; Parry-Billings, M. Properties of glutamine release from muscle and its importance for the immune system. *JPEN J. Parenter. Enter. Nutr.* **1990**, *14*, 63S–67S. [CrossRef] [PubMed]
120. Thomas, S.; Prabhu, R.; Balasubramanian, K.A. Surgical manipulation of the intestine and distant organ damage—Protection by oral glutamine supplementation. *Surgery* **2005**, *137*, 48–55. [CrossRef]

121. Deters, B.J.; Saleem, M. The role of glutamine in supporting gut health and neuropsychiatric factors. *Food Sci. Hum. Wellness* **2021**, *10*, 149–154. [CrossRef]
122. Wu, G. Functional amino acids in growth, reproduction, and health. *Adv. Nutr.* **2010**, *1*, 31–37. [CrossRef] [PubMed]
123. Van der Flier, L.G.; Clevers, H. Stem cells, self-renewal, and differentiation in the intestinal epithelium. *Annu. Rev. Physiol.* **2009**, *71*, 241–260. [CrossRef] [PubMed]
124. Zhang, W.; Liu, H.T. MAPK signal pathways in the regulation of cell proliferation in mammalian cells. *Cell Res.* **2002**, *12*, 9–18. [CrossRef] [PubMed]
125. Wang, B.; Wu, G.; Zhou, Z.; Dai, Z.; Sun, Y.; Ji, Y.; Wu, Z. Glutamine and intestinal barrier function. *Amino Acids* **2014**, *47*, 2143–2154. [CrossRef] [PubMed]
126. Li, N.; Lewis, P.; Samuelson, D.; Liboni, K.; Neu, J. Glutamine regulates Caco-2 cell tight junction proteins. *Am. J. Physiol. Gastrointest. Liv. Physiol.* **2004**, *287*, G726–G733. [CrossRef] [PubMed]
127. Li, N.; Neu, J. Glutamine deprivation alters intestinal tight junctions via a PI3-K/Akt mediated pathway in Caco-2 cells. *J. Nutr.* **2009**, *139*, 710–714. [CrossRef]
128. Ullman, T.A.; Itzkowitz, S.H. Intestinal inflammation and cancer. *Gastroenterology* **2011**, *140*, 1807–1816. [CrossRef] [PubMed]
129. Rhoads, J.M.; Wu, G. Glutamine, arginine, and leucine signaling in the intestine. *Amino Acids* **2009**, *37*, 111–122. [CrossRef]
130. Kaplan, M.H. STAT signaling in inflammation. *JAK-STAT* **2013**, *2*, e24198. [CrossRef]
131. Roth, E.; Oehler, R.; Manhart, N.; Exner, R.; Wessner, B.; Strasser, E.; Spittler, A. Regulative potential of glutamine—Relation to glutathione metabolism. *Nutrition* **2002**, *18*, 217–221. [CrossRef]
132. Fan, T.J.; Han, L.H.; Cong, R.S.; Liang, J. Caspase family proteases and apoptosis. *Acta Biochim. Biophys. Sin.* **2005**, *37*, 719–727. [CrossRef]
133. Ropeleski, M.J.; Riehm, J.; Baer, K.A.; Musch, M.W.; Chang, E.B. Anti-apoptotic effects of L-glutamine-mediated transcriptional modulation of the heat shock protein 72 during heat shock. *Gastroenterology* **2005**, *129*, 170–184. [CrossRef] [PubMed]
134. Martinez, M.R.; Dias, T.B.; Natov, P.S.; Zachara, N.E. Stress-induced O-GlcNAcylation: An adaptive process of injured cells. *Biochem. Soc. Trans.* **2017**, *45*, 237–249. [CrossRef] [PubMed]
135. Rosa, L.; Cutone, A.; Lepanto, M.S.; Paesano, R.; Valenti, P. Lactoferrin: A natural glycoprotein involved in iron and inflammatory homeostasis. *Int. J. Mol. Sci.* **2017**, *18*, 1985. [CrossRef]
136. Buccigrossi, V.; de Marco, G.; Bruzzese, E.; Ombrato, L.; Bracale, I.; Polito, G.; Guarino, A. Lactoferrin Induces Concentration-Dependent Functional Modulation of Intestinal Proliferation and Differentiation. *Pediatr. Res.* **2007**, *61*, 410–414. [CrossRef]
137. Lönnerdal, B. Bioactive Proteins in Human Milk: Health, Nutrition, and Implications for Infant Formulas. *J. Pediatr.* **2016**, *173*, S4–S9. [CrossRef] [PubMed]
138. Wang, B.; Timilsena, Y.P.; Blanch, E.; Adhikari, B. Lactoferrin: Structure, function, denaturation and digestion. *Crit. Rev. Food Sci. Nutr.* **2019**, *59*, 580–596. [CrossRef]
139. Wakabayashi, H.; Yamauchi, K.; Takase, M. Lactoferrin research, technology and applications. *Int. Dairy J.* **2006**, *16*, 1241–1251. [CrossRef]
140. Kruzel, M.L.; Zimecki, M.; Actor, J.K. Lactoferrin in a Context of Inflammation-Induced Pathology. *Front. Immunol.* **2017**, *8*, 1438. [CrossRef]
141. Wakabayashi, H.; Oda, H.; Yamauchi, K.; Abe, F. Lactoferrin for prevention of common viral infections. *J. Infect. Chemother.* **2014**, *20*, 666–671. [CrossRef]
142. Grover, M.; Giouzeppos, O.; Schnagl, R.D.; May, J.T. Effect of human milk prostaglandins and lactoferrin on respiratory syncytial virus and rotavirus. *Acta Paediatr.* **1997**, *86*, 315–316. [CrossRef] [PubMed]
143. Pietrantoni, A.; Ammendolia, M.G.; Superti, F. Bovine lactoferrin: Involvement of metal saturation and carbohydrates in the inhibition of influenza virus infection. *Biochem. Cell Biol.* **2012**, *90*, 442–448. [CrossRef] [PubMed]
144. Saad, K.; Abo-Elela, M.G.M.; El-Baseer, K.A.A.; Ahmed, A.E.; Ahmad, F.A.; Tawfeek, M.S.K.; Houfey, A.A.E.; Aboul_Khair, M.D.; Abdel-Salam, A.M.; Abo-Elgheit, A.; et al. Effects of bovine colostrum on recurrent respiratory tract infections and diarrhea in children. *Medicine* **2016**, *95*, e4560. [CrossRef]
145. Hu, Y.; Meng, X.; Zhang, F.; Xiang, Y.; Wang, J. The in vitro antiviral activity of lactoferrin against common human coronaviruses and SARSCoV-2 is mediated by targeting the heparan sulfate co-receptor. *Emerg. Microbes Infect.* **2021**, *10*, 317–330. [CrossRef]
146. Cutone, A.; Rosa, L.; Lepanto, M.S.; Scotti, M.J.; Berlutti, F.; Bonaccorsi di Patti, M.C.; Musci, G.; Valenti, P. Lactoferrin efficiently counteracts the inflammation-induced changes of the iron homeostasis system in macrophages. *Front. Immunol.* **2017**, *8*, 705. [CrossRef] [PubMed]
147. Widjaja, N.A.; Hamidah, A.; Purnomo, M.T.; Ardianah, E. Effect of lactoferrin in oral nutrition supplement (ONS) towards IL-6 and IL-10 in failure to thrive children with infection. *F1000Research* **2023**, *12*, 897. [CrossRef] [PubMed]
148. Motoki, N.; Mizuki, M.; Tsukahara, T.; Miyakawa, M.; Kubo, S.; Oda, H.; Tanaka, M.; Yamauchi, K.; Abe, F.; Nomiyama, T. Effects of Lactoferrin-Fortified Formula on Acute Gastrointestinal Symptoms in Children Aged 12-32 Months: A Randomized, Double-Blind, Placebo-Controlled Trial. *Front. Pediatr.* **2020**, *8*, 233. [CrossRef]
149. Manzoni, P. Clinical Benefits of Lactoferrin for Infants and Children. *J. Pediatr.* **2016**, *173*, S43–S52. [CrossRef] [PubMed]
150. Fan, P.; Li, L.; Rezaei, A.; Eslamfam, S.; Che, D.; Ma, X. Metabolites of dietary protein and peptides by intestinal microbes and their impacts on gut. *Curr. Protein Pept. Sci.* **2015**, *16*, 646–654. [CrossRef]

151. Bergman, E.N. Energy contributions of volatile fatty acids from the gastrointestinal tract in various species. *Physiol. Rev.* **1990**, *70*, 567–590. [CrossRef]
152. Byrne, C.; Chambers, E.; Morrison, D.; Frost, G. The role of short chain fatty acids in appetite regulation and energy homeostasis. *Int. J. Obes.* **2015**, *39*, 1331–1338. [CrossRef]
153. Kumar, A.; Alrefai, W.A.; Borthakur, A.; Dudeja, P.K. Lactobacillus acidophilus counteracts enteropathogenic E. coli-induced inhibition of butyrate uptake in intestinal epithelial cells. *Am. J. Physiol. Gastrointest. Liver Physiol.* **2015**, *309*, G602–G607. [CrossRef]
154. Takebe, K.; Nio, J.; Morimatsu, M.; Karaki, S.-I.; Kuwahara, A.; Kato, I.; Iwanaga, T. Histochemical demonstration of a Na+ coupled transporter for short-chain fatty acids (slc5a8) in the intestine and kidney of the mouse. *Biomed. Res.* **2005**, *26*, 213–221. [CrossRef]
155. Wong, J.M.W.; De Souza, R.; Kendall, C.W.C.; Emam, A.; Jenkins, D.J.A. Colonic health: Fermentation and short chain fatty acids. *J. Clin. Gastroenterol.* **2006**, *40*, 235–243. [CrossRef]
156. Gill, P.A.; van Zelm, M.C.; Muir, J.G.; Gibson, P.R. Review article: Short chain fatty acids as potential therapeutic agents in human gastrointestinal and inflammatory disorders. *Aliment. Pharmacol. Ther.* **2018**, *48*, 15–34. [CrossRef]
157. Liu, H.; Wang, J.; He, T.; Becker, S.; Zhang, G.; Li, D.; Ma, X. Butyrate: A Double-Edged Sword for Health? *Adv. Nutr.* **2018**, *9*, 21–29. [CrossRef]
158. Kimura, I.; Inoue, D.; Maeda, T.; Hara, T.; Ichimura, A.; Miyauchi, S.; Kobayashi, M.; Hirasawa, A.; Tsujimoto, G. Short-chain fatty acids and ketones directly regulate sympathetic nervous system via G protein–coupled receptor 41 (GPR41). *Proc. Natl. Acad. Sci. USA* **2011**, *108*, 8030–8035. [CrossRef]
159. Singh, N.; Gurav, A.; Sivaprakasam, S.; Brady, E.; Padia, R.; Shi, H.; Thangaraju, M.; Prasad, P.D.; Manicassamy, S.; Munn, D.H. Activation of Gpr109a, receptor for niacin and the commensal metabolite butyrate, suppresses colonic inflammation and carcinogenesis. *Immunity* **2014**, *40*, 128–139. [CrossRef]
160. Meijer, K.; de Vos, P.; Priebe, M.G. Butyrate and other short-chain fatty acids as modulators of immunity: What relevance for health? *Curr. Opin. Clin. Nutr. Metab. Care* **2010**, *13*, 715–721. [CrossRef]
161. Cresci, G.A.; Bush, K.; Nagy, L.E. Tributyrin supplementation protects mice from acute ethanol-induced gut injury. *Alcohol. Clin. Exp. Res.* **2014**, *38*, 1489–1501. [CrossRef]
162. Li, M.; Van Esch, B.C.; Wagenaar, G.T.; Garssen, J.; Folkerts, G.; Henricks, P.A. Pro- and anti-inflammatory effects of short chain fatty acids on immune and endothelial cells. *Eur. J. Pharmacol.* **2018**, *831*, 52–59. [CrossRef] [PubMed]
163. Turner, N.D.; Lupton, J.R. Dietary fiber. *Adv. Nutr.* **2011**, *2*, 151–152. [CrossRef] [PubMed]
164. Flint, H.J.; Scott, K.P.; Louis, P.; Duncan, S.H. The role of the gut microbiota in nutrition and health. *Nat. Rev. Gastroenterol. Hepatol.* **2012**, *9*, 577–589. [CrossRef] [PubMed]
165. Park, J.; Kim, M.; Kang, S.G.; Jannasch, A.H.; Cooper, B.; Patterson, J.; Kim, C.H. Short chain fatty acids induce both effector and regulatory T cells by suppression of histone deacetylases and regulation of the mTOR-S6K pathway. *Mucosal Immunol.* **2015**, *8*, 80. [CrossRef] [PubMed]
166. LeBlanc, J.G.; Chain, F.; Martín, R.; Bermúdez-Humarán, L.G.; Courau, S.; Langella, P. Beneficial effects on host energy metabolism of short-chain fatty acids and vitamins produced by commensal and probiotic bacteria. *Microb. Cell Fact.* **2017**, *16*, 79. [CrossRef]
167. Coppola, S.; Nocerino, R.; Paparo, L.; Bedogni, G.; Calignano, A.; Di Scala, C.; de Giovanni di Santa Severina, A.F.; De Filippis, F.; Ercolini, D.; Berni Canani, R. Therapeutic Effects of Butyrate on Pediatric Obesity: A Randomized Clinical Trial. *JAMA Netw. Open* **2022**, *5*, e2244912. [CrossRef]

Disclaimer/Publisher's Note: The statements, opinions and data contained in all publications are solely those of the individual author(s) and contributor(s) and not of MDPI and/or the editor(s). MDPI and/or the editor(s) disclaim responsibility for any injury to people or property resulting from any ideas, methods, instructions or products referred to in the content.

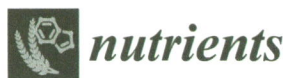 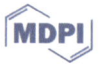

Review

Mexican Plants Involved in Glucose Homeostasis and Body Weight Control: Systematic Review

Montserrat Torres-Vanda [1] and Ruth Gutiérrez-Aguilar [1,2,*]

[1] Laboratorio de Investigación en Enfermedades Metabólicas: Obesidad y Diabetes, Hospital Infantil de México "Federico Gómez", Mexico City 06720, Mexico
[2] División de Investigación, Facultad de Medicina, Universidad Nacional Autónoma de México (UNAM), Mexico City 04510, Mexico
* Correspondence: ruthgutz@unam.mx; Tel.: +52-55-5228-9917 (ext. 4509)

Abstract: Background: Obesity is defined as abnormal or excessive fat accumulation, provoking many different diseases, such as obesity and type 2 diabetes. Type 2 diabetes is a chronic-degenerative disease characterized by increased blood glucose levels. Obesity and type 2 diabetes are currently considered public health problems, and their prevalence has increased over the last few years. Because of the high cost involved in the treatment of both diseases, different alternatives have been sought. However, the general population uses medicinal plants, in the form of tea or infusions, to treat different diseases. Therefore, traditional medicine using medicinal plants has been investigated as a possible treatment for type 2 diabetes and body weight control. Aim of the study: The purpose of this review is to find medicinal plants used in Mexico that could exert their beneficial effect by regulating insulin secretion and body weight control. Material and method: For the development of this review, Mexican plants used in traditional medicine to treat type 2 diabetes and body weight control were searched in PubMed, Google Scholar, and Scopus. The inclusion criteria include plants that presented a significant reduction in blood glucose levels and/or an increase in insulin secretion. Results: We found 306 Mexican plants with hypoglycemic effects. However, plants that did not show evidence of an increase in insulin secretion were eliminated. Finally, only five plants were included in this review: *Momordica charantia* L. (*melón amargo*), *Cucurbita ficifolia bouché* (*chilacayote*), *Coriandrum sativum* L. (*cilantro*), *Persea americana* Mill. (*aguacate*) *Bidens pilosa* (*amor seco*), including 39 articles in total. Here, we summarized the plant extracts (aqueous and organic) that have previously been reported to present hypoglycemic effects, body weight control, increased secretion and sensitivity of insulin, improvement of pancreatic β cells, and glucose tolerance. Additionally, these effects may be due to different bioactive compounds present in the plants' extracts. Conclusion: Both in vivo and in vitro studies are required to understand the mechanism of action of these plant extracts regarding insulin secretion to be used as a possible treatment for type 2 diabetes and body weight control in the future.

Keywords: type 2 diabetes; glucose homeostasis; insulin secretion; body weight control; medicinal plants

---

Citation: Torres-Vanda, M.; Gutiérrez-Aguilar, R. Mexican Plants Involved in Glucose Homeostasis and Body Weight Control: Systematic Review. *Nutrients* 2023, *15*, 2070. https://doi.org/10.3390/nu15092070

Academic Editor: Jacqueline Isaura Alvarez-Leite

Received: 22 February 2023
Revised: 10 March 2023
Accepted: 14 March 2023
Published: 25 April 2023

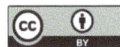

Copyright: © 2023 by the authors. Licensee MDPI, Basel, Switzerland. This article is an open access article distributed under the terms and conditions of the Creative Commons Attribution (CC BY) license (https://creativecommons.org/licenses/by/4.0/).

1. Introduction

Obesity is one of the most serious global public health problems, and it is defined as abnormal or excessive fat accumulation, representing a health risk. In adults, a body mass index (BMI) over 25 is considered overweight, and over 30 is obese [1]. The prevalence of obesity in children and adults has been increasing over the last decades, predicting that one billion people globally, including 1 in 5 women and 1 in 7 men, will be living with obesity by 2030 [2]. In Mexico, 76% of adult women are overweight or obese, while men have a prevalence of 72.1% [3]. Obesity increases the risk of developing different diseases, such as arterial hypertension, dyslipidemia, metabolic syndrome, and type 2 diabetes (T2D) [4].

T2D is a multifactorial metabolic disorder that is mainly influenced by the presence of obesity (80–90% of TD2 patients are overweight or obese), lack of physical activity, poor eating habits, and genetic factors [5]. T2D is characterized by the presence of chronic hyperglycemia, which appears when the body does not effectively use the insulin it produces or, ultimately, when the pancreas does not secrete enough insulin [6].

The prevalence of T2D has gradually been increasing, with a world prevalence of 9.3% [7]. The prevalence of T2D in Mexico has been increasing in the last eight years from 9.2% (2012) to 10.6% (2020) [3]. Therefore, T2D is considered one of the leading causes of death in Mexico, representing a mortality of 15.7% [8].

The high prevalence of obesity and T2D in the Mexican population brings serious consequences on the economy, both individually and collectively [9], since those patients require more frequent medical attention and a greater amount of medicines [10]. Therefore, the general Mexican population resorts to medicinal plants in the form of teas or infusions to ameliorate T2D and control body weight [11].

Medicinal plants have been used empirically (either as part of the diet, infusions, or extracts) to treat and improve T2D symptoms and body weight control. Despite being used empirically, the World Health Organization has guidelines on the safety monitoring of herbal medicines [12]. Different medicinal plants are now approved and recommended for medicinal use after they have been scientifically validated to ensure safety and efficacy, such as *Echinacea purpurea*, *Panax ginseg*, and *Passiflora incarnata*. However, the use of medicinal plants is not yet approved by the FDA [13].

The use of medicinal plants has been reported to have an effect on preventing and restoring pancreatic β cell damage caused by this disease. The positive effects of medicinal plants can be attributed to the content of their chemical compounds, such as flavonoids, polysaccharides, saponins, triterpenes, alkaloids, and phenolic compounds, that could exert their action on glucose homeostasis [14]. In addition, these medicinal plants can improve insulin secretion [14], which is necessary for the proper maintenance of glucose homeostasis.

Consequently, it is very important to study the ethnic plants that offer a beneficial effect on glucose metabolism, as well as their physiological effects. Therefore, these Mexican plants could be used as plausible new treatments for T2D and/or body weight control and could be accessible to the general population. Therefore, in this review, we will focus on describing medicinal plants that could have an action on the stimulation of insulin secretion, as well as body weight control.

2. Methods

2.1. Protocol and Registration

This systematic review was performed according to the Preferred Reporting Items for Systematic Reviews and Meta-Analyses (PRISMA).

2.2. Information Sources and Search Strategy

For the development of this review, Mexican plants used in traditional medicine to treat T2D with hypoglycemic properties, insulin secretion, and body weight control were searched in the databases PubMed, Google Scholar, and Scopus. The bibliographic search was performed using keywords or phrases such as: "antidiabetic Mexican plants", "Mexican plants with hypoglycemic effect", "Mexican plants and type 2 diabetes treatment" "antidiabetic Mexican plants", "antidiabetic Mexican plants and insulin secretion", "antidiabetic Mexican plants and beta cells", "effect of Mexican medicinal plants in insulin secretion", "Mexican plants with glucose lowering effect" and body weight control. Data from publications between 1999 and 2020 were included. The detailed search approach is described in Figure 1.

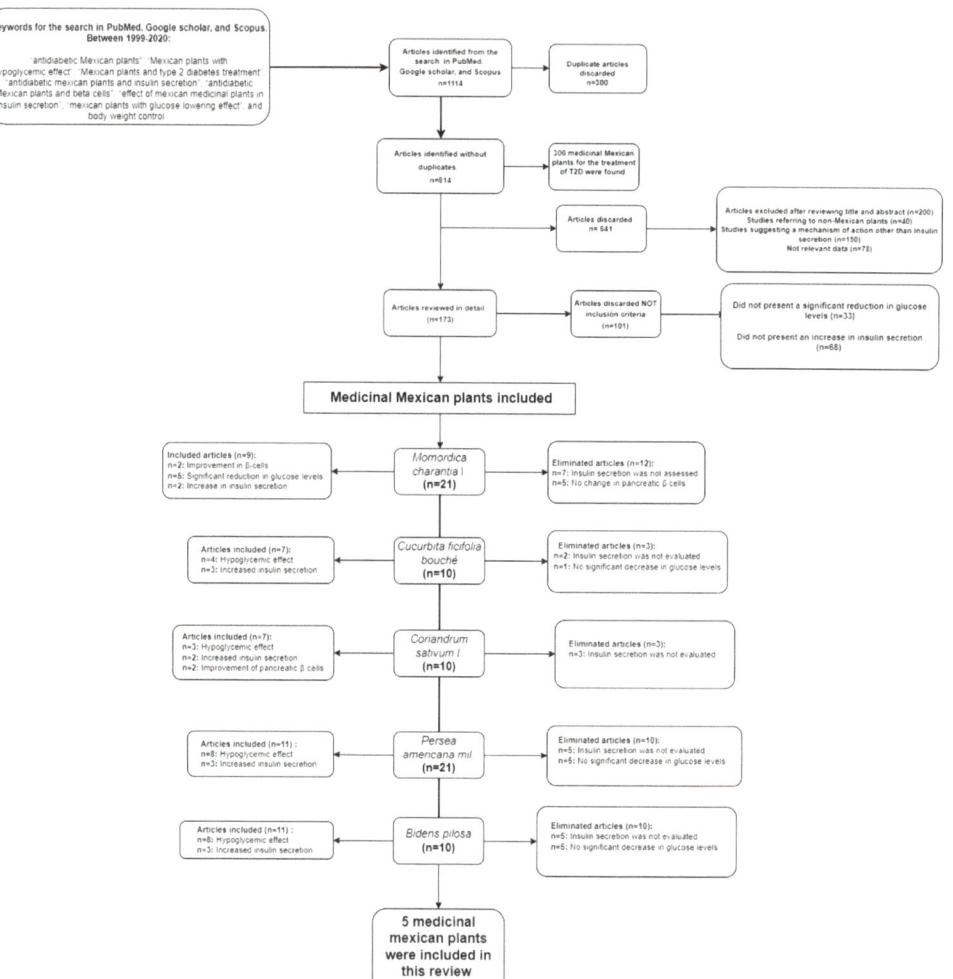

Figure 1. Systematic review flowchart. Identification, eligibility, plants selection, and analysis, using PRISMA (Preferred Reporting Items for Systematic Reviews and Meta-Analysis).

2.3. Eligibility Criteria

The main inclusion criteria for this review were studies that reported a decrease in glucose levels, an increase in insulin secretion, and body weight change using in vivo or in vitro models.

The exclusion criteria were studies suggesting a mechanism of action other than insulin secretion, studies referring to non-Mexican plants, and studies that reported plants that did not have an effect on glucose homeostasis (Figure 1).

2.4. Study Selection

In the screening or identification stage, all bibliographic material was retrieved by screening the titles and abstracts. The duplicated articles were removed. In the eligibility stage, the full texts of the publications were examined to assess the inclusion criteria. The agreement of two people was granted for the papers included in this systematic review.

3. Results

Our initial search identified 1114 publications in Pubmed, Google Scholar, and Scopus; however, 300 papers were duplicated, so they were discarded. Of the 814 non-duplicates, 306 Mexican medicinal plants were found for the treatment of T2D. However, 641 articles were also discarded because they fell within the exclusion criteria, leaving us with 173 articles that were reviewed in detail. Finally, a total of 39 articles were included in this systematic review of the following five plants: *Momordica charantia* L. (*Melón amargo*), *Cucurbita ficifolia bouché* (*chilacayote*), *Coriandrum sativum* L. (*cilantro*), *Persea americana* Mil. (*aguacate*), and *Bidens pilosa* (*amor seco*). In this review, studies in animal models, cell lines, and very few human trials were primarily included. However, other medicinal plants, such as *Psidium guajava*, *Opuntia ficus indica*, and *Aloe vera* have been tested in diabetic patients to evaluate their hypoglycemic effect reducing glucose levels in 10%, 9.2%, and 7.7%, respectively [15–18].

3.1. Momordica charantia L. (Melón amargo)

Momordica charantia L. is a medicinal plant cultivated in tropical and subtropical areas of Asia, South America, Africa, and the Caribbean. In Mexico, it is grown in Oaxaca, Quintana Roo, Chiapas, Tabasco, Veracruz, and Yucatán [19]. It belongs to the *Cucurbitaceae* family and is colloquially known as *Melón amargo* [20] (Figure 2).

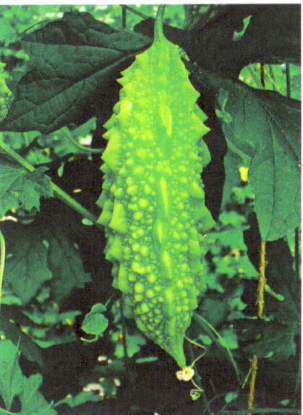

Figure 2. *Momordica charantia* L. (*melón amargo*) plant. Published by Wikimedia Commons licensed by Creative Commons, reprinted from [21]. https://creativecommons.org/licenses/by-sa/3.0/legalcode, accessed on 10 March 2023.

Momordica charantia L. produces an edible fruit that is harvested for cooking. The seeds and skin are also edible [20].

In the articles reviewed for this plant, aqueous or organic extracts from leaves, pulp, or seeds were obtained to perform in vivo and in vitro studies to analyze its hypoglycemic effect.

The effect of the methanolic extract on the leaves of *Momordica charantia* L. was evaluated in a diabetic rat model (Table 1). It was observed that the extract presented hypoglycemic activity (50% glucose levels reduction) and a reduction in triglyceride levels at doses of 200 mg/kg and 400 mg/kg, comparable to glibenclamide. An improvement in the structure of pancreatic β-cells was shown. It was also observed that the diabetic group, treated with the extract, presented an elevation in body weight, reversing the body weight loss caused by diabetes [22].

Table 1. Summary of reviewed articles of *Momordica charantia* L., considering the type of extract, the part of the plant, dose, experimental model, body weight, and physiologic or cellular effects. ↓ Decrease. ↑ Increase.

Plant	Extract	Part of the Plant	Dose	Experimental Model	Physiologic or Cellular Effects	Body Weight	Reference
Momordica charantia L. (melón amargo)	Methanol	Leaves	200 mg/kg 400 mg/kg	Wistar diabetic rats (alloxan)	Both doses showed: ↓ Glucose levels (50%) ↓ Lipids ↑ Antioxidant effect ↑ Structure of pancreatic β cells	- Diabetic rats: ↓ Body weight. - The group treated with the extract: ↑ Body weight, reversing the weight loss caused by diabetes	[22]
	Water	Leaves	100 mg/kg 400 mg/kg	Wistar diabetic rats (alloxan)	Both doses showed: ↓ Glucose (21%) ↓ Lipid levels Insulin secretion was not evaluated	- The diabetic group presented: ↓ Body weight loss of 25.11% - The group threatened with the extract presented: ↑ Body weight of 14.33%	[23]
	Water	Fruit	20 mg/kg	Streptozotocin-induced type 2 diabetic neonatal rats	↓ Glucose levels (33.3%) ↑ Serum insulin levels (33%) ↓ Damage to pancreatic islets		[24]
	Ethanol	Fruit	1 mg/kg 3 mg/kg	Normoglycemic and diabetic rabbits	- 1 mg/kg: ↓ Blood glucose levels (54.8%), ↓ Serum insulin levels (13%) - 3 mg/kg: ↓ Blood glucose levels (61.35%) ↑ Serum insulin levels (17%)	- Normoglycemic rabbits: ↓ Body weight of 4.4% - Diabetic rabbits ↓ Body weight of 1.35% - 1 mg/kg: ↓ Body weight 1.19% - 3 mg/kg: ↓ Body weight of 37%	[25]
	Ethanol	Fruit	250 mg/kg 500 mg/kg	C57BL/6 mice fed a high-fat diet.	Both doses showed: ↑ Insulin sensitivity ↓ Insulin levels (30%) ↓ Glucose blood levels (75%)	- 250 mg/kg: ↓ Body weight (14.8%) compared with the mice fed a high-fat diet - 500 mg/kg: ↓ Body weight (25%) compared to the mice fed with a high-fat diet ↑ SIRT1 levels	[26]
	Acid-ethanol	Pulp (proteins)	in vivo: 1 mg/kg 5 mg/kg 10 mg/kg in vitro: 10 µg/mL	Normoglycemic and diabetic Wistar rats. C2C12 myocytes 3T3-L1 adipocytes	- 10 mg/kg: ↓ Glucose levels in diabetic rats (43%) - The extract: ↑ Plasma insulin concentration. - C2C12 cell line: ↑ Glucose uptake (28%) - 3T3L-1 cell line: ↑ Glucose uptake (35%)		[27]

Table 1. Cont.

Plant	Extract	Part of the Plant	Dose	Experimental Model	Physiologic or Cellular Effects	Body Weight	Reference
	Water	Saponins (pulp)	400 mg/kg, 200 mg/kg, 100 mg/kg	Diabetic Wistar rats	- The three doses presented: ↓ Glucose levels (50%) ↑ Lipid metabolism Regulation of the insulin signaling pathway ↓ Insulin levels (16.6%) Protective effect of pancreatic β cells	- Diabetic group: ↓ body weight compared with normoglycemic rats - Atdministration of the extract: ↑ Body weight	[28]
	Isopropy alcohol	Pulp	Saponins: 20 mg/kg, 40 mg/kg, 80 mg/kg Polysaccharides: 500 mg/kg	Diabetic Kunming mice	- The doses of saponins presented: ↓ Glucose levels (10%) ↓ Insulin resistance returning insulin levels to normal ↑ Proportion of p-AMPK ↑ Antioxidant capacity The dose of 80 mg/kg of saponins presented a better effect	The polysaccharides and saponins extract: ↓ Body weight loss that presents during diabetes	[29]
	Water	Triterpenes (pulp)	20 μM 30 μM	FL83B (Mouse cell line of hepatocytes)	The doses used presented: ↑ Glucose uptake ↑ Phosphorylation of IRS-1 ↑ Insulin sensitivity ↑ AMPK activation ↑ inhibition of PTP-1B		[30]

Another study demonstrated the benefits of the aqueous extract of the leaves of *Momordica charantia* L. (doses 100 and 400 mg/kg), reducing glucose levels by 21%, as well as for triglycerides, HDL, LDL, creatinine, urea levels, and liver enzymes. On the other hand, the diabetic group presented a body loss of 25.11% compared to the normoglycemic group; however, when administering the extract, 14.33% of body weight regained was observed (Table 1) [23]. In another study, the aqueous extract of the whole fruit of *Momordica charantia* L. at a dose of 20 mg/kg in a neonatal diabetic rat model provoked 33.3% of hypoglycemic activity in 2–4 weeks after treatment. Moreover, an increase in serum insulin levels and decreased damage to pancreatic islets was observed [24].

In rabbits, the ethanol extract of the pulp of *Momordica charantia* L. at a dose of 1 mg/kg and 3 mg/kg provoked a decrease in blood glucose of 54.8% and 61.35%, and 13% and 17% increase in serum insulin, respectively. Regarding body weight, the doses presented a decrease of 1.19% and 37%, respectively. However, in normoglycemic control animals, this extract increased the body weight by 4.4% [25]. In C57BL/6 mice fed a high-fat diet, a similar extract was administered (ethanol extract of the pulp) at doses of 250 mg/kg and 500 mg/kg, observing a decrease in glucose blood levels (75%), an increase in insulin sensitivity and a decreased in insulin levels (30%), compared to the obese group. Moreover, the doses of 250 mg/kg and 500 mg/kg presented a decrease of 14 and 25% in body weight, respectively, compared to the mice fed with a high-fat diet. In this experiment, a decrease in fat mass and an increase in expression in SIRT1 (a protein involved in fatty acid beta-oxidation in the liver and insulin sensitivity) was observed (Table 1) [26]. On the other hand, proteins extracted from the pulp of *Momordica charantia* L., administered at doses of 1, 5, and 10 mg/kg in both normoglycemic and diabetic rats, showed an increase in plasma insulin concentrations and a reduction in plasma glucose, reaching a reduction of 43% with the dose of 10 mg/kg in diabetic rats. The effect of this protein extract at a dose of 10 μg/mL was investigated in myocytes (C2C12) and adipocytes (3T3L1), demonstrated an increase in glucose uptake of 28% and 35%, respectively, compared to their baseline control [27] (Table 1).

The hypoglycemic effect of saponins from the hydroalcoholic extract of the pulp of *Momordica charantia* L. was evaluated. The saponins were administered for 4 weeks, using doses of 400, 200, and 100 mg/kg (Table 1). This study showed that saponins could reduce glucose levels (10%) and insulin resistance in diabetic rats [28]. In addition, an improvement in lipid metabolism was demonstrated, preventing oxidative stress and regulating the insulin signaling pathway. In this experiment, the body weight was restored, and a decrease in fasting insulin levels was also obtained, as well as a protective effect of the β cells [28] (Table 1).

In another study, the effect of saponins (doses of 20, 40, and 80 mg/kg) as well as polysaccharides (doses of 500 mg/kg) extracted from the pulp of *Momordica charantia* L. with isopropyl alcohol in diabetic mice reduced glucose levels and insulin resistance (Table 1). In addition, the extracts increased p-AMPK (phosphorylated AMP-activated protein kinase) and improved antioxidant capacity, exhibiting a protective effect on pancreatic β cells. The dose of 80 mg/kg of saponins presented a better effect because it significantly reduced fasting blood glucose levels, improved insulin resistance, and restored body weight [29].

Other compounds found in *Momordica charantia* L. extracts are the triterpenes that are used at 20 and 30 μM in a mouse cell line of hepatocytes (FL83B), increased glucose uptake, and insulin receptor 1 (IRS-1) phosphorylation in insulin-resistant cells, which could indicate the improvement of insulin sensitivity. In addition, the triterpenes favored the translocation of GLUT-4 to the cell surface of insulin-resistant cells, increased AMPK activation and PTP-1B inhibition, improving the effects caused by insulin resistance [30].

In the articles reviewing this plant, the different extracts were compared primarily with glibenclamide (antidiabetic drug), having a similar hypoglycemic effect (50%) and restores body weight loss [22]. In addition, studies comparing the effect of these extracts against metformin (an antidiabetic drug) demonstrated a reduction of blood glucose levels of 50.1% using 300 mg/kg plant extract and 47% for metformin [31–33].

Therefore, *Momordica charantia* L. presents an effect in blood glucose and lipids (triglycerides, HDL, LDL) reduction, an increase in insulin sensitivity and secretion, an improvement in β cells, as well as restoring body weight. These effects can be due to the chemical compounds it presents (saponins, proteins, triterpenes, and polysaccharides) (Table 6).

3.2. Cucurbita ficifolia bouché (Chilacayote)

Cucurbita ficifolia bouché is a medicinal plant native to America. In Mexico, it is grown in Hidalgo, Guerrero, Michoacán, and Veracruz [34]. It belongs to the *Cucurbitaceae* family and is colloquially known as *chilacayote* [35] (Figure 3).

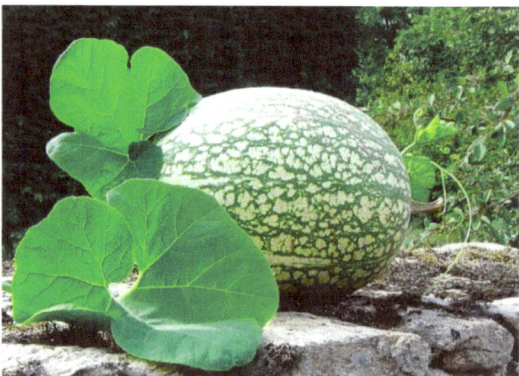

Figure 3. *Cucurbita ficifolia bouché* (*chilacayote*) plant. Published by Wikimedia Commons licensed by Creative Commons, reprinted from [36]. https://creativecommons.org/licenses/by-sa/3.0/legalcode, accessed on 10 March 2023.

The skin, pulp, and seeds are edible. In Mexico, the pulp and seeds are widely used to prepare different dishes and regional sweets [35].

Various investigations have been carried out regarding its hypoglycemic effect, both in vivo and in vitro, mainly using the seeds and pulp of the plant. These studies focus on its effect on insulin secretion and the mechanism for lowering blood glucose levels (Table 2), which are described below.

Table 2. Summary of reviewed articles on *Cucurbita ficifolia bouché*, considering the type of extract, the part of the plant, dose, experimental model, body weight, and physiologic or cellular effects. ↓ Decrease. ↑ Increase.

Plant	Extract	Part of the Plant	Dose	Experimental Model	Physiologic or Cellular Effects	Body Weight	Reference
	Processor	Fruit juice	4 mL/kg	10 patients with T2D	↓ Glucose levels (31%)		[37]
	Chilacayote freeze-dried juice.	Fruit	250 mg/kg 500 mg/kg 750 mg/kg 1000 mg/kg 1250 mg/kg	CD-1 normoglycemic and diabetic mice	All doses showed: ↓ Glucose levels in normoglycemic and diabetic mice (83%) The best dose was 500 mg/kg, without toxic effects		[38]
	Water	Seeds	500 mg/kg	CD-1 normoglycemic and diabetic mice	↓ Glucose levels in all stages of maturity of the fruit It presented a better effect in lowering glucose levels (50%) at 15 days of development of the fruit compared to glibenclamide		[39]
Cucurbita ficifolia bouché (chilacayote)	Methanol	Fruit without seeds	Diabetic: 300 mg/kg 600 mg/kg Normoglycemic: 600 mg/kg	Diabetic and normoglycemic Wistar rats	The two doses presented: ↓ Glucose levels in the diabetic group (60%) ↑ Increase in insulin levels (53%)	- The diabetic group presented: ↓ body weight (25%). - 300 mg/kg: It presented no significant difference in body weight. - 600 mg/kg: ↑ body weight (6%).	[40]
	Methanol	Fruit without seeds	300 mg/kg	Diabetic and normoglycemic Wistar rats	↓ Hyperglycemia (12.5%) ↓ Lipid peroxidation in the pancreas ↑ Insulin levels (36%) in the diabetic group ↑ Active pancreatic β cells		[41]
	Water	Fruit without seeds	0.25 μM of the aqueous extract and D-quiro-inositol	RINmF5 cells (mouse pancreatic β cells)	↑ mRNA of *insulin* (80%) and *Kir6.2* genes ↑ Insulin secretion. Glucose levels were not evaluated		[42]
	Water	Fruit without skin and seeds	*C. ficifolia* (72 μg/mL). D-quiro-inositol (400 μM)	RINmF5 cells (mouse pancreatic β cells)	- D-quiro-inositol: neither the concentration of insulin nor calcium increased - Aqueous extract: ↑ Concentration of calcium and insulin (28.5%)		[43]

A clinical study with 10 patients with T2D, to whom *Cucurbita ficifolia bouché* juice was administered at a dose of 4 mL/kg, showed a 31% decrease in glucose levels after 5 h of intake (Table 2); however, its effect on insulin levels was not evaluated [37]. Another study demonstrated the hypoglycemic effect of lyophilized *Cucurbita ficifolia bouché* fruit juice, both in normoglycemic and diabetic mice, administered intraperitoneally and orally (250, 500, 750, 1000, and 1250 mg/kg). A significant decrease in glucose levels (83%) was obtained in both normoglycemic and diabetic mice, but insulin levels were not measured (Table 2). However, its daily consumption in both cases caused acute toxicity, presenting less toxicity and greater hypoglycemic effects at 500 mg/kg [38].

Recently, *Cucurbita ficifolia bouché* seeds at different stages of ripeness in diabetic and normoglycemic mice at a dose of 500 mg/kg were tested (Table 2). A hypoglycemic effect was observed in all stages of ripeness, having the best effects at 15 days of maturity by reducing 50% of glucose levels. Furthermore, it is suggested that phenolic compounds may be responsible for their hypoglycemic effect, having some effect on insulin secretion [39]. The methanolic extract of *Cucurbita ficifolia bouché* seedless fruit administered in the diabetic group (300 and 600 mg/kg) and in normoglycemic rats (600 mg/kg) was studied. In both groups, a significant decrease in blood glucose levels was observed (60% in the diabetic group). Regarding the diabetic group, a decrease in glycated hemoglobin, body weight (25%), and an increase in plasma insulin (53%) were observed. The administration of 600 mg/kg extract restored the body weight by 6%; however, the dose of 300 mg/kg did not cause a difference in body weight. [40].

In another study, the methanolic extract of the seedless fruit was used in diabetic and normoglycemic rats (Table 2). The rats were fed orally with the extract at a dose of 300 mg/kg, showing a reduction in hyperglycemia (12.5%), pancreatic lipid peroxidation, and an increase in insulin levels in the diabetic group (36%), as well as an increase in the number of active pancreatic β cells [41].

The hypoglycemic effect of the aqueous extract of *Cucurbita ficifolia bouché* seedless pulp and D-quiro-inositol (a compound present in this plant) was evaluated using RINmF5 cells (mouse pancreatic β cells). It was shown that *Insulin* and *Kir6.2* (component of the potassium channel sensitive to ATP) gene expression levels increased in the cells (Table 2). This effect suggests a mechanism of action that involves the expression and secretion of insulin [42]. Based on the previous study, another in vitro investigation (RINmF5 cells) demonstrated that D-quiro-inositol and the extract did not increase insulin or calcium concentration (Table 2). However, the aqueous extract increased the concentration of calcium and insulin. Therefore, the hypoglycemic effect of this plant may be due to other chemical compounds [43], like phenolic compounds (gallic acid, chlorogenic acid), in addition to D-quiro-inositol (Table 6).

In the articles reviewed for this plant, the different extracts have been compared primarily with tolbutamide (83% reduction in blood glucose levels) [38] and not with metformin (anti-diabetic drugs).

3.3. *Coriandrum sativum* L. (Cilantro)

Coriandrum sativum L. is an herbaceous plant widely cultivated in America, Europe, and Eastern countries. In Mexico, it is grown in Puebla, Baja California, Chiapas, Oaxaca, Veracruz, Puebla, Hidalgo, Jalisco, Michoacán, Zacatecas, and Sonora [44]. It belongs to the *Apiaceae* family and is colloquially known as *cilantro* [45] (Figure 4).

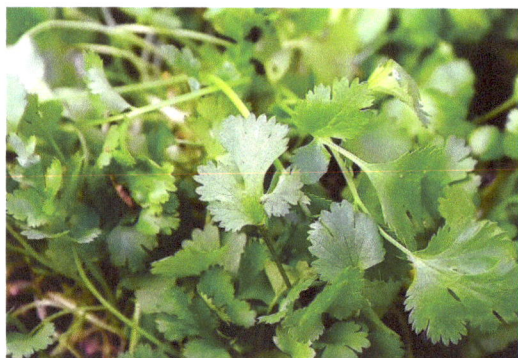

Figure 4. *Coriandrum sativum* L. (*cilantro*). Published by Wikimedia Commons, licensed by Creative Commons, reprinted from [46]. https://creativecommons.org/licenses/by-sa/4.0/legalcode, accessed on 10 March 2023.

The entire plant is edible (leaves and seeds), and it is commonly used as a condiment in different dishes [47].

Various investigations have been carried out to evaluate its hyperglycemic effect and its possible relationship with insulin secretion, as well as body weight control (Table 3). The hypoglycemic effect of the aqueous extract of *Coriandrum sativum* L. seeds, incorporated into the diet (62 ± 5 g/kg) of mice, showed a decrease in blood glucose levels (41%). In addition, extracts using hexane and water, administered at 1 mg/mL in the BRIN–BD11 cell line (rat pancreatic β-cells), presented a higher insulin secretion (50%). On the other hand, the mice in the diabetic group presented a reduction in body weight (21%), while the treated with the extract increased their body weight (4%) compared to the diabetic group (Table 3) [48].

Table 3. Summary of reviewed articles of *Coriandrum sativum* L., considering the type of extract, the part of the plant, dose, experimental model, body weight, and physiologic or cellular effects. ↓ Decrease. ↑ Increase.

Plant	Extract	Part of the Plant	Dose	Experimental Model	Physiologic or Cellular Effects	Body Weight	Reference
Coriandrum sativum L. (cilantro)	Water Water, hexane, ethyl acetate, and methanol for the BRIN–BD11 cell line	Seeds	Mice: the extract was incorporated in the diet (62 ± 5 g/kg) Cell line: 1 mg/mL	Diabetic CD-1 mice and BRIN-BD11 cell line (rat pancreatic β-cells)	The doses used showed: ↓ Blood glucose levels (41%). The aqueous extract, as well as the one made with hexane: ↑ Secretion of insulin (50%) in the BRIN-BD11 cell line	- The diabetic group presented: ↓ Body weight (21%) - The mice treated with the extract: ↓ Body weight (4%)	[48]
	Water	Seeds	20 mg/kg	Normoglycemic and obese (hyperglycemic) rats with limited physical activity	↓ Glucose (20%) ↓ Insulin levels (50%) ↓ Insulin resistance in obese rats The oral administration of the extract caused: ↓ Plasma total cholesterol (48%), HDL (28%), LDL (55%)	The obese rats treated with the extract presented: ↓ Body weight (8%) after 30 days	[49]
	Ethanol	Seeds	100 mg/kg 200 mg/kg 250 mg/kg	Diabetic Wistar rats	-200 and 250 mg/kg: ↓ Blood glucose (33%) ↑ Activity of the pancreatic β cells ↑ Insulin secretion		[50]
	Methanol	Seeds	25 mg/kg 50 mg/kg	Diabetic Wistar rats	Both doses: ↓ Glucose levels (50%) ↓ Dyslipidemia In this article insulin secretion was not evaluated	- 25 mg/kg: ↑ Body weight (48%) - 50 mg/kg: ↑ Body weight (40%)	[51]
	Powder	Seeds	10 g of powder/100 g of food	Diabetic and normoglycemic Wistar rats	↓ Postprandial glucose concentration (44%) ↑ Plasma insulin (40%) in the diabetic group	↓ Fat accumulation	[52]
	Water	Seeds	250 mg/kg 500 mg/kg	Diabetic Wistar rats	Both doses: ↓ Glucose levels (49%), presenting better hypoglycemic effects at the dose of 500 mg/kg The dose of 50 mg/kg: ↓ The total cholesterol level ↑ The high-density lipid cholesterol level		[53]
	Ethanol	Leaves	100 mg/kg	Wistar diabetic rats (alloxan)	↑ Hypoglycemic effect (49%) ↓ triglycerides improvement in the histopathology of pancreatic β cells Insulin secretion was not evaluated	- The diabetic group presented: ↓ Body weight - Administration of the extract: ↑ Body weight	[54]

In another investigation, the aqueous extract of *Coriandrum sativum* L. seeds (20 mg/kg) was administered to normal and obese (hyperglycemic) rats with limited physical activity (Table 3). In obese rats, glucose levels were reduced (20%), as well as insulin levels (50%), improving insulin resistance. Moreover, obese rats treated with the extract presented a decrease in body weight (8%) after 30 days. Moreover, the oral administration of the extract caused a reduction in plasma total cholesterol (48%), HDL (28%) and LDL (55%) [49].

In another study, the ethanolic extract of *Coriandrum sativum* L. seeds, using doses of 100, 200, and 250 mg/kg, was investigated in diabetic rats (Table 3). Doses of 200 and 250 mg/kg reported a reduction in blood glucose (33%), as well as an increase in active pancreatic β cells compared to their diabetic control, improving insulin secretion [50].

Recently, the hypoglycemic effect of polyphenols (extracted with methanol) contained in the seeds of *Coriandrum sativum* L. in an in vivo diabetic model was evaluated, with doses of 25 and 50 mg/kg. The results showed hypoglycemic effects (50%) in addition to improving complications associated with T2D, such as dyslipidemia and body weight loss (48% and 40%, respectively) [51].

The effect of the seed powder of *Coriandrum sativum* L. in diabetic and normoglycemic rats, with a dose of 10 g of powder/100 g of food, produced a lower postprandial glucose concentration (44%) and a reduction in fat accumulation, as well as an increase in plasma insulin (40%) in the diabetic group. This may be due to the high content of antioxidants which helps the preservation of pancreatic β-cells [52]. The aqueous extract of *Coriandrum sativum* L. seeds at different concentrations (250 and 500 mg/kg) (Table 3) demonstrated a greater reduction in blood glucose (49%), as well as in cholesterol levels and an increased high-density lipid cholesterol level in a dose of 500 mg/kg [53].

In diabetic rats where an ethanolic extract of *Coriandrum sativum* L. leaves was administered at a dose of 100 mg/kg, a reduction in glucose (49%) and triglyceride levels was obtained. An improvement in the histopathology of pancreatic β cells was observed, as well as a restoration in body weight; however, insulin secretion was not evaluated (Table 3) [54].

The effects of *Coriandrum sativum* L. extract were evaluated compared to glibenclamide, demonstrating a similar hypoglycemic effect (20%) and improvement in insulin resistance [49]. Moreover, in another study, blood glucose levels were evaluated by comparing the effects of the plant (49% reduction with a dose of 40 mg/kg) with metformin (61% reduction), but neither insulin secretion nor body weight was evaluated in this study [55].

After reviewing the articles referring to this plant, it was observed that *Coriandrum sativum* L. could present a decrease in blood glucose and lipids levels, an increase in insulin sensitivity and secretion, an improvement in β cells, and restore body weight. These effects can be due to the chemical compounds it presents (quercetin and chlorogenic acid quercetin (Table 6).

3.4. Persea americana Mil. (Aguacate)

Persea americana Mil. is a tree native to Central and South America. In Mexico, it is grown in Baja California Sur, Sonora, Michoacán, Jalisco, the State of Mexico, Hidalgo, Veracruz, Puebla, Tabasco, Oaxaca, Morelos, and Guerrero [56]. It belongs to the *Lauraceae* family and is colloquially known as *aguacate* [57] (Figure 5).

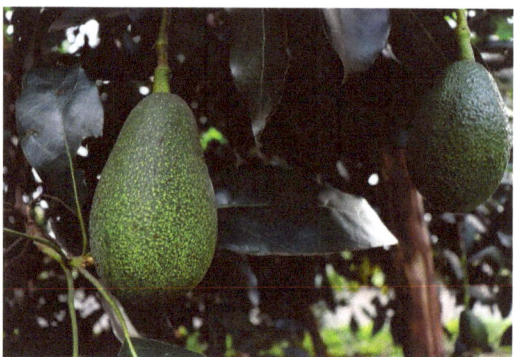

Figure 5. *Persea americana* Mil. (*aguacate*) plant. Reprinted from [58].

The most common edible part of this plant is the pulp; however, the leaves are used as a spice [57].

The aqueous and methanolic extract of *Persea americana* Mil. leaves evaluated in rats with hypercholesterolemia, using a dose of 10 mg/kg (Table 4), indicated a glucose reduction of 16% (aqueous extract) and 11% (methanolic extract), possibly due to an increase in insulin secretion. In these experiments, there were no significant changes in body weight [59]. Ethanolic extract of *Persea americana* Mil. leaves were evaluated in diabetic mice, with doses of 0.490, 0.980, and 1.960 g/kg, showing a greater reduction in glucose levels (64.27%) with the highest dose, suggesting that the hypoglycemic effects of the extract may be due to an increase in insulin secretion, probably by the chemical compounds it contains (flavonoids, saponins, triterpenes); however, in these articles, insulin secretions were not measured (Table 4) [60]. Another group evaluated the effect of the aqueous, ethanolic, and methanolic extract of *Persea americana* Mil. leaves in diabetic rats with a dose of 100 mg/kg (Table 4). The diabetic rats treated with the extract showed an increase in body weight (15.22%). A decrease in glucose levels of 16.3% (aqueous extract), 20.8% (ethanolic extract), and 37.4% (methanolic extract) and recovery of the islets of Langerhans were also observed. Better results were obtained in terms of the hypoglycemic effects of the methanolic extract resembling metformin [61]. Moreover, the hydroalcoholic extract (50% ethanol) of the leaves of *Persea americana* Mil. administered in diabetic and normoglycemic rats, with doses of 0.15 and 0.3 g/kg, produced a reduction in glucose levels of 60% and 71%, respectively (Table 4). In addition, activation of protein kinase B (PKB/Akt) was obtained in the liver and skeletal muscle. In this study, an improvement in pancreatic β cell histology was also obtained; however, it did not show changes in insulin levels. The dose of 0.3 g/kg presented a higher body mass gain compared to the diabetic group, and a lower food intake was also observed [62].

Table 4. Summary of reviewed articles of *Persea americana* Mill., considering the type of extract, the part of the plant, dose, experimental model, body weight, and physiologic or cellular effects. ↓ Decrease. ↑ Increase.

Plant	Extract	Part of the Plant	Dose	Experimental Model	Physiologic or Cellular Effects	Body Weight	Reference
Persea americana Mil. (aguacate)	Water Methanol	Leaves	10 mg/kg	Wistar rats with hypercholesterolemia	↓ Glucose levels with aqueous extract (16%) ↓ Glucose levels with the methanolic extract (11%)	There were no significant changes in body weight	[59]
	Ethanol	Leaves	0.490 g/kg 0.980 g/kg 1.960 g/kg	Diabetic mice	- 1.960 g/kg: ↓ Glucose levels of 64.27% Insulin secretion was not measured		[60]
	Water Ethanol Methanol	Leaves	100 mg/kg	Diabetic Wistar rats	- Aqueous extract: ↓ Glucose levels (16.3%) - Ethanol extract: ↓ Blood glucose levels (20.8%) - Methanol extract: ↓ Glucose levels (37.4%) Recovery of the islets of Langerhans was observed with the three extracts	↑ Body weight (15.22%)	[61]
	Hydroalcoholic extract	Leaves	0.15 g/kg 0.3 g/kg	Diabetic and normoglycemic Wistar rats	The two doses used are presented: ↓ Glucose levels: 0.15 g/kg (60%) 0.3 g/kg (71%) ↑ Activation of protein kinase B (PKB) in liver and skeletal muscle ↑ Pancreatic β-cell was observed. No change in insulin levels	The dose of 0.3 g/kg: ↑ Body mass gain compared to the diabetic group. ↑ Food intake	[62]
	Water	Seed	300 mg/kg 600 mg/kg	Diabetic and normoglycemic Wistar rats	- 300 mg/kg: ↓ Glucose levels (73.23%) - 600 mg/kg: ↓ Glucose levels (78.24%) Protective effect of pancreatic β cells. Insulin secretion was not measured		[63]
	Water	Seed	400 mg/kg 800 mg/kg 1200 mg/kg	Diabetic Wistar rats	The three doses used showed: ↓ Blood glucose levels (51%)	The group threatened with the extract presented: ↑ Body weight (12%) compared with the diabetic untreated group	[64]
	Hot water	Seed	20 g/L 30 g/L 40 g/L	Diabetic Wistar rats	The three doses used are presented: ↑ Hypoglycemic effect similar to glibenclamide (58.9%) ↑ Protective and restorative effect on the pancreas, liver, and kidney tissues	↓ Body weight of diabetic rats The administration of the extract ↑ Body weight loss toward normal	[65]
	Water Methanol	Seed	Aqueous and methanolic extract: 200 mg/kg 300 mg/kg	Diabetic Wistar rats	Both extracts showed: ↓ Glucose levels ↑ Function of the pancreas. Methanolic extract 200 mg/kg: ↓ Glucose levels (70.7%)	↑ Body weight (7.4% aqueous extract or 21.5% methanolic extract) compared to diabetic control group	[66]
	Ethanol	Seeds	300 mg/kg 600 mg/kg 1200 mg/kg	Diabetic Wistar rats	The doses used showed: ↓ Glucose levels (50%) similar to glibenclamide, having a better result with a concentration of 300 mg/kg		[67]
	Ethanol	Pulp	300 mg/kg	Diabetic Wistar rats	Levels of glucose and insulin returned almost to normal levels	The administration of the extract ↑ Body weight	[68]
	Water	Pulp (Avocatin B)	Obese C57BL/6J mice: 100 mg/kg INS-1 cells: 25 µM C2C12 cells: 25 µM Humans (n = 10): 50 mg o 200 mg per day for 60 days	Obese C57BL/6J mice INS-1 cells (pancreatic β cells) C2C12 cells (myocytes) Humans (n = 10)	- Obese mice: ↓ Glucose levels (20%) - INS-1 cells: ↑ Insulin secretion (40%) ↓ insulin resistance - C2C12 cells: ↑ Glucose uptake - Humans: it did not generate discomfort or toxic effects	↓ Body weight (25%) in obese mice ↓ Body weight (6%) in humans	[69]

On the other hand, the aqueous extract of the seed of *Persea americana* Mil. was studied in diabetic and normoglycemic rats, using a dose of 300 and 600 mg/kg, showing a reduction in blood glucose of 73.23% and 78.24%, respectively. Moreover, this extract showed a protective effect of pancreatic β cells; however, insulin levels were not measured [63]. In another study, where the aqueous extract of *Persea americana* Mil. seed was also evaluated, they demonstrated a significant reduction in blood glucose levels (51%) and an increase in body weight (12%) in diabetic rats, with doses of 400, 800, 1200 mg/kg (Table 4) [64].

The administration of the hot water extract of *Persea americana* Mil. seeds was investigated in diabetic rats at doses of 20, 30, and 40 g/L (Table 4), showing a hypoglycemic effect similar to gibenclamide, with a decrease of 58.9% of blood glucose levels. During the 21 days of the experiment, the body weight of diabetic rats was reduced; however, the administration of the extract restored the body weight loss to normal. In addition, histopathological studies showed a protective and restorative effect on the liver, pancreas, and kidney tissues [65]. Subsequently, another study evaluated the aqueous and methanolic extract of *Persea americana* Mil. seed in diabetic rats, with doses of 200 and 300 mg/kg (Table 4). The aqueous and methanolic extracts presented an increase in body weight of 7.4% and 21.5%, respectively, compared with the control diabetic group (without the extract). A decrease in glucose levels and improvement in liver function were also obtained, with favorable results with the methanolic extract at a dose of 200 mg/kg (glucose reduction of 70.7%) having similar effects to insulin administration [66]. Recently, the hypoglycemic effect of the ethanolic extract of *Persea americana* Mil. seeds was studied in diabetic rats, with doses of 300, 600, and 1200 mg/kg (Table 4), obtaining a decrease of 50% in blood glucose levels, similar to the effects with glibenclamide [67].

In another study, ethanolic extract from *Persea americana* Mil. pulp was investigated in diabetic rats at a dose of 300 mg/kg (Table 4). It was observed that the levels of glucose, body weight, glycosylated hemoglobin, urea, serum creatinine, and insulin in plasma reverted almost to normal levels [68].

On the other hand, avocatin B, a compound exclusively found in avocados (in seeds, pulp, and peel), can act as an inhibitor of fatty acid oxidation. Therefore, its influence on improving insulin resistance was evaluated in an animal model of obese rats (100 mg/kg), in a β cell line (INS-1) at a dose of 25 μM, and in a skeletal muscle cell line (C2C12) with a dose of 25 μM (Table 4). The results showed an improvement in insulin resistance and an increase in the secretion of insulin (40%) in INS-1 cells, a reduction in glucose levels in obese mice (20%), as well as a decreased in body weight (25%) the supplemented obese mice between baseline and day 30 of treatment. Moreover, an enhancement of glucose uptake by C2C12 cells was observed. On the other hand, a pilot study was carried out with humans (n = 10), administering 50 mg or 200 mg per day for 60 days of avocatin B, observing that its consumption had no effect on blood markers of kidney, liver, and muscle toxicity (total bilirubin, alanine aminotransferase, creatinine, and creatine phosphokinase), concluding that the supplementation with avocatin B does not generate discomfort or harmful effects. Insulin secretion and glucose levels were not measured in humans because the objective was to assert avocatin B toxicity in humans. However, it was reported that 200 mg of avocatin B per day reduced body weight by 6% [69].

In the articles reviewed of this plant, the different extracts were compared primarily with glibenclamide having a similar hypoglycemic effect (58.9%), restoring body weight loss and a protective effect in the pancreas [65]. On the other hand, there have been studies where the hypoglycemic effects of the plant (reduction of 79% with a dose of 53.3 mg/kg) have been compared with metformin (reduction of 80%) [70].

After reviewing the articles referring to this plant, it was observed that *Persea americana* Mil. can present a decrease in blood glucose and lipids levels, an increase in insulin sensitivity and secretion, an improvement in β cells, and restore body weight. These effects can be due to the chemical compounds it presents (avocatin B and saponins) (Table 6).

3.5. Bidens pilosa (Amor seco)

Bidens pilosa is a medicinal plant belonging to the *Asteraceae* family, colloquially known as *amor seco*, native to America [71]. In Mexico, it is cultivated in Aguascalientes, Durango, Guanajuato, Guerrero, Hidalgo, Jalisco, Michoacán, Morelos, Puebla, Querétaro, Tabasco, Tlaxcala, Veracruz, and Zacatecas [72]. It is widely used as a herbal remedy to treat diseases such as T2D and type 1 diabetes, leukemia, ulcers, gastric neoplasia, and inflammation [73] (Figure 6).

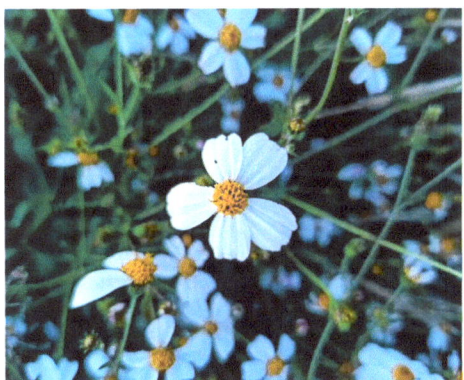

Figure 6. *Bidens pilosa* (*amor seco*) plant. Published by Wikimedia Commons, licensed by Creative Commons, reprinted from [74]. https://creativecommons.org/licenses/by-sa/4.0/legalcode, accessed on 10 March 2023.

This plant is widely used as fodder for domestic animals. It also has an edible flower that is used in salads; the shoots and leaves are used as potherbs [71].

Its antidiabetic effects, as well as its protective effect on pancreatic β cells (Table 5), have been investigated using extracts from the leaves, flowers, and seeds of *Bidens pilosa* in both in vivo and in vitro models.

Table 5. Summary of reviewed articles on *Bidens pilosa*, considering the type of extract, the part of the plant, dose, experimental model, body weight, and physiologic or cellular effects. ↓ Decrease. ↑ Increase.

Plant	Extract	Part of the Plant	Dose	Experimental Model	Physiologic or Cellular Effects	Body Weight	Reference
Bidens pilosa (amor seco)	Water	Whole plant	10 mg/kg 50 mg/kg 250 mg/kg	C57BL/KsJ-db/db mice	The doses showed: ↑ Glucose tolerance (50%) ↑ Increased insulin levels (20%) The dose of 50 mg/kg presented the most similar effect to glibenclamide	The group treated with the extract presented: ↓ Body weight (13%)	[75]
	Ethanol–water	Stem	Extract: 1 g/kg Polyenes mixture: 0.5 g/kg and 0.25 g/kg	C5BL/Ks-db/db mice	A dose of 1 g/kg: ↓ Blood glucose levels (33%) ↓ Blood glucose levels with a concentration of 0.5 g/kg (41%) ↓ Blood glucose levels with a concentration of 0.25 g/kg (25%) Insulin secretion was not measured	No significant differences in body weight were observed; however, the administration of the polyenes mixture reduced food intake	[76]
	Water	Branches	Diabetic rats: 70 mg/mL 90 mg/mL 110 mg/mL Normoglycemic rats: 90 mg/mL	Diabetic and normoglycemic Wistar rats	- Diabetic rats: ↓ Glucose levels with a dose of 70 mg/mL (18.4%) - Normoglycemic rats: ↓ Glucose levels with a dose of 90 mg/mL (33.58%) Insulin levels were not measured		[77]
	DMSO	Cytopiloyne	db/db mice: 0.1 mg/kg 0.5 mg/kg 2.5 mg/kg RIN-m5F cells: 7 µM 14 µM 28 µM	db/db mice RIN-m5F (pancreatic β cells)	The doses used are presented: In vivo model: ↓ Postprandial blood glucose levels (61%) ↑ Insulin levels (54%) ↑ Protected pancreatic β-cells. In vitro: ↑ Intracellular insulin concentration with a dose of 28 µM ↑ PKC-α activation with increasing dose ↑ Insulin transcript at 28 µM dose.		[78]
	Bidens pilosa formulation (capsule)		Humans (n = 10) 400 mg	Diabetic and normoglycemic humans	↓ Fasting glucose levels (39%) ↑ Increasing insulin levels (20%) in normoglycemic subjects		[79]

The antidiabetic effect of the aqueous extract of the whole plant of *Bidens pilosa* was evaluated in vivo (C57BL/KsJ-db/db mice), with doses of 10, 50, and 250 mg/kg (Table 5). A greater decrease in glucose (50%) and increase in serum insulin (40%) was observed in a dose-dependent manner. Furthermore, the effect of this extract on glucose tolerance was evaluated in db/db mice with a dose of 50 mg/kg, resulting in an improvement in glucose tolerance, such as glibenclamide. A 0.9% reduction in glycated hemoglobin was also obtained, and in histological studies of the pancreas, the extract showed a protective effect on pancreatic β cells. Moreover, the group treated with the extract presented a decrease in body weight (13%) compared with the control group [75]. In another study, the aqueous ethanol extract from the stem of *Bidens pilosa* (1 g/kg) was investigated in C5BL/Ks-db/db mice (T2D model), obtaining blood glucose reduction (33%) (Table 5). In addition, the polyenes mixture presented a dose-dependent reduction in blood glucose levels for 0.5 g/kg (41%) compared to 0.25 mg/kg (25%). However, its effect on insulin secretion was not investigated in this article. On the other hand, no significant differences in body weight were observed; however, the administration of the polyenes mixture reduced food intake [76]. In a more recent study, the hypoglycemic effect of the aqueous extract of *Bidens pilosa* branches was evaluated in diabetic rats (doses of 70, 90, and 110 mg/mL) and normoglycemic rats (doses of 90 mg/mL) (Table 5). A significant reduction in blood glucose levels (18.4%) was obtained with a dose of 70 mg/mL in the diabetic group and a dose of 90 mg/mL in normoglycemic rats (33.58% reduction). Insulin levels were not evaluated in this article; however, it is suggested that it can improve insulin secretion due to the compounds it contains (saponins, tannins, and polyphenols) [77].

A polyacetylene compound from *Bidens pilosa*, called cytopiloyne, was administered in db/db mouse model with doses of 0.1, 0.5, and 2.5 mg/kg (Table 5). This compound exhibited a reduction in postprandial blood glucose levels (61%), an increase in blood insulin (54%), an improvement in glucose tolerance, a reduction in glycosylated hemoglobin levels, and protection of pancreatic β cells. To learn more about the mechanism of action of cytopiloyne, we evaluated its effect on insulin mRNA transcription in the RIN-m5F cell line (pancreatic β cells) at concentrations of 7, 14, and 28 μM. Insulin transcript increased two-fold at a dose of 28 μM cytopiloyne, as well as the intracellular insulin concentration. Moreover, an increase in the mobilization of calcium and diacylglycerols was demonstrated. Cytopiloyne increased PKC-α activation, which is involved in insulin secretion from pancreatic β cells and is activated by diacylglycerols and calcium. This indicated that cytopiloyne enhances β-cell insulin secretion and expression through the regulation of PKC-α by calcium and diacylglycerols [78].

The hypoglycemic effect of *Bidens pilosa* has also been tested in a pilot study in diabetic and normoglycemic humans (n = 10) with a dose of 400 mg (Table 5). A decrease in fasting glucose levels (39%) was observed, as well as glycated hemoglobin levels and increased serum insulin (20%) in normoglycemic subjects. Moreover, it was observed that the mixture of the formulation of *Bidens pilosa* and antidiabetic drugs caused better glycemic control in diabetic patients. These results could be due to an improvement in the function of pancreatic β cells [79].

In the articles reviewed for this plant, the different extracts were compared primarily with glibenclamide, having a similar hypoglycemic effect (50%) [75]. On the other hand, there have not been studies where it has been compared with metformin.

After reviewing the articles referring to this plant, it was observed that *Bidens pilosa* could present a lowering in blood glucose, an increase in insulin secretion, and glucose tolerance. These effects can be due to the chemical compounds it presents (cytopiloyne and tanins) (Table 6).

Table 6. Summary of the effects, compounds, and toxicity of the five reviewed plants. ↓ Decrease. ↑ Increase.

Plant	*Momordica charantia* L. (Melón amargo)	*Cucurbita ficifolia* bouché. (Chilacayote)	*Coriandrum sativum* L. (Cilantro)	*Persea americana* Mil. (Aguacate)	*Bidens pilosa.* (Amor seco)
Effects	↓ Glucose levels ↑ Insulin secretion ↑ Insulin sensitivity ↑ Enhancement of pancreatic β cells ↓ Lipids (serum) ↑ Restore body weight	↓ Glucose levels ↑ Insulin secretion ↑ Enhancement of pancreatic β cells ↓ Lipids (serum) ↑ Restore body weight	↓ Glucose levels ↑ Insulin secretion ↑ Insulin sensitivity ↑ Enhancement of pancreatic β cells ↓ Lipids (serum) ↑ Restore body weight	↓ Glucose levels ↑ Insulin secretion ↑ Insulin sensitivity ↑ Enhancement of pancreatic β cells ↓ Lipids (serum) ↑ Restore body weight	↓ Glucose levels ↑ Insulin secretion ↑ Glucose tolerance ↑ Enhancement of pancreatic β cells ↑ Restore body weight
Compounds involved.	- Saponins - Proteins - Triterpenes - Polysaccharides	- D-quiro-inositol - Phenolic compounds (gallic acid, chlorogenic acid)	- Antioxidants (quercetin) - Polyphenols (chlorogenic acid quercetin)	- Avocatin B - Saponins	- Cytopiloyne - Polyphenols (tannins)
Toxicity	- The proteins, triterpenes, and polysaccharides of *Momordica charantia* L. have not shown toxicity - The toxicity of saponins from *Momordica charantia* L. has not been evaluated. However, an LD 50 (oral, rat) of 960 mg/kg is recommended	- Gallic acid: LD50 (oral, rat) 5000 mg/kg - Chlorogenic acid: it does not present toxicity -Inositol: LD50 (oral, mouse) 10,000 mg/kg	- Quercetin: LD50 (oral, rat) 161 mg/kg LD50 (oral, mouse) 160 mg/kg - Chlorogenic acid: it does not present toxicity	- Avocatin B: the oral dose of 100 mg/kg in rats does not present toxicity In humans, the 200 mg dose is not toxic either - Persin: LD50 of 751.6 mg/kg administered intraperitoneally in rats - The toxicity of saponins from *Persea americana* Mil. has not been evaluated. However, it is recommended an LD 50 (oral, rat) of 960 mg/kg	- Tannins: LD50 (oral, rat) 2260 mg/kg - Cytopiloyne: at doses of 2.5 mg/kg orally in mice, they do not present toxicity

4. Discussion

Mexican plants have been used for many centuries for the treatment of T2D and, recently, for body weight control. In México, the Federal Commission for the Protection against Sanitary Risk (COFEPRIS) allowed the use of 18 medicinal plants as herbal medicine [80]. For example, *Echinacea purpurea* is approved in Mexico, Belgium, Bulgaria, Croatia, and Denmark with a dose of 100 mg [81]. Another example is *Panax ginseg*, which is approved in Mexico, Austria, Belgium, Denmark, France, Germany, Ireland, Portugal, and Spain with a dose of 100 mg or 300 mg [82]. Moreover, *Passiflora incarnata* is also approved in Mexico, Germany, Austria, and Belgium with a dose of 200 mg [83]. For herbal compounds commercialization, the advertising and marketing must include therapeutic indication and symptomatic effect; in no case could these products be advertised as curatives [84].

However, there are many other medicinal plants that have scarce scientific studies demonstrating the physiological and molecular mechanism of action of these plants over glucose homeostasis and body weight. Therefore, the need to review the literature and describe the state of the art of these plants is necessary to ultimately propose future routes to study their mechanism of action and their plausible use to treat these diseases.

4.1. Momordica charantia L. (Melón amargo)

When reviewing the articles referring to *Momordica charantia* L., its antidiabetic effects may be due to the chemical compounds present in its aqueous or organic extracts such as proteins [27] saponins [28,29], triterpenes [30], and polysaccharides [29] (Table 2).

The proteins contained in *Momordica charantia* L. were found to increase plasma insulin levels and glucose uptake, suggesting that it may also have an effect on improving insulin sensitivity. However, the type of proteins that were extracted from *Momordica charantia* L. was not mentioned; therefore, more studies are needed to identify the active compounds that promote the beneficial effects mentioned above [27]. Regarding saponins, their hypoglycemic action is caused by the improvement of insulin response [29], increasing insulin levels, and improving pancreatic β-cell function [28]. However, it is important to consider that saponins can present toxicity and irritability in the intestine when ingested in high amounts (lethal dose (LD) 960 mg/kg) [85] (Table 2).

T2D has been shown to be associated with increased free radical formation and decreased antioxidant potential, leading to oxidative stress induced by hyperglycemia and free fatty acids, causing insulin resistance and pancreatic β-cell dysfunction [86]. In the articles reviewed, both the saponins [28] and the triterpenes [30] of *Momordica charantia* L. presented an antioxidant effect improving and preserving pancreatic β cells; this is in conjunction with its hypoglycemic action and increased insulin production.

It is important to highlight that in the reviewed articles, it was also observed that the extracts used from this plant had similar effects to the pharmacological controls [24] with glibenclamide, a sulfonylurea that increases the secretion of insulin by stimulating pancreatic β cells [87]. Therefore, it is suggested that this plant could present a mechanism of action similar to sulfonylureas. On the other hand, it has been investigated that the inhibition of PTP-1B plays an important role in the signaling of metabolic pathways and that it may be a possible therapeutic target for T2D. This protein participates in the negative regulation of insulin receptor signaling [88]. In one of the reviewed articles, it is reported that *Momordica charantia* L. triterpenes exerted an inhibiting effect on PTP-1B, improving the effects caused by insulin resistance [30], which may represent a possible treatment for T2D.

Moreover, *Momordica charantia* L. has the effect of restoring body weight, which could be a consequence of its positive influence on lipid metabolism (decrease in serum triglycerides, cholesterol, and LDL levels) [22,23,25,28,29]. On the other hand, one of the articles reviewed mentioned that the extract of this plant could reduce fat mass and increases SIRT1 levels, which can increase hepatic gluconeogenesis and fatty acid use, contributing to the loss of fat mass [26]. In addition, these effects have been associated with the inhibition of pancreatic lipase (which breaks down fats so they can be absorbed in the intestines) or modulating appetite, influencing weight gain or loss [89].

In addition, *Momordica charantia* L. has the effect of restoring body weight, decreasing blood glucose and lipids levels, increasing insulin secretion, improving insulin sensitivity, and the histology of pancreatic β cells (Table 2). Therefore, this plant is a good candidate to further study its beneficial effects on glucose homeostasis and body weight control.

4.2. Cucurbita ficifolia bouché (Chilacayote)

Cucurbita ficifolia bouché presented similar effects to *Momordica charantia* L. because they belong to the same family (*Cucurbitaceae*). Both plants can reduce blood glucose levels [37–41], increase the concentration of insulin [35,40–43], and improve the functioning of pancreatic β cells [41]. Moreover, *Cucurbita ficifolia bouché* increases intracellular calcium concentration in in vitro models [43] (Table 2).

Cucurbita ficifolia bouché contains phenolic compounds, mainly gallic acid, chlorogenic acid, and quercetin (Table 6). These compounds have an antioxidant effect, preventing the death of pancreatic β cells and allowing the recovery of those partially destroyed [41]. On the other hand, it has been reported that phenolic compounds can increase insulin secretion by stimulating GLP-1 (incretin) secretion [90]. Incretin hormones are peptides released from the gastrointestinal tract in response to food ingestion. These hormones enhance insulin secretion and regulate glucose homeostasis [91]. Moreover, gallic acid has been reported to reduce glucose levels in diabetic rats due to its insulin-releasing effect [92]. On the other hand, chlorogenic acid has been associated with an increase in insulin sensitivity, improvement in glucose tolerance, and an increase in insulin secretion [93]. Therefore, these compounds can potentiate the hypoglycemic effect of *Cucurbita ficifolia bouché* by different mechanisms.

On the other hand, it has been suggested that the active principle of this plant may be the compound called D-quiro-inositol. Inositol molecules, particularly D-quiro-inositol, have been suggested to be important mediators of insulin action [94]. D-quiro-inositol is normally present in the urine and blood, but it is at greatly reduced levels or absent in T2D patients, which has been associated with a decrease in insulin sensitivity [95]. The possible mechanism of action of this compound has been investigated using aqueous extracts from the fruit of *Cucurbita ficifolia bouché* [42,43]. These studies proposed that its hypoglycemic effects may be mediated by an increase in the expression of mRNA for insulin and for the major subunit of the ATP-sensitive K^+ channel (Kir6.2), a protein present in pancreatic β-cells, which plays an important role in insulin secretion [43] and mediate the increase in intracellular calcium and insulin secretion [43] It is important to consider that D-quiro-inositol is found in a higher concentration, mainly in the ripe fruit; however, hypoglycemic capacity has also been shown in diabetic patients with the immature fruit used in doses of 4 mL/kg [37], as well as when using immature fruit seeds in diabetic mouse models (dose of 500 mg/kg) [39]. D-quiro-inositol has also been associated with body weight control by reducing BMI in obese patients [96] and restoring body weight during T2D, which can be due to its positive effects in insulin secretion and hypoglycemic effects [41]. Therefore, this suggests that the hypoglycemic effect of *Cucurbita ficifolia bouché* not only depends on D-quiro-inositol but also on other compounds, such as phenolics, which are found in both ripe and unripe fruit [39]. On the other hand, D-quiro-inositol has an oral LD50 toxicity (mouse) of 10,000 mg/kg [97] (Table 6).

For many of the articles reported on this plant, the antidiabetic effect of *Cucurbita ficifolia bouché* was compared with pharmacological controls such as tolbutamide (sulfonylurea). This drug acts on the pancreas, stimulating functional pancreatic β cells and causing an increase in insulin secretion [98]. Considering the above, the extracts of *Cucurbita ficifolia bouché* presented similar results to those observed with tolbutamide (stimulates the secretion of insulin by the pancreas) [40]. This suggests that they might have a similar mechanism of action.

On the other hand, it is important to consider the toxicity of the compounds of this plant, which are mainly: gallic acid (LD50 (oral, rat) 5000 mg/kg), chlorogenic acid (LD50 (intraperitoneal, rat) 4000 mg/kg), and inositol (LD50 (oral, mouse) 10,000 mg/kg) (Table 6).

4.3. Coriandrum sativum L. (Cilantro)

Coriandrum sativum L., such as *Momordica charantia* L. and *Cucurbita ficifolia bouché*, presented an improvement in pancreatic β cells [50], which can be attributed to its content of antioxidants, especially the flavonoid quercetin (a phenolic compound) present in plants and foods [52] (Table 6).

Quercetin supplementation has been shown to help normalize blood glucose concentration [99]. In addition, it has been shown to improve antioxidant status [50], prevent oxidative damage, help pancreatic islet regeneration, and increase insulin secretion [50]. Quercetin can be obtained from the powder of its seeds [52]. Coriander does not present high toxicity; however, quercetin has an LD50 (oral, rat) of 161 mg/kg (Table 6) [52]. Therefore, it would be important to know the concentration of this compound in coriander to determine a dose of extract that does not represent toxicity for animal models or humans. *Coriandrum sativum* L. also has polyphenols, especially chlorogenic acid, which may be responsible for its hypoglycemic effect [51] since it has been associated with an increase in insulin sensitivity, improvement in glucose tolerance, and increase in insulin secretion [93]. On the other hand, one of the reviewed articles suggests that *Coriandrum sativum* L. improves insulin sensitivity [49], similar to *Momordica charantia* L. [30]. However, it is important to consider that although *Coriandrum sativum* L. extract was able to lower blood glucose and insulin resistance indicators in obese rats, they were subjected to physical activity. This could be a variable that could have influenced the hypoglycemic results of the extract [49]. It is also important to consider that the effects of *Coriandrum sativum* L. in increasing insulin concentration [50] are dose-dependent. At a dose of 20 mg/kg, it does not present a significant increase in insulin secretion [49], while at higher doses (200 mg/kg), the concentration of this hormone significantly increases [50].

On the other hand, *Coriandrum sativum* L. restored body weight loss during diabetes, which can be because of its ability to improve insulin sensitivity and decrease lipids and glucose levels [48,51,52]. In addition, this plant has effects on weight loss in an obese animal model; this can be due to its chemical compounds, such as quercetin [49]. This compound has been associated with a decrease in body weight, food intake, plasma cholesterol, and fat accumulation [100].

Considering the previous studies, we can suggest that the antidiabetic effects of *Coriandrum sativum* L. can mainly be explained by the protective effect on pancreatic β cells of the flavonoids and polyphenols present in the seeds, causing an improvement in insulin secretion. However, it is important to consider that toxicity, in particular of quercetin, presents an LD50 (oral, rat) 161 mg/kg and an LD50 (oral, mouse) 160 mg/kg, while chlorogenic acid has an LD50 (intraperitoneal, rat) 4000 mg/kg (Table 6).

4.4. Persea americana Mil. (Aguacate)

Persea americana Mil. can cause a hypoglycemic effect [60,62–65,67,68], as well as an increase in insulin sensitivity [69], an improvement in pancreatic β-cell function and histology [63,65,66], and an increase in insulin levels [68,69] (Table 4).

Studies have suggested that flavonoids, present in *Persea americana* Mil. could produce a decrease in serum glucose levels and an increase in glucose uptake by peripheral tissues via protein kinase B (PKB/Akt) [101,102]. Activation of this enzyme can increase glucose transport by translocating GLUT-4 from the cytosol to the plasma membrane, thereby increasing glucose uptake in skeletal muscle, adipocytes, liver, and other tissues [103].

On the other hand, a compound present in *Persea americana* Mil., called avocatin B, has recently been investigated. Avocatin B is a mixture of avocadene and avocadin, two 17-carbon polyhydric fatty alcohols originally discovered in avocado seeds. However, it has been reported that up to 200 mg of avocatin B may be present in avocado pulp [69]. This compound is capable of increasing insulin production both in vivo (obese rats) and in vitro (INS-1 cells). Although little is known about its mechanism of action, it has been proposed that it is capable of inhibiting the oxidation of fatty acids, which in turn causes an increase in the use of glucose and a decrease in insulin resistance [69].

In the reviewed articles, *Persea americana* Mil. restored the body weight loss caused by diabetes [61,62,64–66,68]. In one of the articles, it was mentioned that this plant could also cause body weight loss in a model of obese mice; this may be due to the benefits that avocatin B could present in glucose and fat metabolism [69].

On the other hand, it is important to consider that toxicological studies in which *Persea americana* Mil. pulp has been administered orally have established an LD50 of 15,000 mg/kg in rats. This effect may be related to the presence in *Persea americana* Mil. seeds and leaves of a compound called persin, which has a toxic effect on rats and mice, in whom an LD50 of 751.6 mg/kg administered intraperitoneally is reported [66]. Persin is also found in *Persea americana* Mil. pulp but in a lower concentration, and although a toxic effect on humans has not been demonstrated [69], it is important to consider its toxicity to avoid an adverse effect in the future experiments.

Therefore, the hypoglycemic effect of avocado may be due to the stimulating effect on pancreatic β-cells, making them capable of secreting more insulin, or to a protective effect on pancreatic β-cells. This may be due to the chemical compounds present mainly in its leaves (flavonoids) and pulp (avocatin B) (Table 6). In addition, it is important to consider that avocatin B, both at high doses (1200 mg/kg) and at lower doses (10 mg/kg), produces a decrease in blood glucose levels and has not shown toxic effects. Additionally, it is important to consider that *Persea americana* Mil. has effects on insulin secretion in both in vivo and in vitro models.

4.5. Bidens pilosa (Amor seco)

Bidens pilosa can lower blood glucose levels [76–79] and increase insulin concentration [75,79]. In addition, it improves glucose tolerance and pancreatic β-cell function [75,78] (Table 5).

This plant has polyphenolic compounds, in particular flavonoids and tannins. These compounds also exert antioxidant activity, preserving and improving the function of pancreatic β cells [77]. It has also been reported that tannins and flavonoids have the property of slowing down the absorption of sugars in the intestine, which limits and regulates their passage into the blood [90].

Bidens pilosa also showed a reduction in glucose levels similar to that shown by glibenclamide (sulfonylurea). Sulfonylureas have been reported to have hypoglycemic effects by stimulating insulin production through pancreatic β cells. *Bidens pilosa* presented a reduction in glucose levels [77] and an increase in serum insulin levels similar to those presented by glibenclamide [75].

Recently, a polyacetylene, called cytopiloyne, present in *Bidens pilosa* has been identified [78]. It has been observed that this compound is capable of stimulating insulin secretion. Its mechanism of action is not yet fully understood. However, cytopiloyne has been proposed to improve pancreatic β-cell function and intracellular calcium flux, thereby enhancing insulin synthesis and secretion [104]. Cytopiloyne has also been proposed to increase PKC-α activation, which enhances insulin secretion and expression in pancreatic β cells [78].

Bidens pilosa also presented the effect on body weight loss in a model of db/db mice [75], probably due to its chemical compounds, specifically its polyenes [76]. Polyenes have been associated with a reduction in fat accumulation, adipocyte size and/or body weight [105].

It is worth mentioning that, as in the case of *Cucurbita ficifolia bouché*, experiments have been carried out in diabetic patients using a formulation of *Bidens pilosa*, presenting hypoglycemic effects and an increase in insulin secretion. However, this study was performed on a small population of 10 patients. In addition, the composition and elaboration of the plant formulation are not mentioned [79].

On the other hand, it must be considered that tannins present an LD50 (oral, rat) of 2260 mg/kg [106]. As for cytopiloine, it has been observed that in doses of 2.5 mg/kg orally in mice, it does not present toxicity [78] (Table 6).

5. Conclusions

In this review, five Mexican medicinal plants used to treat T2D were selected. It was observed that both aqueous and organic extracts of different plants could have hypoglycemic effects, increasing insulin secretion and sensitivity, improving the function of pancreatic β cells and glucose tolerance, as well as regulating body weight. These effects may be due to the different chemical compounds present in these plants, such as saponins, phenolic compounds, antioxidants, tannins, triterpenes, avocatin B, cytopiloyne, etc. However, it is important to further study the toxicology of the different plants and their chemical compounds to determine the recommended doses for their hypoglycemic and body weight control effect.

However, for most of these plants, the mechanism of action by which they exert their hypoglycemic effect is not fully understood. Therefore, it is necessary to further study the different extracts in both in vivo and in vitro models to continue validating the evidence for its implication in glucose homeostasis and body weight control.

In addition, it is important to investigate the active principle of these plants that helps modulate glucose homeostasis, insulin secretion, and body weight control, as well as its mechanism of action. In the future, these plants could be proposed as a possible treatment for T2D and obesity, impacting a more economical and accessible option for patients with these diseases.

Author Contributions: Conceptualization, R.G.-A. and M.T.-V.; methodology, M.T.-V. and R.G.-A.; investigation, M.T.-V.; resources, R.G.-A.; data curation, M.T.-V.; writing—original draft preparation, M.T.-V.; writing—review and editing, M.T.-V. and R.G.-A.; visualization, R.G.-A.; supervision, R.G.-A.; funding acquisition, R.G.-A. All authors have read and agreed to the published version of the manuscript.

Funding: This research and APC was funded by Hospital Infantil de México Federico Gómez HIM/2014/056 SSA.1132.

Institutional Review Board Statement: Not applicable.

Informed Consent Statement: Not applicable.

Data Availability Statement: No new data were created or analyzed in this study. Data sharing is not applicable to this article.

Conflicts of Interest: The authors declare no conflict of interest.

References

1. World Health Organization (WHO). *Overweight and Obesity in the Western Pacific Region*; WHO: Geneva, Switzerland, 2017; Volume 4.
2. De Pauw, R.; Claessens, M.; Gorasso, V.; Drieskens, S.; Faes, C.; Devleesschauwer, B. Past, Present, and Future Trends of Overweight and Obesity in Belgium Using Bayesian Age-Period-Cohort Models. *BMC Public Health* **2022**, *22*, 1309. [CrossRef]
3. Instituto Nacional de Salud Pública. *Informe de Resultados de La Encuesta Nacional de Salud y Nutrición-Continua 2021*; ENSANUT: Mexico City, Mexico, 2021.
4. Forouhi, N.G.; Wareham, N.J. Epidemiology of Diabetes. *Medicine* **2014**, *42*, 698–702. [CrossRef] [PubMed]
5. Khan, M.A.B.; Hashim, M.J.; King, J.K.; Govender, R.D.; Mustafa, H.; Al Kaabi, J. Epidemiology of Type 2 Diabetes—Global Burden of Disease and Forecasted Trends. *J. Epidemiol. Glob. Health* **2019**, *10*, 107. [CrossRef] [PubMed]
6. *OMS: Organización Mundial de la Salud Diabetes OMS*; WHO Media Center: Geneva, Switzerland, 2017.
7. Saeedi, P.; Petersohn, I.; Salpea, P.; Malanda, B.; Karuranga, S.; Unwin, N.; Colagiuri, S.; Guariguata, L.; Motala, A.A.; Ogurtsova, K.; et al. Global and Regional Diabetes Prevalence Estimates for 2019 and Projections for 2030 and 2045: Results from the International Diabetes Federation Diabetes Atlas, 9th Edition. *Diabetes Res. Clin. Pract.* **2019**, *157*, 107843. [CrossRef] [PubMed]
8. Instituto Nacional de Estadística y Geografía (INEGI). *Diabetes En México*; INEGI: Aguascalientes, Mexico, 2020; pp. 1–5.
9. Salas-Zapata, L.; Palacio-Mejía, L.S.; Aracena-Genao, B.; Hernández-Ávila, J.E.; Nieto-López, E.S. Direct Service Costs of Diabetes Mellitus Hospitalisations in the Mexican Institute of Social Security. *Gac. Sanit.* **2018**, *32*, 209–215. [CrossRef]
10. De los Ángeles Rodríguez Bolaños, R.; Shigematsu, L.M.R.; Ruíz, J.A.J.; Márquez, S.A.J.; Ávila, M.H. Direct Costs of Medical Care for Patients with Type 2 Diabetes Mellitus in Mexico: Micro-Costing Analysis. *Rev. Panam. Salud Publica/Pan Am. J. Public Health* **2010**, *28*, 412–420. [CrossRef]
11. Acosta-Recalde, P.; Vera, G.Z.; Morinigo, M.; Maidana, G.M.; Samaniego, L. Uso de Plantas Medicinales y Fitoterápicos En Pacientes Con Diabetes Mellitus Tipo 2. *Memorias Inst. Investig. Ciencias Salud* **2018**, *16*, 6–11. [CrossRef]
12. World Health Organization (WHO). *WHO Guidelines on Safety Monitoring of Herbal Medicines in Pharmacovigilance Systems*; World Health Organization: Geneva, Switzerland, 2004.
13. Principe, E.; Jose, A.S. Propagation Management of Herbal and Medicinal Plants. *Res. Inf. Ser. Ecosyst.* **2002**, *14*, 1–12.
14. Meneses, O. *Caracterización Morfológica, Genética y Antidiabética de Tres Especies de Plantas Medicinales*; UAEH: Biblioteca Digital: Hidalgo, Mexico, 2006.
15. König, A.; Schwarzinger, B.; Stadlbauer, V.; Lanzerstorfer, P.; Iken, M.; Schwarzinger, C.; Kolb, P.; Schwarzinger, S.; Mörwald, K.; Brunner, S.; et al. Guava (*Psidium guajava*) Fruit Extract Prepared by Supercritical CO_2 Extraction Inhibits Intestinal Glucose Resorption in a Double-Blind, Randomized Clinical Study. *Nutrients* **2019**, *11*, 1512. [CrossRef]
16. Marmitt, D.J.; Shahrajabian, M.H.; Goettert, M.I.; Rempel, C. Clinical Trials with Plants in Diabetes Mellitus Therapy: A Systematic Review. *Expert Rev. Clin. Pharmacol.* **2021**, *14*, 735–747. [CrossRef]
17. López-Romero, P.; Pichardo-Ontiveros, E.; Avila-Nava, A.; Vázquez-Manjarrez, N.; Tovar, A.R.; Pedraza-Chaverri, J.; Torres, N. The Effect of Nopal (*Opuntia ficus indica*) on Postprandial Blood Glucose, Incretins, and Antioxidant Activity in Mexican Patients with Type 2 Diabetes after Consumption of Two Different Composition Breakfasts. *J. Acad. Nutr. Diet.* **2014**, *114*, 1811–1818. [CrossRef]
18. Zhang, Y.; Liu, W.; Liu, D.; Zhao, T.; Tian, H. Efficacy of Aloe Vera Supplementation on Prediabetes and Early Non-Treated Diabetic Patients: A Systematic Review and Meta-Analysis of Randomized Controlled Trials. *Nutrients* **2016**, *8*, 388. [CrossRef] [PubMed]
19. Biblioteca Digital de la Medicina Tradicional Mexicana. *Momordica charantia*. 2009. Available online: http://www.medicinatradicionalmexicana.unam.mx/apmtm/termino.php?l=3&t=momordica-charantia (accessed on 10 April 2021).
20. Vera Saltos, A.P.; Manzaba Intriago, M.R. Efecto De La Relación Pulpa–Mucílago De *Melón amargo* (*Momordica charantia*) En La Concentración Final De Una Leche Fermentada. Bachelor's Thesis, Escuela Superior Politécnica Agropecuaria De Manabí Manuel Félix López (Espammfl) Espam, Calceta, Ecuador, 2019.
21. Zell, H. Momordica_charantiae. Available online: https://commons.wikimedia.org/wiki/File:Momordica_charantia_003.JPG (accessed on 10 March 2023).
22. Ofuegbe, S.; Falayi, O.; Ogunpolu, B.; Oyagbemi, A.; Temidayo, O.; Yakubu, M.; Oguntibeju, O.; Adedapo, A. Antidiabetic and Anti-Oxidant Effects of Methanol Leaf Extract of *Momordica charantia* Following Alloxan-Induced Hyperglycaemia in Rats. *J. Herb. Drugs* **2019**, *10*, 103–116.
23. Oyesola, O.; Shallie, P.; Osonuga, I.; Soetan, O.; Owoeye, I. *Momordica charantia* Improves Biochemical Indices in Alloxan-Induced Diabetic Rat Model. *Natl. J. Physiol. Pharm. Pharmacol.* **2020**, *10*, 1. [CrossRef]

24. Abdollahi, M.; Zuki, A.B.Z.; Rezaeizadeh, A.; Goh, Y.M.; Noordin, M.M. Effects of *Momordica charantia* Aqueous Extract on Renal Histopathological Changes Associated with Streptozotocin-Induced Diabetes Mellitus Type II in Neonatal Rats. *J. Med. Plants Res.* **2011**, *5*, 1779–1787.
25. Mushtaq, W.; Tariq, M.; Ishtiaq, M.; Asghar, R.; Hussain, T.; Bashir, T. Role of *Momordica charantia* L. As Herbal Medicine to Cure Hyperglycemia in Vivo on Induced Diabetic Model Animals. *Pak. J. Bot.* **2016**, *48*, 1651–1656.
26. Ae Yoon, N.; Park, J.; Yeon Jeong, J.; Rashidova, N.; Ryu, J.; Seob Roh, G.; Joon Kim, H.; Jae Cho, G.; Sung Choi, W.; Hoon Lee, D.; et al. Anti-Diabetic Activity of Ethanol Extract from *Bitter melon* in Mice Fed High-Fat Diet. *Dev. Reprod.* **2019**, *23*, 129–138. [CrossRef]
27. Yibchok-anun, S.; Adisakwattana, S.; Yao, C.Y.; Sangvanich, P.; Roengsumran, S.; Hsu, W.H. Slow Acting Protein Extract from Fruit Pulp of *Momordica charantia* with Insulin Secretagogue and Insulinomimetic Activities. *Biol. Pharm. Bull.* **2006**, *29*, 1126–1131. [CrossRef]
28. Jiang, S.; Xu, L.; Xu, Y.; Guo, Y.; Wei, L.; Li, X.; Song, W. Antidiabetic Effect of *Momordica charantia* Saponins in Rats Induced by High-Fat Diet Combined with STZ. *Electron. J. Biotechnol.* **2020**, *43*, 41–47. [CrossRef]
29. Wang, Q.; Wu, X.; Shi, F.; Liu, Y. Comparison of Antidiabetic Effects of Saponins and Polysaccharides from *Momordica charantia* L. in STZ-Induced Type 2 Diabetic Mice. *Biomed. Pharmacother.* **2019**, *109*, 744–750. [CrossRef]
30. Chang, C.-I.; Chou, C.-H.; Liao, M.-H.; Chen, T.M.; Cheng, C.H.; Anggriani, R.; Tsai, C.P.; Tseng, H.I.; Cheng, H.L. *Bitter melon* Triterpenes Work as Insulin Sensitizers and Insulin Substitutes in Insulin-Resistant Cells. *J. Funct. Foods* **2015**, *13*, 214–224. [CrossRef]
31. Islam, M.; Islam, M.S.; Zannah, S.; Sadik, G.; Rashid, M. *Momordica charantia* (*Bitter melon*) in Combination with Metformin Potentiates Hypoglycemic and Hypolipidemic Effects in Alloxan-Induced Diabetic Rats. *Bangladesh Pharm. J.* **2018**, *21*, 109–117. [CrossRef]
32. Pramesthi, A.D.E.D.; Ardana, M.; Indriyanti, N. Drug-Herb Interaction between Metformin and *Momordica charantia* in Diabetic Mice. *Mol. Cell. Biomed. Sci.* **2019**, *3*, 81. [CrossRef]
33. Poonam, T.; Prem Prakash, G.; Vijay Kumar, L. Interaction of *Momordica charantia* with Metformin in Diabetic Rats. *Am. J. Pharmacol. Toxicol.* **2013**, *8*, 102–106. [CrossRef]
34. Biblioteca Digital de la Medicina Tradicional Mexicana. *Cucurbita ficifolia bouché*. 2009. Available online: http://www.medicinatradicionalmexicana.unam.mx/apmtm/termino.php?l=3&t=cucurbita-ficifolia. (accessed on 10 April 2021).
35. Andrade-Cetto, A.; Heinrich, M. Mexican Plants with Hypoglycaemic Effect Used in the Treatment of Diabetes. *J. Ethnopharmacol.* **2005**, *99*, 325–348. [CrossRef]
36. Hans, B. *Cucurbita ficifolia bouché*. Cucurbita ficifolia Courge de Siam. Available online: https://commons.wikimedia.org/wiki/File:Cucurbita_ficifolia_Courge_de_Siam.jpg (accessed on 10 March 2023).
37. Acosta-Patiño, J.L.; Jiménez-Balderas, E.; Juárez-Oropeza, M.A.; Díaz-Zagoya, J.C. Hypoglycemic Action of *Cucurbita ficifolia* on Type 2 Diabetic Patients with Moderately High Blood Glucose Levels. *J. Ethnopharmacol.* **2001**, *77*, 99–101. [CrossRef]
38. Alarcon-Aguilar, F.; Hernandez-Galicia, E.; Campos-Sepulveda, A.; Xolalpa-Molina, S.; Rivas-Vilchis, J.; Vazquez-Carrillo, L.; Roman-Ramos, R. Evaluation of the Hypoglycemic Effect of *Cucurbita ficifolia bouché* (*Cucurbitaceae*) in Different Experimental Models. *J. Ethnopharmacol.* **2002**, *82*, 185–189. [CrossRef]
39. Moya-Hernández, A.; Bosquez-Molina, E.; Verde-Calvo, J.R.; Blancas-Flores, G.; Trejo-Aguilar, G.M. Hypoglycemic Effect and Bioactive Compounds Associated with the Ripening Stages of the *Cucurbita ficifolia bouché* Fruit. *J. Sci. Food Agric.* **2020**, *100*, 5171–5181. [CrossRef]
40. Xia, T.; Wang, Q. Antihyperglycemic Effect of *Cucurbita ficifolia* Fruit Extract in Streptozotocin-Induced Diabetic Rats. *Fitoterapia* **2006**, *77*, 530–533. [CrossRef]
41. Xia, T. Hypoglycaemic Role of *Cucurbita ficifolia* (*Cucurbitaceae*) Fruit Extract in Streptozotocin-Induced Diabetic Rats. *J. Sci. Food Agric.* **2007**, *1243*, 1237–1243. [CrossRef]
42. Miranda-Pérez, M.E.; Escobar-villanueva, M.D.C.; Ortega, C.; Sánchez-muñoz, F.; Almanza-pérez, J.C.; Alarcón-, F.J. *Cucurbita ficifolia bouché* Fruit Acts as an Insulin Secretagogue in RINm5F Cells. *Ibcj* **2012**, *3*, 8–14.
43. Miranda-Perez, M.E.; Ortega-Camarillo, C.; Del Carmen Escobar-Villanueva, M.; Blancas-Flores, G.; Alarcon-Aguilar, F.J. *Cucurbita ficifolia bouché* Increases Insulin Secretion in RINm5F Cells through an Influx of Ca^{2+} from the Endoplasmic Reticulum. *J. Ethnopharmacol.* **2016**, *188*, 159–166. [CrossRef] [PubMed]
44. Bioblioteca Digital de la Medicina Tradicional Mexicana, *Coriandrum sativum*. 2009. Available online: http://www.medicinatradicionalmexicana.unam.mx/apmtm/termino.php?l=3&t=coriandrum-sativum (accessed on 15 March 2021).
45. Ceballos, A.; Giraldo, G. El Cilantro (*Coriandrum sativum* L.) Como Fuente Potencial de Antioxidantes Naturales. *Vector* **2011**, *6*, 85–93. Available online: http://200.21.104.25/Vector/Downloads/Vector6_11.Pdf (accessed on 10 March 2023).
46. Stang, D. *Coriandrum sativum* L. Available online: https://commons.wikimedia.org/wiki/File:Coriandrum_sativum_4zz.jpg (accessed on 10 March 2023).
47. Rodríguez, H. La Cocina Tradicional y La Salud. 2015, Volume 16, pp. 1–11. Available online: https://www.revista.unam.mx/vol.16/num5/art36/ (accessed on 4 April 2021).
48. Gray, A.M.; Flatt, P.R. Insulin-Releasing and Insulin-like Activity of the Traditional Anti-Diabetic Plant *Coriandrum sativum* (Coriander). *Br. J. Nutr.* **1999**, *81*, 203–209. [CrossRef] [PubMed]

49. Aissaoui, A.; Zizi, S.; Israili, Z.H.; Lyoussi, B. Hypoglycemic and Hypolipidemic Effects of *Coriandrum sativum* L. in Meriones Shawi Rats. *J. Ethnopharmacol.* **2011**, *137*, 652–661. [CrossRef]
50. Eidi, M.; Eidi, A.; Saeidi, R.; Molanaei, S.; Sadeghipour, A.; Bahar, M.; Bahar, K. Effect of Coriander Seed (*Coriandrum sativum* L.) Ethanol Extract on Insulin Release from Pancreatic Beta Cells in Streptozotocin-Induced Diabetic Rats. *Phyther. Res.* **2009**, *23*, 404–406. [CrossRef]
51. Mechchate, H.; Es-safi, I.; Amaghnouje, A.; Boukhira, S.; Alotaibi, A.; Al-zharani, M.; Nasr, F.; Noman, O.M.; Conte, R.; Amal, E.H.E.Y.; et al. Antioxidant, Anti-Inflammatory and Antidiabetic Proprieties of LC-MS/MS Identified Polyphenols from Coriander Seeds. *Molecules* **2021**, *26*, 487. [CrossRef] [PubMed]
52. Deepa, B.; Anuradha, C.V. Antioxidant Potential of *Coriandrum sativum* L. Seed Extract. *Indian J. Exp. Biol.* **2011**, *49*, 30–38.
53. Naqvi, K.J.; Ali, M.; Ahamad, J. Antidiabetic Activity of Aqueous Extract of *Coriandrum sativum* L. Fruits in Streptozotocin Induced Rats. *Int. J. Pharm. Pharm. Sci.* **2012**, *4*, 239–240.
54. Sudha, T.S. The Combined Effect of Trigonella Foenum Seeds and *Coriandrum sativum* Leaf Extracts in Alloxan Induced Diabetes Mellitus Wister Albino Rats. *Bioinformation* **2019**, *15*, 716–722. [CrossRef]
55. Das, S.; Chaware, S.; Narkar, N.; Tilak, A.V.; Raveendran, S.; Rane, P. Antidiabetic Activity of *Coriandrum sativum* in Streptozotocin Induced Diabetic Rats. *Int. J. Basic Clin. Pharmacol.* **2019**, *8*, 925. [CrossRef]
56. Biblioteca Digital de la Medicina Tradicional Mexicana. *Persea americana*. 2009. Available online: http://www.medicinatradicionalmexicana.unam.mx/apmtm/termino.php?l=3&t=persea-americana (accessed on 10 March 2022).
57. Angel, O.T.M. Valor nutrimental de la pulpa fresca de aguacate Hass. In Proceedings of the V World Avocado Congress (Actas V Congreso Mundial del Aguacate), Málaga, Spain, 19–24 October 2003; pp. 741–748.
58. Safari Travel Plus *Persea americana* Mil. Available online: https://commons.wikimedia.org/wiki/File:Avocado_On_Tree.jpp. (accessed on 10 March 2023).
59. Brai, B.I.C.; Odetola, A.A.; Agomo, P.U. Hypoglycemic and Hypocholesterolemic Potential of *Persea americana* Leaf Extracts. *J. Med. Food* **2007**, *10*, 356–360. [CrossRef]
60. Kumala, S.; Faculty, P.; Sawah, S. The Effect of Avocado (*Persea americana* Mill.) Leaves Extract towards The Mouse's Blood Glucose Decrease with The Glucose Tolerance Method. *Int. J. Pharm. Sci. Res.* **2013**, *4*, 661–665.
61. Kouamé, N.M.; Koffi, C.; N'Zoué, K.S.; Yao, N.A.R.; Doukouré, B.; Kamagaté, M. Comparative Antidiabetic Activity of Aqueous, Ethanol, and Methanol Leaf Extracts of *Persea americana* and Their Effectiveness in Type 2 Diabetic Rats. *Evidence-Based Complement. Altern. Med.* **2019**, *2019*, 5984570. [CrossRef]
62. Lima, C.R.; Vasconcelos, C.F.B.; Costa-Silva, J.H.; Maranhão, C.A.; Costa, J.; Batista, T.M.; Carneiro, E.M.; Soares, L.A.L.; Ferreira, F.; Wanderley, A.G. Anti-Diabetic Activity of Extract from *Persea americana* Mill. Leaf via the Activation of Protein Kinase B (PKB/Akt) in Streptozotocin-Induced Diabetic Rats. *J. Ethnopharmacol.* **2012**, *141*, 517–525. [CrossRef]
63. Edem, D.O.; Ekanem, I.S.; Ebong, P.E. Effect of aqueous extracts of alligator pear seed (*Persea americana* Mill.) on Blood Glucose and Histopathology of Pancreas in Alloxan-Induced Diabetic Rats. *Pak. J. Pharm. Sci.* **2009**, *22*, 272–276. [PubMed]
64. Alhassan, A.; Sule, M.S.; Atiku, M.K.; Wudil, A.M.; Abubakar, H.; Mohammed, S.A. Effects of Aqueous Avocado Pear (*Persea americana*) Seed Extract on Alloxan Induced Diabetes Rats. *Greener J. Med. Sci.* **2012**, *2*, 5–11. [CrossRef]
65. Ezejiofor, A.N.; Okorie, A.; Orisakwe, O.E. Hypoglycaemic and Tissue-Protective Effects of the Aqueous Extract of *Persea americana* Seeds on Alloxan-Induced Albino Rats. *Malays. J. Med. Sci.* **2013**, *20*, 31–39.
66. Ejiofor, C.C.; Ezeagu, I.E.; Ayoola, M. Hypoglycaemic and Biochemical Effects of the Aqueous and Methanolic Extract of *Persea americana* Seeds on Alloxan-Induced Albino Rats. *Eur. J. Med. Plants* **2018**, *26*, 1–12. [CrossRef]
67. Nardi, L.; Lister, I.N.; Girsang, E.; Fachrial, E. Hypoglycemic Effect of Avocado Seed Extract (*Persean americana* Mill.) from Analysis of Oral Glucose Tolerance Test On *Rattus norvegicus* L. *Am. Sci. Res. J. Eng. Technol. Sci.* **2020**, *65*, 49–56.
68. Mahadeva, R.; Adinew, B. Remnant B-Cell-Stimulative and Anti-Oxidative Effects of *Persea americana* Fruit Extract Studied in Rats Introduced into Streptozotocin—Induced Hyperglycaemic State. *Afr. J. Tradit. Complement. Altern. Med.* **2011**, *8*, 210–217. [CrossRef]
69. Ahmed, N.; Tcheng, M.; Roma, A.; Buraczynski, M.; Jayanth, P.; Rea, K.; Akhtar, T.A.; Spagnuolo, P.A. Avocatin B Protects Against Lipotoxicity and Improves Insulin Sensitivity in Diet-Induced Obesity. *Mol. Nutr. Food Res.* **2019**, *63*, e1900688. [CrossRef] [PubMed]
70. Ojo, O.A.; Amanze, J.C.; Oni, A.I.; Grant, S.; Iyobhebhe, M.; Elebiyo, T.C.; Rotimi, D.; Asogwa, N.T.; Oyinloye, B.E.; Ajiboye, B.O.; et al. Antidiabetic Activity of Avocado Seeds (*Persea americana* Mill.) in Diabetic Rats via Activation of PI3K/AKT Signaling Pathway. *Sci. Rep.* **2022**, *12*, 2919. [CrossRef] [PubMed]
71. Yang, W.-C. Botanical, Pharmacological, Phytochemical, and Toxicological Aspects of the Antidiabetic Plant *Bidens pilosa* L. *Evid.-Based Complement. Altern. Med.* **2014**, *2014*, 698617. [CrossRef] [PubMed]
72. Biblioteca Digital de la Medicina Tradicional Mexicana. *Bidens pilosa*. 2009. Available online: http://www.medicinatradicionalmexicana.unam.mx/apmtm/termino.php?l=3&t=mozote (accessed on 9 June 2021).
73. Arroyo, J.; Bonilla, P.; Ráez, E.; Barreda, A.; Huamán, O. Efecto Quimioprotector de *Bidens pilosa* En El Cáncer de Mama Inducido En Ratas TT—*Bidens pilosa* Chemoprotective Effect on Induced Breast Cancer in Rats. *An. Fac. Med.* **2010**, *71*, 153–160. [CrossRef]
74. Fonseca Mata, J.C. Bidens pilosa. Available online: https://commons.wikimedia.org/wiki/File:Bidens_pilosa_-_Asteraceae.jpg (accessed on 10 March 2023).

75. Hsu, Y.-J.; Lee, T.-H.; Chang, C.L.-T.; Huang, Y.-T.; Yang, W.-C. Anti-Hyperglycemic Effects and Mechanism of *Bidens pilosa* Water Extract. *J. Ethnopharmacol.* **2009**, *122*, 379–383. [CrossRef]
76. Ubillas, R.; Mendez, C.; Jolad, S.; Luo, J.; King, S.; Carlson, T.; Fort, D. Antihyperglycemic Acetylenic Glucosides from *Bidens pilosa*. *Planta Med.* **1999**, *66*, 82–83. [CrossRef] [PubMed]
77. Gnagne, A.S.; Coulibaly, K.; Fofie, N.B.Y.; Bene, K.; Zirihi, G.N. Hypoglycemic Potential of Aqueous Extracts of *Ageratum conyzoides* L., *Anthocleista djalonensis* A. Chev. and *Bidens Pilosa* L., Three Plants from the Ivorian Pharmacopoeia. *Eur. Sci. J.* **2018**, *14*, 360. [CrossRef]
78. Chang, C.L.-T.; Liu, H.-Y.; Kuo, T.-F.; Hsu, Y.-J.; Shen, M.-Y.; Pan, C.-Y.; Yang, W.-C. Antidiabetic Effect and Mode of Action of Cytopiloyne. *Evid.-Based Complement. Altern. Med.* **2013**, *2013*, 685642. [CrossRef]
79. Lai, B.-Y.; Chen, T.-Y.; Huang, S.-H.; Kuo, T.-F.; Chang, T.-H.; Chiang, C.-K.; Yang, M.-T.; Chang, C.L.-T. *Bidens pilosa* Formulation Improves Blood Homeostasis and β-Cell Function in Men: A Pilot Study. *Evid.-Based Complement. Altern. Med.* **2015**, *2015*, 832314. [CrossRef]
80. Comisión Federal para la Protección contra los Riesgos Sanitarios. *Liberación de 18 Plantas Medicinales Para Su Uso Legal*; COFEPRIS: Mexico City, Mexico, 2018.
81. Committee on Herbal Medicinal Products (HMPC). Assessment Report on *Echinacea purpurea* (L.) Moench. Herba Recens. *Eur. Med. Agency* **2014**, *44*, 1–73.
82. Committee on Herbal Medicinal Products (HMPC). Assessment Report on *Panax ginseng*. *Eur. Med. Agency* **2014**, *44*, 5.
83. Committee on Herbal Medicinal Products (HMPC). Assessment Report on *Passiflora incarnata* L., Herba. *Eur. Med. Agency* **2014**, *44*, 1.
84. Rodríguez-Hernández, A.A.; Flores-Soria, F.G.; Patiño-Rodríguez, O.; Escobedo-Moratilla, A. Sanitary Registries and Popular Medicinal Plants Used in Medicines and Herbal Remedies in Mexico (2001–2020): A Review and Potential Perspectives. *Horticulturae* **2022**, *8*, 377. [CrossRef]
85. Ahumada, A.; Ortega, A.; Chito, D.; Benítez, R. Saponinas de Quinua *(Chenopodium quinoa Willd.)*: Un Subproducto Con Alto Potencial Biológico. *Rev. Colomb. Cienc. Quím.-Farm.* **2016**, *45*, 438–469. [CrossRef]
86. Bano, G. Glucose Homeostasis, Obesity and Diabetes. *Best Pract. Res. Clin. Obstet. Gynaecol.* **2013**, *27*, 715–726. [CrossRef]
87. Rosas-Saucedo, J.; Rosas-Guzmán, J.; Mesa-Pérez, J.A.; González-Ortiz, M.; Martínez-Abundis, E.; González-Suárez, R.; Sinay, I.; Lyra, R. Sulfonilureas. Estado Actual de Su Empleo En América Latina. Documento de Posición de La Asociación Latinoamericana de Diabetes. *Alad* **2019**, *9*, 19000375. [CrossRef]
88. López-Zelada, K.A.; Garibay-Díaz, J.C.; Escobar-Arriaga, E.; León-Rodríguez, E.; De La Peña-López, R.; Esparza-López, J.; De Jesús Ibarra-Sánchez, M. El Silenciamiento de PTP1B Disminuye La Proliferación Celular En Cultivos Primarios de Cáncer de Mama. *Gac. Mex. Oncol.* **2014**, *13*, 144–151.
89. Marrelli, M.; Conforti, F.; Araniti, F.; Statti, G.A. Effects of Saponins on Lipid Metabolism: A Review of Potential Health Benefits in the Treatment of Obesity. *Molecules* **2016**, *21*, 1404. [CrossRef]
90. Serra Bisbal, J.J.; Melero Lloret, J.; Martínez Lozano, G.; Fagoaga, C. Especies Vegetales Como Antioxidantes de Alimentos. *Nereis. Interdiscip. Ibero-Am. J. Methods Model. Simul.* **2020**, *12*, 71–90. [CrossRef]
91. Martínez, M. Incretinas e Incretinomiméticos: Actualización En Liraglutida, Una Nueva Opción Terapéutica Para Pacientes Con Diabetes Mellitus Tipo 2. *Med. Gen.* **2010**, *127*, 169–185.
92. Huang, D.-W.; Chang, W.-C.; Wu, J.S.-B.; Shih, R.-W.; Shen, S.-C. Gallic Acid Ameliorates Hyperglycemia and Improves Hepatic Carbohydrate Metabolism in Rats Fed a High-Fructose Diet. *Nutr. Res.* **2016**, *36*, 150–160. [CrossRef]
93. Meng, S.; Cao, J.; Feng, Q.; Peng, J.; Hu, Y. Roles of Chlorogenic Acid on Regulating Glucose and Lipids Metabolism: A Review. *Evid.-Based Complement. Altern. Med.* **2013**, *2013*, 801457. [CrossRef]
94. Larner, J. D-Chiro-Inositol in Insulin Action and Insulin Resistance—Old-Fashioned Biochemistry Still at Work. *IUBMB Life* **2001**, *51*, 139–148. [CrossRef]
95. Larner, J. D-Chiro-Inositol-Its Functional Role in Insulin Action and Its Deficit in Insulin Resistance. *Int. J. Exp. Diabetes Res.* **2002**, *3*, 47–60. [CrossRef] [PubMed]
96. Saleem, F.; Rizvi, S.W. New Therapeutic Approaches in Obesity and Metabolic Syndrome Associated with Polycystic Ovary Syndrome. *Cureus* **2017**, *9*, e1844. [CrossRef] [PubMed]
97. Favela Inositol. *Faga Lab*; Favela Pro: Sinaloa, Mexico, 2020; pp. 8001–8003.
98. Sánchez, P.L. Sulfonilureas En El Tratamiento Del Paciente Con Diabetes Mellitus Tipo 2. *Endocrinol. Nutr.* **2008**, *55*, 17–25. [CrossRef]
99. Vessal, M.; Hemmati, M.; Vasei, M. Antidiabetic Effects of Quercetin in Streptozotocin-Induced Diabetic Rats. *Comp. Biochem. Physiol.-C Toxicol. Pharmacol.* **2003**, *135*, 357–364. [CrossRef]
100. Carrasco-Pozo, C.; Cires, M.J.; Gotteland, M. Quercetin and Epigallocatechin Gallate in the Prevention and Treatment of Obesity: From Molecular to Clinical Studies. *J. Med. Food* **2019**, *22*, 753–770. [CrossRef]
101. Cazarolli, L.H.; Folador, P.; Pizzolatti, M.G.; Mena Barreto Silva, F.R. Signaling Pathways of Kaempferol-3-Neohesperidoside in Glycogen Synthesis in Rat Soleus Muscle. *Biochimie* **2009**, *91*, 843–849. [CrossRef]
102. Tzeng, Y.M.; Chen, K.; Rao, Y.K.; Lee, M.J. Kaempferitrin Activates the Insulin Signaling Pathway and Stimulates Secretion of Adiponectin in 3T3-L1 Adipocytes. *Eur. J. Pharmacol.* **2009**, *607*, 27–34. [CrossRef] [PubMed]

103. Ždychová, J.; Komers, R. Emerging Role of Akt Kinase/Protein Kinase B Signaling in Pathophysiology of Diabetes and Its Complications. *Physiol. Res.* **2005**, *54*, 1–16. [CrossRef] [PubMed]
104. Kuo, T.-F.; Yang, G.; Chen, T.-Y.; Wu, Y.-C.; Minh, H.T.N.; Chen, L.-S.; Chen, W.-C.; Huang, M.-G.; Liang, Y.-C.; Yang, W.-C. Bidens Pilosa: Nutritional Value and Benefits for Metabolic Syndrome. *Food Front.* **2020**, *2*, 32–45. [CrossRef]
105. Liang, Y.C.; Yang, M.T.; Lin, C.J.; Chang, C.L.T.; Yang, W.C. Bidens Pilosa and Its Active Compound Inhibit Adipogenesis and Lipid Accumulation via Down-Modulation of the C/EBP and PPARγ Pathways. *Sci. Rep.* **2016**, *6*, 24285. [CrossRef] [PubMed]
106. Roth, C. *Ficha de Seguridad*; Agrovin: Alcazar de San Juan, Spain, 2010; Volume 2.

Disclaimer/Publisher's Note: The statements, opinions and data contained in all publications are solely those of the individual author(s) and contributor(s) and not of MDPI and/or the editor(s). MDPI and/or the editor(s) disclaim responsibility for any injury to people or property resulting from any ideas, methods, instructions or products referred to in the content.

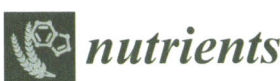

Review

Bioactivity of Macronutrients from *Chlorella* in Physical Exercise

Karenia Lorenzo [1], Garoa Santocildes [1,2], Joan Ramon Torrella [1], José Magalhães [3], Teresa Pagès [1], Ginés Viscor [1], Josep Lluís Torres [2] and Sara Ramos-Romero [1,*]

[1] Physiology Section, Department of Cell Biology, Physiology and Immunology, Faculty of Biology, University of Barcelona, 08028 Barcelona, Spain
[2] Department of Biological Chemistry, Institute of Advanced Chemistry of Catalonia (IQAC-CSIC), 08034 Barcelona, Spain
[3] Laboratory of Metabolism and Exercise (LaMetEx), Research Centre in Physical Activity, Health and Leisure (CIAFEL), Faculty of Sport, University of Porto, 4200-450 Porto, Portugal
* Correspondence: sara.ramosromero@ub.edu; Tel.: +34-934-021-556

Abstract: *Chlorella* is a marine microalga rich in proteins and containing all the essential amino acids. *Chlorella* also contains fiber and other polysaccharides, as well as polyunsaturated fatty acids such as linoleic acid and alpha-linolenic acid. The proportion of the different macronutrients in *Chlorella* can be modulated by altering the conditions in which it is cultured. The bioactivities of these macronutrients make *Chlorella* a good candidate food to include in regular diets or as the basis of dietary supplements in exercise-related nutrition both for recreational exercisers and professional athletes. This paper reviews current knowledge of the effects of the macronutrients in *Chlorella* on physical exercise, specifically their impact on performance and recovery. In general, consuming *Chlorella* improves both anaerobic and aerobic exercise performance as well as physical stamina and reduces fatigue. These effects seem to be related to the antioxidant, anti-inflammatory, and metabolic activity of all its macronutrients, while each component of *Chlorella* contributes its bioactivity via a specific action. *Chlorella* is an excellent dietary source of high-quality protein in the context of physical exercise, as dietary proteins increase satiety, activation of the anabolic mTOR (mammalian Target of Rapamycin) pathway in skeletal muscle, and the thermic effects of meals. *Chlorella* proteins also increase intramuscular free amino acid levels and enhance the ability of the muscles to utilize them during exercise. Fiber from *Chlorella* increases the diversity of the gut microbiota, which helps control body weight and maintain intestinal barrier integrity, and the production of short-chain fatty acids (SCFAs), which improve physical performance. Polyunsaturated fatty acids (PUFAs) from *Chlorella* contribute to endothelial protection and modulate the fluidity and rigidity of cell membranes, which may improve performance. Ultimately, in contrast to several other nutritional sources, the use of *Chlorella* to provide high-quality protein, dietary fiber, and bioactive fatty acids may also significantly contribute to a sustainable world through the fixation of carbon dioxide and a reduction of the amount of land used to produce animal feed.

Keywords: algae; fatty acid; protein; fiber; physical activity

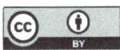

1. Introduction

Algae, as well as the products made from them, are in increasing demand worldwide because of their nutritional value and practical contributions. Microalgae (unicellular algae) are a source of high-quality proteins, similar to those found in milk, eggs, and meat, with a low fat content [1]. They also include other bioactive components, specifically polyunsaturated fatty acids (PUFAs), polysaccharide fibers, polyphenols, carotenoids, phycobiliproteins, vitamins, and sterols [2–4]. In addition to the nutritional benefits provided by these, the viability of cultivating microalgae in specific installations as an alternative source for CO_2 fixation, thereby capturing this greenhouse gas without occupying soil, makes them particularly promising for the sustainability of the planet. Microalgae are used in the pharmaceutical, cosmetic, and food industries; however, the European Commission only lists two species in their Novel Food Catalogue: *Arthrospira* (also called Spirulina, a cyanobacterium) and *Chlorella* (a green alga). (In this paper, we use the terms "*Chlorella*" when referring to the genus of this living organism, and "spirulina" and "chlorella" when referring generically to biomass preparations of these microalgae. We will also use the terms "spirulina" and "chlorella" when referring to studies or reports in which the particular species used is not specified.)

Chlorella was first described by Beijerinck in 1890. Its name is derived from 'chloros' (from Greek, meaning green) and the suffix 'ella' (from Latin, meaning small). Nowadays, more than 20 species and over 100 strains of *Chlorella* have been described [5], belonging to 2 classes of Chlorophyta: Chlorophyceae and Trebouxiophyceae. *Chlorella* is a spherical/ellipsoidal cell with a 2–10 μm diameter that reproduces via asexual autospores. The main habitats where *Chlorella* lives are both fresh water and seawater, although it can also be found in soil, living independently as well as in symbiosis with lichens or protozoa [6]. The biochemical compositions of *Chlorella* vary greatly between species and even strains and also depend on the culture conditions, including nutritional and environmental factors. The general growth and protein production of this microalga increase with the rising nitrogen content of its medium, while nitrogen limitation augments the proportion of starch or lipids in *Chlorella* [6]. In general, the macronutrient composition of *Chlorella* biomass is over 60% dry weight of protein (including all the essential amino acids) and more than 10% of both lipids and carbohydrates (Table 1) [7]. Moreover, *Chlorella* contains many different components with functional activities (Table 1).

Table 1. Most relevant biochemical composition of *Chlorella*.

	Main Components
Macronutrients	
Proteins	All the essential amino acids
Carbohydrates	α- and β-glucans, fiber
Lipids	PUFAs (linoleic acid, alpha-linolenic acid)
Micronutrients	
Minerals	Na^+, K^+, Fe^{2+}, Ca^{2+}, Mg^{2+}, Mn^{2+}, Zn^{2+}, Co^{2+}
Vitamins	A, B_1, B_2, B_6, B_{12}, C, E, K_1, folic and pantothenic acids, niacin
Pigments	Chlorophylls, carotenoids, lutein

Spirulina is the other microalga approved for human consumption [4]. Preparations of chlorella and spirulina have different proportions of common components. The polysaccharide (β-glucans and arabinomannans) composition of *Chlorella* spp. has been better defined than that of Spirulina [4]. *Chlorella* contains β-glucans (polymers of β-D-glucose linked through 1–3 β-glycosidic bonds, 6–9% of dry weight) [8] and arabinomannans (oligomers of arabinose and mannose) [9] as well as other less known saccharides with hypolipidemic activity [10]. As well as these lipidemic functions, up to 50% of *Chlorella* dry weight can consist of triacylglycerols (TAGs) when it has been exposed to high light or nitrogen deficiency conditions [11]. Peptides from the enzymatic hydrolysis of *Chlorella* can also have health benefits, such as hypoglycemic, anti-inflammatory, and blood pressure-lowering activities (e.g., inhibition of angiotensin I-converting enzyme, ACE) [4,12,13]. Therefore, because of its nutritional value and bioactive compounds, *Chlorella* is an interesting microalga for human consumption; however, if it is not properly processed, it could be poorly digested and induce side effects because, in its naturally occurring form it contains a cellulose cell wall. So, chlorella must be mechanically broken down during production for human consumption to avoid gastrointestinal issues, including nausea, vomiting, and stomach problems. Other side effects related to chlorella intake include renal and allergy problems [14]. Despite this, in the context of human health and disease, chlorella has been shown to have cardiovascular benefits, as revealed by its capacity to lower total cholesterol, low-density lipoprotein cholesterol, systolic blood pressure, diastolic blood pressure, and fasting blood glucose in healthy individuals and patients with non-alcoholic fatty liver disease, hypertension, hypercholesterolemia, and dyslipidemia [15]. At the doses used to elicit these responses, chlorella is considered to be safe [16].

In addition to its macronutrients, chlorella also contains phenolic compounds with radical scavenging capacity and α-amylase/glycosidase inhibitory activity [12], as well as other components such as vitamins (e.g., vitamin B_9 or folate) [17] and carotenoids (e.g., astaxanthin) [18] that may contribute to its antioxidant and anti-inflammatory activities [19]). Moreover, it incorporates chlorophyll and other minerals with some biological functions [7]. Taken together, it seems that the functional activity of chlorella intake could be complementary or synergistic with other health-related habits, such as consuming a balanced diet, getting adequate sleep, or taking physical exercise.

Physical exercise represents a stressful activity for the body's cells, tissues, and organs, which dysregulates whole-body homeostasis in a progressive and reversible way. However, as a consequence of its regular and systematic practice, different cellular signaling pathways become activated and generate systemic and local chronic adaptations. These promote physiological, biochemical, and morphological adjustments of the organism to the exercise [20], such as a gain of muscle mass and strength and improvements in cardiovascular health and functional capacity [21].

Besides their role as biochemical triggers and mechanical platforms for strength production, skeletal muscle fibers are nowadays also considered to be essential pleotropic sources of several compounds and molecules crucial for muscle-to-organ/tissue crosstalk communication [22]. Myokines, for example, are specific cytokines, small peptides, growth factors, and metallopeptidases produced and released by skeletal muscle, with both paracrine and endocrine effects, that promote communication between muscle cells and other target organs or tissue cells [21]. It has been shown that regular exercise increases the production and secretion of myokines, such as irisin, insulin-like growth factor 1 (IGF-1), brain-derived neurotrophic factor (BDNF), meteorin-like protein (Metrnl), fibroblast growth factor, β-aminoisobutyric acid (BAIBA), the interleukins (ILs) IL-15, IL-7, IL-6, and decorin, whilst reducing the production and release of myostatin. These myokines are the drivers of the most beneficial effects of exercise in terms of health-related outcomes and chronic adaptive responses to training [23,24]. This is because their regulation is directly related, among other things, to increased protein synthesis and reduced muscle protein breakdown, increased lipid oxidation, browning of white adipose tissue, increased insulin sensitivity, increased myogenesis, and satellite cell activation (for a review, see [25]). Furthermore, it is known that, both during and after conventional exercise models, contracting muscles increase ROS production in a way that positively impacts muscle cellular signaling and adaptive responses, thereby strengthening cells to deal better with the demands of physical exercise and to mitigate several deleterious consequences associated with pathological conditions [20,22]. Regarding health-related benefits, regular exercise has been defined as a prophylactic but also a therapeutic, non-pharmacological "polypill", able to prevent around 26 different chronic diseases and reduce all-cause mortality [23,24,26], by reducing the incidence of cardiovascular diseases; through the regulation of blood lipids, hypertension, and arterial fitness [22]; and by protecting against atherosclerosis, type 2 diabetes, and breast and colon cancer [23]. Moreover, regular exercise is a consensual treatment tool against different pathological risk factors or situations, such as obesity (by helping practitioners to lose weight, reducing the metabolic risk factor, and improving adipose tissue health [22,27]), ischemic heart disease, heart failure, type 2 diabetes, chronic obstructive pulmonary disease, chronic low-grade systemic inflammation, and non-alcoholic fatty liver disease [23]. Furthermore, physical exercise has been considered crucial to mental health, helping in the management of depression and anxiety and in the therapeutic challenge against neurodegenerative disorders such as Alzheimer's or Parkinson's disease [28,29]. Apart from preventing and treating pathological situations, regular physical exercise can improve cardiovascular fitness and aerobic capacity, thereby slowing biological aging through a reduction of age-related sarcopenia and thus increasing quality of life and potentially life expectancy.

Chlorella, as well as spirulina and other microalgae, is progressively being introduced into human and animal nutrition as a wholesome source of nutrients that is complementary or an alternative to animal-derived foodstuffs. Whereas research on the properties of edible microalgae in the context of health and disease has been summarized many times, the important area of sports nutrition has not been systematically reviewed to date. Therefore, the present paper aims to contribute to the advancement of research on the use of new environmentally friendly and health-promoting foodstuffs in this area. Taken together, it is reasonable to assume that microalgae and their bioactive compounds are interesting nutritional sources to improve exercise performance and post-exercise recovery, as well as enhance the beneficial clinical features of physical exercise [1]. This paper reviews the available evidence supporting the benefits of the edible microalgae *Chlorella* in the context of physical exercise; however, the role played by chlorella's multiple components in these effects is still an active area of research.

2. Methods

We searched the literature using the PUBMED and Google Scholar databases in June 2022. A variety of combinations of words and terms were entered as the search criteria, including, but not limited to, "chlorella", "physical activity", "training", "exercise", "algae", "fatty acid", "protein", "fiber", "polysaccharides", and "PUFAs".

Both animal and human studies are included in this review. Additionally, healthy subjects as well as animals or humans with any stated medical condition are included. Manuscripts published before 1992 and non-English language publications were excluded. We also excluded from the analysis studies with no exercise protocol or those with no direct or indirect relationship with physical exercise.

Nineteen papers that evaluated supplementation with chlorella or some of its macronutrients in the context of physical exercise are included in this review. Some features of these articles that discuss chlorella supplementation, such as participants, supplementation, exercise protocols, and findings, are summarized in Table 2.

Table 2. Studies involving the effects of *Chlorella* administration on physical parameters.

Subjects	Supplementation Protocol	Exercise Protocols and Tests	Results
ICR mice, male Healthy	*C. vulgaris* (Hot water extract) Dosage: 0.05–0.15 g/kg/day Intervention: 1 week	Training: – Forced swimming test (6′, measured the total duration of immobility.	↓ Immobility time, BUN, CK, and LDH No effect: Glc, TP [30]
ICR mice, male 4 weeks old Healthy	*C. vulgaris* (Hydrolyzed) Dosage: 10 mL/kg/day Intervention: 2 weeks	Training: – Forced swimming test (6′, measured the total duration of immobility.	↑ IFN-γ, IL-2 (in Molt-4 cells) ↓ Immobility time, BUN [31]
BALB/c mice, male 6 weeks old Healthy	Chlorella powder in chow Dosage: 0.5%, 1 mg/kg/day Intervention: 2 weeks	Training: – Forced swimming test (Measured the maximum swimming time).	↑ Swimming time, FFA, Glc, TG, and lactic acid. ↓ Oxidoreductase activity and the leukotriene synthesis pathway [32]
Men and women ≈21 years old Healthy	Chlorella tablets Dosage: 15 tablets, 2 times/day Intervention: 4 weeks	Training: – Maximal exercise test (Incremental cycling to exhaustion).	↑ VO$_2$ peak [33]

Table 2. Cont.

Subjects	Supplementation Protocol	Exercise Protocols and Tests	Results
Sprague-Dawley rats, male 12 weeks old Healthy	Chlorella powder in chow Dosage: 0.5% Intervention: 6 weeks	Training: HIIE (14 × 20″ swim, with a 10″ pause between series, bearing a weight, 4 days/week, for 6 week). Exercise performance test (Maximal number of HIIE).	↑ number HIIE sessions, the expression of MCT1, MCT4, and PPARγ coactivator-1α, and the activities of LDH, CS, and COX in the red region of gastrocnemius. No effect: MCT1 expression and LDH, CS, and COX activities in the white region of gastrocnemius [34]
OLETF rats, male 20 weeks old Type 2 diabetics	Chlorella powder in chow Dosage: 0.5% Intervention: 8 week	Training: Aerobic exercise (running on the treadmill for 1 h, 25 m/min, 5 days/week, during 8 weeks).	↑ insulin sensitivity index concomitant with muscle PI3K activity, Akt phosphorylation, and GLUT4 translocation levels ↓ fasting blood glucose, insulin levels, and total glucose AUC during the OGTT [35]
Men ≈23 years old Overweight	*C. vulgaris* tablets Dosage: 300 mg, 4 times/day Intervention: 1 week	Training: – Acute eccentric exercise protocol (20′ treadmill run at a speed of 9 km/h with a negative 10% slope, 1 week after supplementation)	↓ IL-6 levels and insulin resistance, 24 h after acute eccentric exercise test [36]

Legend. HIIE: high-intensity intermittent exercise; MCT: monocarboxylate transporter; LDH: lactate dehydrogenase; CS: citrate synthase; COX: cytochrome-c oxidase; ICR: Institute of Cancer Research; CVE: extracts of *C. vulgaris*; BUN: blood urea nitrogen; CK: creatine kinase; Glc: glucose; TP: total protein; HCV: *Chlorella vulgaris* by malted barley; CPK: creatine phosphokinase; IFN-γ: interferon gamma; IL-2: interleukin 2; OLETF: Otsuka Long-Evans Tokushima Fatty; AUC: area under the curve; OGTT: oral glucose tolerance test; PI3K: phosphatidylinositol-3 kinase; Akt: protein kinase B; GLUT4: glucose transporter 4; BALB/c: albino, laboratory-bred strain; FFA: free fatty acid; TG: triglyceride; HR: heart rate; PPAR: peroxisome proliferator-activated receptor.

3. *Chlorella* spp. and Physical Exercise

The use of chlorella as a nutritional source of specific bioactive compounds in the context of novel foods or as a supplement has been shown to enhance physical exercise performance in humans and other mammals (Table 2). For example, through the improved expression of monocarboxylate transporters (MCT) 1 and 4, peroxisome proliferator-activated receptor gamma (PPAR-γ) coactivator-1α, and the activities of lactic dehydrogenase (LDH), phosphofructokinase, citrate synthase, and cytochrome oxidase (COX) in the red region of rat muscle, chlorella synergistically enhances the ability to perform maximum numbers of high-intensity intermittent training (HIIT) sessions as a result of training [34]. These biochemical effects increased the ability to produce ATP in skeletal muscle via the glycolytic and oxidative pathways, resulting in a significant improvement in exercise performance. Additionally, diverse chlorella preparations can influence the magnitude of intense exercise-related muscle damage and physical stamina. Hot water extracts from *Chlorella vulgaris* decrease blood urea nitrogen (BUN), creatine kinase, and LDH in the blood serum of mice after a forced swimming test [30]. Additionally, hydrolyzed *C. vulgaris* reduces the immobility time in forced swimming tests in mice while reducing BUN [31]. Despite numerous studies that link chlorella intake with improvements in different aspects of physical exercise, there is still a lack of consensus about the main mechanism(s) via which these effects are produced. In general, chlorella intake has been shown to have mainly antioxidant, immunomodulatory, metabolic, and antihypertensive effects [7]. All together, these effects could act synergistically to improve exercise performance.

The capacity of the bioactive compounds present in *Chlorella* to scavenge free radicals could be one of the main mechanisms underlying its biological activities. *C. vulgaris* supplementation improves several oxidative stress markers, such as malondialdehyde (MDA), total antioxidant capacity (TAC), and lipid peroxidation in rats in which oxidative stress has been induced [37], as well as increasing the activities of some antioxidant enzymes, such as superoxide dismutase (SOD) and catalase (CAT) in smokers [38]. Additionally, some of its bioactive compounds, like astaxanthin, modulate signaling pathways related to oxidative stress, such as those involving mitogen-activated protein kinases (MAPK), phosphatidylinositol-3 kinase/protein kinase B (PI3K/Akt), and nuclear factor erythroid 2-related factor 2/antioxidant response element (Nrf2/ARE) [39]. Altogether, the data suggest that *Chlorella* has potential as an antioxidant during and after physical exercise. However, the role of antioxidants in exercise training is still controversial. Antioxidant supplementation can reduce the advantages induced by training, as some chronic exercise adaptations related to performance are mediated by both ROS and reactive nitrogen species (RNS), namely enhancements in antioxidant capacity, mitochondrial biogenesis, cellular defense mechanisms, and insulin sensitivity [40]. In general, it seems that physiological doses of ROS/RNS are beneficial when it comes to improving exercise performance-related "machinery", while exaggerated production may be detrimental. Therefore, more studies are needed to ascertain adequate chlorella doses that support antioxidant benefits related to exercise intensity and duration without compromising ROS/RNS-related cellular signaling adaptations and, ultimately, performance.

Similarly to the production of ROS/RNS, physical exercise also increases the concentration of a number of pro-inflammatory cytokines in the blood [23], depending on the intensity, duration, and predominant mode of the imposed muscle contractions. Specifically, IL-6 is the first cytokine present in the bloodstream during physical exercise; in turn, it activates the production of other cytokines, such as IL-1 and IL-10, and inhibits the release of TNF-α. Data regarding *Chlorella vulgaris* show that it reduces the production of IL-6 and TNF-α in vitro, as well as reducing NO and prostaglandin E2 (PGE$_2$) release, which suggests that this microalga has significant anti-inflammatory activity [41]. The activity of *Chlorella vulgaris* on serum IL-6 levels has also been related to a reduction of insulin resistance after one session of intense acute eccentric exercise in overweight men [36]. This ability of chlorella to modulate insulin signaling pathways seems to also be related to its activity on muscle sirtuin 1 (SIRT1) [34], as increased expression of SIRT1 improves insulin sensitivity and attenuates insulin resistance [42]. A combination of chronic intake of chlorella and endurance training further increased PI3K activity, Akt phosphorylation, and glucose transporter type 4 (GLUT4) translocation in the skeletal muscle of diabetic rats [35]. This combined treatment may produce larger beneficial effects on improving glycemic control via the enhancement of skeletal muscle glucose uptake.

The effects of chlorella on glucose metabolism may also be interesting for exercise performance under several specific conditions. During moderate to intense or prolonged exercise, liver glycogen stores and gluconeogenesis help to maintain blood glucose levels in the body and sustain the glycolytic flux in the active musculature. Surprisingly, chlorella intake preserved liver glycogen stores and performance during a swimming test, as it prompted an energy shift from carbohydrate to free fatty acid utilization [32].

Glucose metabolism is linked to blood pressure as insulin resistance is a main upstream event leading to hypertension [43]. However, there are other factors that can also modulate blood pressure, such as nitric oxide (NO) levels. Local NO production by the vascular endothelium improves the flow-mediated dilation (FMD) that affects arterial function by decreasing peripheral vascular resistance, thus impacting general vascular health [44]. Chlorella supplementation increases NO production [45] and the expression of endothelial nitric oxide synthase (eNOS) in men, thereby augmenting blood flow to muscles [46], which could eventually enhance performance. The vasodilatation induced by NO would lead to greater muscle perfusion and O$_2$ delivery, theoretically speeding up VO$_2$ kinetics and improving muscle performance and recovery [47]. Accordingly, supplementation with chlorella leads to a significant increase in peak oxygen uptake, suggesting that chlorella increases endurance in young individuals [33]. Moreover, the antihypertensive effects of chlorella are significant not only in healthy young subjects but also in middle-aged and elder individuals, as reported by Otsuki et al. [45,48]. The antihypertensive effect of chlorella seems to be related to the activation of NO production by endothelial cells, which triggers vasodilatation, as well as the improvement of glucose metabolism.

Although the beneficial effects of chlorella on exercise performance might involve synergies between its bioactive features, they might also be related to some specific bioactive compounds that are present in it. So, discriminative knowledge of the benefits of each *Chlorella*-derived product as a positive ergogenic effector could be an interesting subject for the functional food industry, as well as for the consumer.

4. Bioactive Macronutrients from *Chlorella* and Physical Exercise

4.1. Benefits of Proteins and Peptides from Chlorella for Physical Exercise

Chlorella species have a great potential to be used as an alternative protein source because over 80% of them are digestible by humans and comparable both quantitatively and qualitatively to other conventional vegetable proteins [49]. In terms of quantity, proteins range from 51% to 58% in *C. vulgaris*, and 57% for *C. pyrenoidosa* on a dry weight basis in growth conditions that are rich in nitrogen. In the absence of nitrogen, the amount of proteins present can decrease by up to 20% w/w on a dry weight basis [49–51]. The current trend of increasing atmospheric CO_2 may also lead to an increase in the protein content of these species [51]. In terms of quality, most microalgae contain all of the essential amino acids that mammals are unable to synthesize and therefore must obtain from their food intake [50]. Specifically, the essential amino acid index (EAAI) of *C. pyrenoidosa* indicates that all essential amino acids are present at substantial concentrations [52]. Compared to other macronutrients, protein intake increases satiety, activation of the anabolic mTOR (mammalian target of rapamycin) pathway in skeletal muscle, and the thermic effects of meals [53]. As plant-based diets seem to be a good option for enhancing athletic performance while also improving general physical and environmental health [54], a regular intake of *Chlorella* or its isolated proteins could be an environmentally friendly choice of dietary supplement for people undergoing training.

Apart from its protein content, *Chlorella* also contains bioactive peptides that may be of interest in terms of exercise performance. Bioactive peptides usually contain 3–16 amino acid residues, and their activities are mainly based on their amino acid composition and sequence [55]. Some bioactive peptides are antioxidants, as they scavenge ROS and free radicals or prevent oxidative damage by interrupting the radical chain reaction of oxidation. This antioxidant activity of peptides mainly depends on the hydrophobic amino acids they contain, specifically some aromatic amino acids and their histidine content [56]. A peptide from *C. ellipsoidea* (LNGDVW, 702.2 Da) has demonstrated great efficiency in scavenging various free radicals in vitro and therefore has the potential to be a good dietary supplement for the prevention of oxidative stress [57]. Another peptide from *C. vulgaris* (VECYGPNRPQF, 1309 Da) can efficiently quench a variety of free radicals, including hydroxyl, superoxide, peroxyl, 2,2-diphenyl-1-picrylhydrazyl (DPPH), and 2,2'-azino-bis(3-ethylbenzothiazoline-6-sulfonic acid) (ABTS) radicals, and also has significant protective effects on DNA and against cellular damage caused by hydroxyl radicals [58]. So, the intake of certain peptides from *Chlorella* with a tested antioxidant capacity could improve the detrimental oxidative stress potentially induced by particular high-intensity bouts of exercise or periods of exacerbated exercise regimens and training schedules [40].

Most analyses show that the highest proportions of amino acids in marine algae, and specifically in most *Chlorella* species, are glutamic and aspartic acids [6,59]. Besides the organoleptic properties of glutamate (one of the main components of the savory flavor, contributing to the basic umami taste), it also has bioactive activities that are potentially interesting in the context of exercise. Dietary supplementation with glutamic acid increases intramuscular free amino acid (FAA) concentrations and decreases the mRNA levels of genes involved in protein degradation in the skeletal muscle of growing pigs [60]. Moreover, when combined with leucine, it improves the FAA profile and mRNA levels of amino acid transporters in muscle, including neutral amino acid transporter 2 (ASCT2), large neutral amino acid transporter (LAT1), sodium-coupled neutral amino acid transporter 2 (SNAT2), low-affinity intestinal transporter of glycine and imino acids (PAT-1), and high-affinity renal transporter of glycine, proline, and hydroxyproline (PAT2) [61]. Meanwhile, aspartate, the other main amino acid in chlorella, enhances the ability of muscle to utilize free fatty acids during moderate exercise, thereby sparing glycogen and improving the biochemical capacity of the muscle for the oxidation of fatty acids through β-oxidation [62]. Chlorella products also contain high levels of arginine, a pivotal amino acid for the production of NO and the regulation of the immune system [7]. L-arginine supplementation in combination with other components improves tolerance of aerobic and anaerobic physical exercise in untrained and moderately trained subjects [63]. Moreover, supplementation with L-arginine together with physical training seems to be an important stimulus that induces significant improvements in exercise performance and redox status in rats [64].

Numerous papers have provided evidence that *Chlorella*-derived bioactive peptides have notably beneficial effects on human health. This evidence suggests that various amino acids and their metabolites play important roles in the skeletal muscle and have a significant overall ergogenic effect on exercise.

4.2. Benefits of Polysaccharides from Chlorella for Physical Exercise

A key part of the bioactivity of chlorella might be associated with its polysaccharides [65]. Polysaccharides with different structural features from various *Chlorella* species present a variety of biological activities, such as immunomodulatory, antioxidant, hypolipidemic, antitumor, or anti-asthmatic [66].

Research into the bioactivity of polysaccharides extracted from *C. pyrenoidosa* has focused on their effects on immunity and their antioxidant activities [66]. The polysaccharide fractions from *C. pyrenoidosa*, consisting mainly of the D-arabinose, D-glucose, D-xylose, D-galactose, D-mannose, and L-rhamnose moieties, have in vitro antitumor [67] and antioxidant capacity, specifically against superoxide and hydroxyl radicals [66]. α and β-Glucans, polysaccharides present in *C. pyrenoidosa* and *C. sorokiniana* [65], can modulate ROS production, the expression of the ROS-generating enzyme dual oxidase 2 (DUOX-2), and the immune factors TNF-α, IL-1β, and COX-2, thereby contributing to maintaining low levels of oxidative stress and pro-inflammatory molecules [68].

Dietary fiber consists of complex polysaccharides that are poorly or non-digestible by humans. High-fiber diets improve glycemic control, blood lipids, body weight, and inflammation [69]. *C. vulgaris* contains dietary fiber in highly variable proportions, ranging from 5.6% to 26.0% w/w on a dry weight basis [70]. In *Chlorella*-derived products, more than 65% of their carbohydrate content is dietary fiber from the *Chlorella* cell wall [7]. Soluble dietary fiber is mainly composed of resistant or functional oligosaccharides, such as fructo-oligosaccharides (FOS), galacto-oligosaccharides (GOS), and inulin, and viscous dietary fibers with a high molecular weight (glucan, pectins, and gums) [71]. Several studies suggest that both resistant oligosaccharides and viscous dietary fibers can effectively increase the bacterial diversity of the human gut microbiota and the abundance of bifidobacteria, lactobacilli, Prevotellaceae, and *Faecalibaculum* spp. [72]. Recent research has revealed a connection between the profile and diversity of the gut microbiota and the host's physical performance [73]. Fiber intake promotes gut microbial diversity and increases the proportion of species, such as *Faecalibacterium prausnitzii*, *Lactobacillus* spp., *Bifidoacterium* spp., Firmicutes, and Bacteroidetes, that produce SCFAs [74]. SCFAs, including acetate, butyrate, and propionate, exert a wide range of metabolic functions, including anabolic regulation, insulin sensitivity, and modulation of inflammation, when absorbed into systemic circulation [75]. In vitro, *C. pyrenoidosa* increases the abundance of the genera *Prevotella*, *Ruminococcus*, and *Faecalibacterium*, as well as the production of butyrate and propionate [76]. Meanwhile, *C. pyrenoidosa* polysaccharides (CPPs) reduce *Escherichia-Shigella*, *Fusobacterium*, and *Klebsiella* and increase *Parabacteroides*, *Phascolarctobacterium*, and *Bacteroides* [77]. At the phylum level, CPPs increase the abundance of Bacteroidetes, leading to a lower Firmicutes/Bacteroidetes ratio [77], which seems to be closely related to body weight control and to the maintenance of intestinal barrier integrity, as precursors of low-grade inflammation, which are both important aspects affecting exercise performance. Other *Chlorella* species, such as *C. vulgaris* and *C. protothecoides,* increase propionate-producing bacteria in vitro [78]. In rats, a CPP treatment increased the growth of *Coprococcus, Turicibacter,* and *Lactobacillus* and the concentrations of acetate, propionate, and butyrate [10,79]. *C. vulgaris* also modulates *Lactobacillus* spp. metabolism, thereby increasing growth and the production of L-lactic acid while reducing the production of D-lactic acid [79]. Increasing the proportion of *Lactobacillus plantarum* in the gut seems to augment muscle mass, enhance energy harvesting, and have health promotion, performance improvement, and anti-fatigue effects [80].

Other aspects of physical performance can also be directly improved by SCFAs [73]. SCFAs can be used as carbon and energy sources for liver and muscle cells, thus improving endurance performance by maintaining blood glucose levels [81]. SCFAs also appear to regulate neutrophil function and migration, inhibit inflammatory cytokines, and control the redox environment in cells, which may help to enhance muscle renewal and adaptability, improve exercise performance, and delay symptoms of fatigue [81]. However, the efficacy of chlorella supplementation depends on the gut microbiota of the host [82], so future studies should focus on the underlying mechanisms implicated in the crosstalk between *Chlorella* polysaccharides, gut microbiota, and exercise performance in order to maximize the metabolic benefits of polysaccharides from *Chlorella*.

4.3. Benefits of Fatty Acids from Chlorella for Physical Exercise

Chlorella synthesizes high levels of unsaturated fatty acids in response to some environmental factors, such as temperature, pH, light, air composition (mainly nitrogen and phosphorous limitations), salinity, and nutrients [83]. The lipid composition of *C. vulgaris* includes about 23–34% of saturated fatty acids (SFAs), 15–25% of monounsaturated fatty acids (MUFAs), and 42–62% of PUFAs (of which over 30% are ω3 PUFAs) by weight as a percentage of the unfractionated total lipids [84,85]. The major PUFAs in *C. vulgaris* are linoleic acid (LA, C18:2 ω6; over 23%) and alpha-linolenic acid (ALA, C18:3 ω3; over 21%) [84]. LA is considered an essential fatty acid because higher animals, including humans, cannot synthesize it [86]. The proportions of total unsaturated fatty acids and PUFAs in *C. vulgaris* are the highest of the green microalgae [84], and they can be increased under favorable growing conditions. This makes it suitable for industrial and nutritional purposes [87].

Incorporating specific nutrients or dietary supplements to enhance exercise performance and recovery is a common strategy used by recreational practitioners and, particularly, by professional athletes. Moreover, supplementation with unsaturated fatty acids has been shown to have a number of biological effects on health and is related to diseases [88]. Many studies have evaluated the impact of unsaturated fatty acid supplementation, mainly with ω3 PUFAs, on exercise performance, because of their antioxidant effects [89]. As mentioned before, particular conditions of physical exercise, specifically those involving extremely intense exercise, very concentrated training, or periods of competition, as well as exercise sessions with a high predominance or proportion of eccentric contractions, can result in increased oxidative damage to cellular constituents. This is because such exercise increases the production of ROS/RNS in skeletal muscle above a physiological threshold [90]. Under these conditions, instead of being positive triggers of adaptive cellular signaling pathways, high levels of ROS cause functional oxidative damage to proteins, lipids, and other cell components that could exacerbate atrophy, sarcopenia, and myopathy factors in muscle. The persistence of greatly elevated levels of ROS at the local level may also reduce muscle reparation and differentiation of myoblasts and myotubes [91]. However, it has been shown that the MUFAs in chlorella reduce lipid peroxidation and oxidative stress damage [88]. Additionally, ω3 ALA is an antioxidant fatty acid that enhances eNOS activity and inhibits superoxide and peroxynitrite formation, thereby contributing to endothelial protection among other possible activities [92]. The effect of ω3 ALA on endothelial function can also be related to its activity on SIRT3 impairment, which in turn restores the mitochondrial redox balance in endothelial cells [93].

The antioxidant potential and free radical scavenging activity of ω3 ALA can also protect against cellular damage, apoptosis, and inflammation [94,95]. Inflammatory responses have been observed in athletes who engage in long-duration exercise, such as marathons or triathlons [96]. Inflammation is a physiological response to tissue damage that increases the expression of TNF-α, IL-1β, and IL-6 via NFḳB. After muscle injury, NFḳB increases the expression of RING-finger protein-1 (MuRF1), eventually promoting muscle wasting [97,98]. ω3 ALA intake seems to reduce plasma concentrations of IL-6 and other molecules related to inflammatory signaling, such as C-reactive protein, E-selectin, ICAM-1, and soluble vascular cell adhesion molecule 1 (VCAM-1), thereby helping to control the inflammatory response [99]. Several epidemiological studies show that ω6 LA also reduces the inflammatory response, despite its pro-inflammatory effect in vitro [100]. An adequate proportion of these two principal PUFAs (ω6 LA and ω3 ALA) in chlorella seems important to arrive at the desired anti-inflammatory effect, as a high ω6 diet can inhibit the anti-inflammatory and inflammation-resolving effects of the ω3 fatty acids [100].

A reduction of plasma IL-6 by ω3 ALA has also been reported during resistance training in older men [101]. This action may be based on the stimulation of muscle protein synthesis and enhancement of muscle mass via mTOR signaling, as described for ω3 PUFAs [102]. Insulin signaling plays a key role in mTOR activation, so PUFA supplementation might alleviate anabolic resistance [103] and improve the action of insulin, as skeletal muscle is the major site of insulin-stimulated glucose disposal [104]. Interestingly, metabolic benefits in terms of muscle glycemia have been reported for ω6 LA rather than ω3 PUFA [105], and there is an inverse association between the serum proportion ω6 LA and both fasting plasma glucose and post-load glucose [106]. ω3 ALA is also active at the metabolic level, as it increases the activity of carnitine palmitoyl transferase I and FA translocase [107]. The activity of these enzymes increases maximal fat oxidation in mitochondria, thus supporting the assumption that ω3 ALA intake may be used as a nutritional support to increase aerobic performance with substantial reliance on lipid-based metabolism and, at the same time, a glycogen sparing effect [107]. Dietary ω3 ALA and ω6 LA are oxidized much more rapidly than other biologically active fatty acids, such as docosahexaenoic acid (DHA) and arachidonic acid [108]. Specifically, ω3 ALA has been shown to have the highest rate of β-oxidation among the unsaturated fatty acids tested [86], so ω3 ALA could serve better than other fatty acids, as an energy substrate during long-term exercise bouts when carbohydrate reserves are depleted.

The dietary lipid profile determines the tissue phospholipid composition, which modulates not only insulin signaling but also the fluidity and rigidity of the cell membrane [109,110]. The administration of ω3 ALA maintains the integrity of the membrane in red blood cells (RBCs) when exposed to oxidative damage, and reduces lipid peroxidation [95]. The inclusion of ω3 PUFAs in the phospholipids of the RBC membrane increases the loss of deformability induced by exercise, thus improving performance by enhancing oxygen transport to the skeletal muscle [111]. However, most studies of ω3 PUFAs and RBC deformability have used fish oil, which is rich in ALA-derived ω3 PUFAs, mainly eicosapentaenoic acid (EPA) and docosahexaenoic acid (DHA), but not with the major fatty acids found in *Chlorella* (LA and ALA). Additionally, there is some concern about the adequate dosage of ω3 fatty acids, as excessive incorporation into plasma and tissue lipids may increase their susceptibility to lipid peroxidation, which is much more evident in athletes who may undergo high levels of oxidative stress [111]. So, further studies are still needed to provide better knowledge of the effects of fatty acids from *Chlorella* on cell membrane dynamics and the implications in the context of physical exercise.

5. Discussion

Chlorella is a low-fat, rich source of high-quality protein that has been authorized for human consumption by different regulatory agencies, including the European Food Safety

Authority (EFSA). Chlorella also contains other bioactive macronutrients, such as fiber and unsaturated fatty acids. The proportion of each macronutrient stored in chlorella biomass can be maximized by modulating the growing conditions of this microalgae, which makes it an interesting option for the food industry as well as offering an opportunity to improve public health through better nutrition [6]. The intake of chlorella as part of a regular diet or as a supplement for humans and other mammals has been associated with many activities related to the improvement of exercise performance and recovery, such as glycemia and lipid balance and immunomodulation (Figure 1) [112].

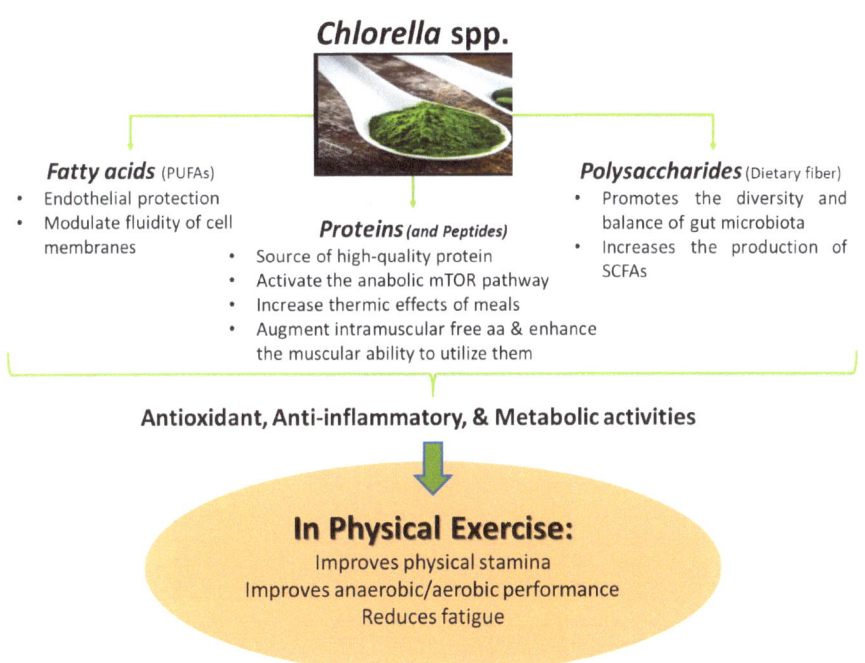

Figure 1. Effects of *Chlorella* and its macronutrients on physical exercise.

In general, chlorella intake improves anaerobic and aerobic exercise performance as well as physical stamina and reduces the onset of fatigue [30,32–34]. One of the primary bases for all these benefits could be the antioxidant capacity of its macronutrients, such as peptides, polysaccharides, and fatty acids. This antioxidant capacity of chlorella also confers it an interesting anti-inflammatory capacity that could be useful in some exercise conditions and regimens [41]. Moreover, the effects of chlorella on endurance seem to be related to its activities at the metabolic level, improving glycemic control via the enhancement of muscle glucose uptake and sparing of glycogen stores, and augmenting blood flow to the muscles by increasing NO production and vasodilatation [34,35,45]. Chlorella is used in humans at doses of a few grams per day and is considered safe at doses of up to 10–15 g per day [16]. Cardiovascular benefits have been shown at a dose of 4 g per day, while a lower dose of 1.5 g per day was ineffective in patients with type-2 diabetes mellitus [113].

Besides the activities (antioxidant, anti-inflammatory, and metabolic) common to all the macronutrients in chlorella, each of them makes different specific contributions that improve exercise performance. The high content of protein in chlorella makes it a good dietary recommendation in physical exercise contexts, as it increases satiety, activation of the anabolic mTOR pathway in skeletal muscle, and the thermic effects of meals [53]. Proteins from *Chlorella* also increase the amount of intramuscular free amino acids and enhance the ability of the muscles to utilize them during moderate exercise, thereby sparing glycogen and improving the biochemical capacity of the muscle for fatty acid oxidation through β-oxidation [60,61]. The carbohydrates from *Chlorella* contribute to the benefits of dietary fiber, which promotes the right balance of gut microbiota and increases its diversity; two factors also related to the exercise performance of the host [73]. This prebiotic effect of chlorella also increases the production of SCFAs, which can be used as carbon and energy sources by liver and muscle cells, thus improving endurance by maintaining blood glucose levels [81]. Finally, lipids from *Chlorella*, mainly ω3 ALA and ω6 LA, can modify tissue phospholipid composition, contributing to the fluidity and rigidity of the cell membranes, which are important aspects of physical performance [111].

This review summarizes the still limited information available on chlorella and physical exercise in humans and other animals. The main strength of this work lies in the conclusion that all the studies reviewed underscore the positive effects of chlorella on physical performance. The main limitation of the review lies in the difficulty of establishing possible mechanisms of action, as chlorella is a complex mixture of bioactive components with different activities. More accurate mechanistic suggestions can be made when looking at individual components. Therefore, an important section of this review examines the role of proteins and peptides, polysaccharides (fiber), and unsaturated fatty acids, the main bioactive components of chlorella, whether or not they have been isolated from this and other microalgae. This is a limitation because it is always difficult to extrapolate such results to the whole mixture. Furthermore, the doses used in the different studies may differ considerably from those in supplements. Moreover, cooperative or opposite effects may be as important as those attributed to the individual components.

Despite the increasing evidence linking chlorella consumption to the improvement of different aspects of physical exercise, there is a lack of consensus about the significance of the different mechanism(s) proposed. The observations made related to the bioactivity of chlorella in the context of physical exercise require verification by new mechanistic studies in animal models. In addition, research is needed on adequate dosages to be administered under different exercise conditions and regimens and to ascertain if a personalized prescription is required. Moreover, as the efficacy of chlorella supplementation on gut microbiota will also depend on the previous status of the host, which is in turn modulated by his or her engagement in physical exercise, new studies should address these complex interrelationships. As microalgae, particularly chlorella, are rich sources of high-quality proteins and peptides, they are good candidates for functional components in sports nutrition, while it is also being demonstrated that other components in chlorella contribute to sports performance. In particular, the cell wall is a source of prebiotic polysaccharides. Prebiotics help to maintain a balanced intestinal microbiota and are important actors in the prevention of non-communicable diseases such as diabetes. Recently, beneficial effects of exercise on the gut microbiota have been revealed [114], and still more recent studies are exploring the inverse relationship: the influence of the gut microbiota on exercise performance via the action of gut fermentation-derived short-chain fatty acids and the stimulation of various pathways of lactate metabolism (same reference). Polysaccharides in chlorella preparations are released from the cell wall by enzymatic treatments. To maximize the prebiotic potential of chlorella-derived products, future efforts should be devoted to the optimization of hydrolysis conditions.

The evidence available to date shows that chlorella, as well as spirulina and maybe other microalga, can effectively be used as supplements or even meal replacements to improve sports performance or simply to maximize the benefits of moderate exercise in the normal population. Microalgae may be one of the foodstuffs of the future, since they are a source of high-quality protein and many other bioactive components, and they may also significantly contribute to a sustainable world through their contribution to the fixation of carbon dioxide and a reduction in the amount of land used for the production of animal feed.

6. Conclusions

Chlorella improves anaerobic and aerobic exercise performance, physical stamina, and reduces the onset of fatigue. These benefits could be attributed to the antioxidant, anti-inflammatory, and metabolic activities common to its macronutrients (peptides, polysaccharides, and fatty acids). Moreover, each macronutrient brings to Chlorella some particular functions that could be related to the improvement of physical exercise and performance.

Proteins from *Chlorella* increase the amount of intramuscular free amino acids and enhance the ability of the muscles to utilize them, thereby sparing glycogen and improving the biochemical capacity for fatty acid β-oxidation. Some carbohydrates derived from *Chlorella* cell walls, help to maintain a balanced gut microbiota and increase its diversity. This prebiotic effect of chlorella results in an increased production of SCFAs, which can be used as carbon and energy sources. Thus, carbohydrate-derived SCFAs improve endurance by maintaining blood glucose levels. Finally, lipids such as ω3 ALA and ω6 LA can contribute to physical performance by favorably modifying the fluidity and rigidity of the cell membranes.

Author Contributions: Writing—original draft preparation, K.L. and G.S.; writing—review and editing, S.R.-R., J.M. and J.R.T.; supervision, T.P., G.V. and J.L.T.; funding acquisition, S.R.-R., G.V. and J.L.T. All authors have read and agreed to the published version of the manuscript.

Funding: This work was supported by the Spanish Ministry of Science and Innovation (grant number PID2020-117009RB-I00).

Data Availability Statement: Not applicable.

Conflicts of Interest: The authors declare no conflict of interest.

References

1. Koyande, A.K.; Chew, K.W.; Rambabu, K.; Tao, Y.; Dinh-Toi, C.; Show, P.-L. Microalgae: A potential alternative to health supplementation for humans. *Food Sci. Hum. Wellness* **2019**, *8*, 16–24. [CrossRef]
2. de Jesus Raposo, M.F.; Miranda Bernardo de Morais, A.M.; Santos Costa de Morais, R.M. Emergent sources of prebiotics: Seaweeds and microalgae. *Mar. Drugs* **2016**, *14*, 27. [CrossRef] [PubMed]
3. Udayan, A.; Arumugam, M.; Pandey, A. Nutraceuticals from algae and cyanobacteria. In *Algal Green Chemistry: Recent Progress in Biotechnology*; Rastogi, R.P., Madamwar, D., Pandey, A., Eds.; Elsevier: Amsterdam, The Netherlands, 2017; pp. 65–89. [CrossRef]
4. Ramos-Romero, S.; Torrella, J.R.; Pages, T.; Viscor, G.; Torres, J.L. Edible Microalgae and Their Bioactive Compounds in the Prevention and Treatment of Metabolic Alterations. *Nutrients* **2021**, *13*, 563. [CrossRef] [PubMed]
5. Wu, H.L.; Hseu, R.S.; Lin, L.P. Identification of Chlorella spp. isolates using ribosomal DNA sequences. *Bot. Bull. Acad. Sin.* **2001**, *42*, 115–121.
6. Richmond, A.; Hu, Q. *Handbook of Microalgal Culture: Applied Phycology and Biotechnology*; John Wiley & Sons: Hoboken, NJ, USA, 2013.
7. Bito, T.; Okumura, E.; Fujishima, M.; Watanabe, F. Potential of *Chlorella* as a dietary supplement to promote human health. *Nutrients* **2020**, *12*, 2524. [CrossRef]
8. Schulze, C.; Wetzel, M.; Reinhardt, J.; Schmidt, M.; Felten, L.; Mundt, S. Screening of microalgae for primary metabolites including β-glucans and the influence of nitrate starvation and irradiance on β-glucan production. *J. Appl. Phycol.* **2016**, *28*, 2719–2725. [CrossRef]
9. Pieper, S.; Unterieser, I.; Mann, F.; Mischnick, P. A new arabinomannan from the cell wall of the chlorococcal algae *Chlorella vulgaris*. *Carbohydr. Res.* **2012**, *352*, 166–176. [CrossRef]
10. Wan, X.-z.; Ai, C.; Chen, Y.-h.; Gao, X.-x.; Zhong, R.-t.; Liu, B.; Chen, X.-h.; Zhao, C. Physicochemical characterization of a polysaccharide from green microalga *Chlorella pyrenoidosa* and its hypolipidemic activity via gut microbiota regulation in rats. *J. Agric. Food Chem.* **2020**, *68*, 1186–1197. [CrossRef]
11. Becker, E.W. Microalgae for human and animal nutrition. In *Handbook of Microalgal Culture*; Richmon, A., Ed.; John Wiley & Sons: Oxford, UK, 2013; pp. 461–503. [CrossRef]
12. Fernando, I.P.S.; Ryu, B.; Ahn, G.; Yeo, I.-K.; Jeon, Y.-J. Therapeutic potential of algal natural products against metabolic syndrome: A review of recent developments. *Trends Food Sci. Technol.* **2020**, *97*, 286–299. [CrossRef]
13. Suetsuna, K.; Chen, J.-R. Identification of antihypertensive peptides from peptic digest of two microalgae, *Chlorella vulgaris* and *Spirulina platensis*. *Mar. Biotechnol.* **2001**, *3*, 305–309. [CrossRef]
14. Tiberg, E.; Dreborg, S.; Bjorksten, B. Allergy to green-algae (*Chlorella*) among children. *J. Allergy Clin. Immunol.* **1995**, *96*, 257–259. [CrossRef]

15. Fallah, A.A.; Sarmast, E.; Habibian Dehkordi, S.; Engardeh, J.; Mahmoodnia, L.; Khaledifar, A.; Jafari, T. Effect of *Chlorella* supplementation on cardiovascular risk factors: A meta-analysis of randomized controlled trials. *Clin. Nutr.* **2018**, *37*, 1892–1901. [CrossRef]
16. Ferreira de Oliveira, A.P.; Arisseto Bragotto, A.P. Microalgae-based products: Food and public health. *Future Foods* **2022**, *6*, 100157. [CrossRef]
17. Woortman, D.V.; Fuchs, T.; Striegel, L.; Fuchs, M.; Weber, N.; Brück, T.B.; Rychlik, M. Microalgae a auperior source of folates: Quantification of folates in halophile microalgae by stable isotope dilution assay. *Front. Bioeng. Biotechnol.* **2020**, *7*, 481. [CrossRef]
18. Liu, J.; Sun, Z.; Gerken, H.; Liu, Z.; Jiang, Y.; Chen, F. *Chlorella zofingiensis* as an alternative microalgal producer of astaxanthin: Biology and industrial potential. *Mar. Drugs* **2014**, *12*, 3487–3515. [CrossRef]
19. Gómez-Zavaglia, A.; Prieto Lage, M.A.; Jiménez-Lopez, C.; Mejuto, J.C.; Simal-Gandara, J. The potential of seaweeds as a source of functional ingredients of prebiotic and antioxidant value. *Antioxidants* **2019**, *8*, 406. [CrossRef]
20. Bouviere, J.; Fortunato, R.S.; Dupuy, C.; Werneck-de-Castro, J.P.; Carvalho, D.P.; Louzada, R.A. Exercise-Stimulated ROS Sensitive Signaling Pathways in Skeletal Muscle. *Antioxidants* **2021**, *10*, 537. [CrossRef]
21. Zunner, B.E.M.; Wachsmuth, N.B.; Eckstein, M.L.; Scherl, L.; Schierbauer, J.R.; Haupt, S.; Stumpf, C.; Reusch, L.; Moser, O. Myokines and Resistance Training: A Narrative Review. *Int. J. Mol. Sci.* **2022**, *23*, 3501. [CrossRef]
22. Louzada, R.A.; Bouviere, J.; Matta, L.P.; Werneck-de-Castro, J.P.; Dupuy, C.; Carvalho, D.P.; Fortunato, R.S. Redox Signaling in Widespread Health Benefits of Exercise. *Antioxid. Redox Signal.* **2020**, *33*, 745–760. [CrossRef]
23. Petersen, A.M.; Pedersen, B.K. The anti-inflammatory effect of exercise. *J. Appl. Physiol.* **2005**, *98*, 1154–1162. [CrossRef]
24. Fiuza-Luces, C.; Garatachea, N.; Berger, N.A.; Lucia, A. Exercise is the Real Polypill. *Physiology* **2013**, *28*, 330–358. [CrossRef] [PubMed]
25. Bilski, J.; Pierzchalski, P.; Szczepanik, M.; Bonior, J.; Zoladz, J.A. Multifactorial Mechanism of Sarcopenia and Sarcopenic Obesity. Role of Physical Exercise, Microbiota and Myokines. *Cells* **2022**, *11*, 160. [CrossRef] [PubMed]
26. Pedersen, B.K.; Saltin, B. Exercise as medicine—Evidence for prescribing exercise as therapy in 26 different chronic diseases. *Scand. J. Med. Sci. Sport.* **2015**, *25*, 1–72. [CrossRef] [PubMed]
27. Atakan, M.M.; Kosar, S.N.; Guzel, Y.; Tin, H.T.; Yan, X. The Role of Exercise, Diet, and Cytokines in Preventing Obesity and Improving Adipose Tissue. *Nutrients* **2021**, *13*, 1459. [CrossRef] [PubMed]
28. Deslandes, A.; Moraes, H.; Ferreira, C.; Veiga, H.; Silveira, H.; Mouta, R.; Pompeu, F.; Coutinho, E.S.; Laks, J. Exercise and Mental Health: Many Reasons to Move. *Neuropsychobiology* **2009**, *59*, 191–198. [CrossRef] [PubMed]
29. Ruegsegger, G.N.; Booth, F.W. Health Benefits of Exercise. *Cold Spring Harb. Perspect. Med.* **2018**, *8*, a029694. [CrossRef]
30. An, H.J.; Choi, H.M.; Park, H.S.; Han, J.G.; Lee, E.H.; Park, Y.S.; Um, J.Y.; Hong, S.H.; Kim, H.M. Oral administration of hot water extracts of *Chlorella vulgaris* increases physical stamina in mice. *Ann. Nutr. Metab.* **2006**, *50*, 380–386. [CrossRef]
31. Kim, N.H.; Kim, K.Y.; Jeong, H.J.; Kim, H.M.; Hong, S.H.; Um, J.Y. Effects of hydrolyzed *Chlorella vulgaris* by malted barley on the immunomodulatory response in ICR mice and in Molt-4 cells. *J. Sci. Food Agric.* **2010**, *90*, 1551–1556. [CrossRef]
32. Mizoguchi, T.; Arakawa, Y.; Kobayashi, M.; Fujishima, M. Influence of *Chlorella* powder intake during swimming stress in mice. *Biochem. Biophys. Res. Commun.* **2011**, *404*, 121–126. [CrossRef]
33. Umemoto, S.; Otsuki, T. Chlorelladerived multicomponent supplementation increases aerobic endurance capacity in young individuals. *J. Clin. Biochem. Nutr.* **2014**, *55*, 143–146. [CrossRef]
34. Horii, N.; Hasegawa, N.; Fujie, S.; Uchida, M.; Miyamoto-Mikami, E.; Hashimoto, T.; Tabata, I.; Iemitsu, M. High-intensity intermittent exercise training with chlorella intake accelerates exercise performance and muscle glycolytic and oxidative capacity in rats. *Am. J. Physiol. Regul. Integr. Comp. Physiol.* **2017**, *312*, R520–R528. [CrossRef]
35. Horii, N.; Hasegawa, N.; Fujie, S.; Uchida, M.; Iemitsu, K.; Inoue, K.; Iemitsu, M. Effect of combination of chlorella intake and aerobic exercise training on glycemic control in type 2 diabetic rats. *Nutrition* **2019**, *63–64*, 45–50. [CrossRef]
36. Samadi, M.; Shirvani, H.; Shafeie, A.A. Effect of *Chlorella vulgaris* supplementation with eccentric exercise on serum interleukin 6 and insulin resistance in overweight men. *Sport Sci. Health* **2020**, *16*, 543–549. [CrossRef]
37. Vijayavel, K.; Anbuselvam, C.; Balasubramanian, M.P. Antioxidant effect of the marine algae *Chlorella vulgaris* against naphthalene-induced oxidative stress in the albino rats. *Mol. Cell. Biochem.* **2007**, *303*, 39–44. [CrossRef]
38. Lee, S.H.; Kang, H.J.; Lee, H.J.; Kang, M.H.; Park, Y.K. Six-week supplementation with *Chlorella* has favorable impact on antioxidant status in Korean male smokers. *Nutrition* **2010**, *26*, 175–183. [CrossRef]
39. Zhu, X.; Chen, Y.; Chen, Q.; Yang, H.; Xie, X. Astaxanthin promotes Nrf2/ARE signaling to alleviate renal fibronectin and collagen IV accumulation in diabetic rats. *J. Diabetes Res.* **2018**, *2018*, 6730315. [CrossRef]
40. Merry, T.L.; Ristow, M. Do antioxidant supplements interfere with skeletal muscle adaptation to exercise training? *J. Physiol.* **2016**, *594*, 5135–5147. [CrossRef]
41. Sibi, G.; Rabina, S. Inhibition of Pro-inflammatory Mediators and Cytokines by *Chlorella Vulgaris* Extracts. *Pharmacogn. Res.* **2016**, *8*, 118–122. [CrossRef]
42. Sun, C.; Zhang, F.; Ge, X.; Yan, T.; Chen, X.; Shi, X.; Zhai, Q. SIRT1 improves insulin sensitivity under insulin-resistant conditions by repressing PTP1B. *Cell Metab.* **2007**, *6*, 307–319. [CrossRef]
43. Tran, L.T.; Yuen, V.G.; McNeill, J.H. The fructose-fed rat: A review on the mechanisms of fructose-induced insulin resistance and hypertension. *Moll. Cell. Biochem.* **2009**, *332*, 145–159. [CrossRef]

44. Thijssen, D.H.J.; Black, M.A.; Pyke, K.E.; Padilla, J.; Atkinson, G.; Harris, R.A.; Parker, B.; Widlansky, M.E.; Tschakovsky, M.E.; Green, D.J. Assessment of flow-mediated dilation in humans: A methodological and physiological guideline. *Am. J. Physiol. Heart Circ. Physiol.* **2011**, *300*, H2–H12. [CrossRef] [PubMed]
45. Otsuki, T.; Shimizu, K.; Maeda, S. Changes in arterial stiffness and nitric oxide production with Chlorelladerived multicomponent supplementation in middleaged and older individuals. *Clin. Biochem. Nutr.* **2015**, *57*, 228–232. [CrossRef] [PubMed]
46. Ichimura, M.; Kato, S.; Tsuneyama, K.; Matsutake, S.; Kamogawa, M.; Hirao, E.; Miyata, A.; Mori, S.; Yamaguchi, N.; Suruga, K.; et al. Phycocyanin prevents hypertension and low serum adiponectin level in a rat model of metabolic syndrome. *Nutr. Res.* **2013**, *33*, 397–405. [CrossRef] [PubMed]
47. Meirelles, C.M.; Matsuura, C.; Silva, R.S., Jr.; Guimarães, F.F.; Gomes, P.S.C. Acute Effects of L-Arginine Supplementation on Oxygen Consumption Kinetics and Muscle Oxyhemoglobin and Deoxyhemoglobin during Treadmill Running in Male Adults. *Int. J. Exerc. Sci.* **2019**, *12*, 444–455. [PubMed]
48. Otsuki, T.; Shimizu, K.; Zempo-Miyaki, A.; Maeda, S. Changes in salivary flow rate following Chlorella derived multicomponent supplementation. *J. Clin. Biochem. Nutr.* **2016**, *59*, 45–48. [CrossRef]
49. Becker, E.W. Micro-algae as a source of protein. *Biotechnol. Adv.* **2007**, *25*, 207–210. [CrossRef]
50. Barkia, I.; Saari, N.; Manning, S.R. Microalgae for high-value products towards human health and nutrition. *Mar. Drugs* **2019**, *17*, 304. [CrossRef]
51. Molino, A.; Iovine, A.; Casella, P.; Mehariya, S.; Chianese, S.; Cerbone, A.; Rimauro, J.; Musmarra, D. Microalgae Characterization for Consolidated and New Application in Human Food, Animal Feed and Nutraceuticals. *Int. J. Environ. Res. Public Health* **2018**, *15*, 2436. [CrossRef]
52. Waghmare, A.G.; Salve, M.K.; LeBlanc, J.G.; Arya, S.S. Concentration and characterization of microalgae proteins from Chlorella pyrenoidosa. *Bioresour. Bioprocess.* **2016**, *3*, 16. [CrossRef]
53. Morales, F.E.; Tinsley, G.M.; Gordon, P.M. Acute and Long-Term Impact of High-Protein Diets on Endocrine and Metabolic Function, Body Composition, and Exercise-Induced Adaptations. *J. Am. Coll. Nutr.* **2017**, *36*, 295–305. [CrossRef]
54. Lynch, H.; Johnston, C.; Wharton, C. Plant-Based Diets: Considerations for Environmental Impact, Protein Quality, and Exercise Performance. *Nutrients* **2018**, *10*, 1841. [CrossRef]
55. Li, Y.W.; Li, B. Characterization of structure-antioxidant activity relationship of peptides in free radical systems using QSAR models: Key sequence positions and their amino acid properties. *J. Theor. Biol.* **2013**, *318*, 29–43. [CrossRef]
56. Ngo, D.H.; Vo, T.S.; Ngo, D.N.; Wijesekara, I.; Kim, S.K. Biological activities and potential health benefits of bioactive peptides derived from marine organisms. *Int. J. Biol. Macromol.* **2012**, *51*, 378–383. [CrossRef]
57. Ko, S.C.; Kim, D.; Jeon, Y.J. Protective effect of a novel antioxidative peptide purified from a marine Chlorella ellipsoidea protein against free radical-induced oxidative stress. *Food Chem. Toxicol.* **2012**, *50*, 2294–2302. [CrossRef]
58. Sheih, I.C.; Wu, T.-K.; Fang, T.J. Antioxidant properties of a new antioxidative peptide from algae protein waste hydrolysate in different oxidation systems. *Bioresour. Technol.* **2009**, *100*, 3419–3425. [CrossRef]
59. Wells, M.L.; Potin, P.; Craigie, J.S.; Raven, J.A.; Merchant, S.S.; Helliwell, K.E.; Smith, A.G.; Camire, M.E.; Brawley, S.H. Algae as nutritional and functional food sources: Revisiting our understanding. *J. Appl. Phycol.* **2017**, *29*, 949–982. [CrossRef]
60. Hu, C.J.; Li, F.N.; Duan, Y.H.; Zhang, T.; Li, H.W.; Yin, Y.L.; Wu, G.Y.; Kong, X.F. Dietary supplementation with arginine and glutamic acid alters the expression of amino acid transporters in skeletal muscle of growing pigs. *Amino Acids* **2019**, *51*, 1081–1092. [CrossRef]
61. Hu, C.; Li, F.; Duan, Y.; Kong, X.; Yan, Y.; Deng, J.; Tan, C.; Wu, G.; Yin, Y. Leucine alone or in combination with glutamic acid, but not with arginine, increases biceps femoris muscle and alters muscle AA transport and concentrations in fattening pigs. *J. Anim. Physiol. Anim. Nutr.* **2019**, *103*, 791–800. [CrossRef]
62. Lancha, A.H.J.; Recco, M.B.; Abdallat, D.S.P.; Curi, R. Effect of Aspartate, Asparagine, and Carnitine Supplementation in the Diet on Metabolism of Skeletal Muscle During a Moderate Exercise. *Physiol. Behav.* **1995**, *57*, 367–371. [CrossRef]
63. Sureda, A.; Pons, A. Arginine and Citrulline Supplementation in Sports and Exercise: Ergogenic Nutrients? *Med. Sport. Sci.* **2013**, *59*, 18–28.
64. Silva, E.P., Jr.; Borges, L.S.; Mendes-da-Silva, C.; Hirabara, S.M.; Lambertucci, R.H. L-arginine supplementation improves rats' antioxidant system and exercise performance. *Free Radic. Res.* **2017**, *51*, 281–293. [CrossRef] [PubMed]
65. Yuan, Q.; Li, H.; Wei, Z.; Lv, K.; Gao, C.; Liu, Y.; Zhao, L. Isolation, structures and biological activities of polysaccharides from Chlorella: A review. *Int. J. Biol. Macromol.* **2020**, *163*, 2199–2209. [CrossRef] [PubMed]
66. Chen, Y.X.; Liu, X.Y.; Xiao, Z.; Huang, Y.F.; Liu, B. Antioxidant activities of polysaccharides obtained from Chlorella pyrenoidosa via different ethanol concentrations. *Int. J. Biol. Macromol.* **2016**, *91*, 505–509. [CrossRef] [PubMed]
67. Sheng, J.; Yu, F.; Xin, Z.; Zhao, L.; Zhu, X.; Hu, Q. Preparation, identification and their antitumor activities in vitro of polysaccharides from Chlorella pyrenoidosa. *Food Chem.* **2007**, *105*, 533–539. [CrossRef]
68. De Felice, B.; Damiano, S.; Montanino, C.; Del Buono, A.; La Rosa, G.; Guida, B.; Santillo, M. Effect of beta- and alpha-glucans on immune modulating factors expression in enterocyte-like Caco-2 and goblet-like LS 174T cells. *Int. J. Biol. Macromol.* **2020**, *153*, 600–607. [CrossRef]
69. Reynolds, A.N.; Akerman, A.P.; Mann, J. Dietary fibre and whole grains in diabetes management: Systematic review and meta-analyses. *PLoS Med.* **2020**, *17*, e1003053. [CrossRef]

70. Matos, A.P.; Feller, R.; Moecke, E.H.S.; de Oliveira, J.V.; Furigo, A.; Derner, R.B.; Sant'Anna, E.S. Chemical Characterization of Six Microalgae with Potential Utility for Food Application. *J. Am. Oil Chem. Soc.* **2016**, *93*, 963–972. [CrossRef]
71. Guan, Z.W.; Yu, E.Z.; Feng, Q. Soluble Dietary Fiber, One of the Most Important Nutrients for the Gut Microbiota. *Molecules* **2021**, *26*, 6802. [CrossRef]
72. Mao, G.; Li, S.; Orfila, C.; Shen, X.; Zhou, S.; Linhardt, R.J.; Ye, X.; Chen, S. Depolymerized RG-I-enriched pectin from citrus segment membranes modulates gut microbiota, increases SCFA production, and promotes the growth of *Bifidobacterium* spp., *Lactobacillus* spp. and *Faecalibaculum* spp. *Food Funct.* **2019**, *10*, 7828–7843. [CrossRef]
73. Marttinen, M.; Ala-Jaakkola, R.; Laitila, A.; Lehtinen, M.J. Gut Microbiota, Probiotics and Physical Performance in Athletes and Physically Active Individuals. *Nutrients* **2020**, *12*, 2936. [CrossRef]
74. Simpson, H.L.; Campbell, B.J. Review article: Dietary fibre-microbiota interactions. *Aliment. Pharm. Ther.* **2015**, *42*, 158–179. [CrossRef]
75. Blaak, E.E.; Canfora, E.E.; Theis, S.; Frost, G.; Groen, A.K.; Mithieux, G.; Nauta, A.; Scott, K.; Stahl, B.; van Harsselaar, J.; et al. Short chain fatty acids in human gut and metabolic health. *Benef. Microbes* **2020**, *11*, 411–455. [CrossRef]
76. van der Linde, C.; Barone, M.; Turroni, S.; Brigidi, P.; Keleszade, E.; Swann, J.R.; Costabile, A. An In Vitro Pilot Fermentation Study on the Impact of Chlorella pyrenoidosa on Gut Microbiome Composition and Metabolites in Healthy and Coeliac Subjects. *Molecules* **2021**, *26*, 2330. [CrossRef]
77. Lv, K.L.; Yuan, Q.X.; Li, H.; Li, T.T.; Ma, H.Q.; Gao, C.H.; Zhang, S.Y.; Liu, Y.H.; Zhao, L.Y. Chlorella pyrenoidosa Polysaccharides as a Prebiotic to Modulate Gut Microbiota: Physicochemical Properties and Fermentation Characteristics In Vitro. *Foods* **2022**, *11*, 725. [CrossRef]
78. Jin, J.B.; Cha, J.W.; Shin, I.S.; Jeon, J.Y.; Cha, K.H.; Pan, C.H. Supplementation with Chlorella vulgaris, Chlorella protothecoides, and Schizochytrium sp. increases propionate-producing bacteria in in vitro human gut fermentation. *J. Sci. Food Agric.* **2020**, *100*, 2938–2945. [CrossRef]
79. Ścieszka, S.; Klewicka, E. Influence of the Microalga Chlorella vulgaris on the Growth and Metabolic Activity of Lactobacillus spp. Bacteria. *Foods* **2020**, *9*, 959. [CrossRef]
80. Chen, Y.M.; Wei, L.; Chiu, Y.S.; Hsu, Y.J.; Tsai, T.Y.; Wang, M.F.; Huang, C.C. Lactobacillus plantarum TWK10 Supplementation Improves Exercise Performance and Increases Muscle Mass in Mice. *Nutrients* **2016**, *8*, 205. [CrossRef]
81. Mach, N.; Fuster-Botella, D. Endurance exercise and gut microbiota: A review. *J. Sport Health Sci.* **2017**, *6*, 179–197. [CrossRef]
82. Nishimoto, Y.; Nomaguchi, T.; Mori, Y.; Ito, M.; Nakamura, Y.; Fujishima, M.; Murakami, S.; Yamada, T.; Fukuda, S. The Nutritional Efficacy of Chlorella Supplementation Depends on the Individual Gut Environment: A Randomised Control Study. *Front. Nutr.* **2021**, *8*, 648073. [CrossRef]
83. Batista, A.P.; Gouveia, L.; Bandarra, N.M.; Franco, J.M.; Raymundo, A. Comparison of microalgal biomass profiles as novel functional ingredient for food products. *Algal Res.* **2013**, *2*, 164–173. [CrossRef]
84. Yao, L.; Gerde, J.A.; Lee, S.L.; Wang, T.; Harrata, K.A. Microalgae lipid characterization. *J. Agric. Food Chem.* **2015**, *63*, 1773–1787. [CrossRef] [PubMed]
85. Santos-Sanchez, N.F.; Valadez-Blanco, R.; Hernandez-Carlos, B.; Torres-Arino, A.; Guadarrama-Mendoza, P.C.; Salas-Coronado, R. Lipids rich in ω-3 polyunsaturated fatty acids from microalgae. *Appl. Microbiol. Biotechnol.* **2016**, *100*, 8667–8684. [CrossRef] [PubMed]
86. Baker, E.J.; Miles, E.A.; Burdge, G.C.; Yaqoob, P.; Calder, P.C. Metabolism and functional effects of plant-derived omega-3 fatty acids in humans. *Prog. Lipid Res.* **2016**, *64*, 30–56. [CrossRef] [PubMed]
87. Chen, W.; Sommerfeld, M.; Hu, Q.A. Microwave-assisted Nile red method for in vivo quantification of neutral lipids in microalgae. *Bioresour. Technol.* **2011**, *102*, 135–141. [CrossRef] [PubMed]
88. Lunn, J.; Theobald, H.E. The health effects of dietary unsaturated fatty acids. *Nutr. Bull.* **2006**, *31*, 178–224. [CrossRef]
89. Gammone, M.A.; Riccioni, G.; Parrinello, G.; D'Orazio, N. Omega-3 Polyunsaturated Fatty Acids: Benefits and Endpoints in Sport. *Nutrients* **2018**, *11*, 46. [CrossRef]
90. Pingitore, A.; Lima, G.P.P.; Mastorci, F.; Quinones, A.; Iervasi, G.; Vassalle, C. Exercise and oxidative stress: Potential effects of antioxidant dietary strategies in sports. *Nutrition* **2015**, *31*, 916–922. [CrossRef]
91. Barbieri, E.; Sestili, P. Reactive oxygen species in skeletal muscle signaling. *J. Signal. Transduct.* **2012**, *2012*, 982794. [CrossRef]
92. Zhang, W.; Fu, F.; Tie, R.; Liang, X.Y.; Tian, F.; Xing, W.J.; Li, J.; le Ji, L.; Xing, J.L.; Sun, X.; et al. Alpha-linolenic acid intake prevents endothelial dysfunction in high-fat diet-fed streptozotocin rats and underlying mechanisms. *Vasa Eur. J. Vasc. Med.* **2013**, *42*, 421–428. [CrossRef]
93. Li, G.; Wang, X.; Yang, H.; Zhang, P.; Wu, F.; Li, Y.; Zhou, Y.; Zhang, X.; Ma, H.; Zhang, W.; et al. α-Linolenic acid but not linolenic acid protects against hypertension: Critical role of SIRT3 and autophagic flux. *Cell Death Dis.* **2020**, *11*, 83. [CrossRef]
94. Simopoulos, A.P. Omega-3 fatty acids and antioxidants in edible wild plants. *Biol. Res.* **2004**, *37*, 263–277. [CrossRef]
95. Pal, M.; Ghosh, M. Prophylactic effect of alpha-linolenic acid and alpha-eleostearic acid against MeHg induced oxidative stress, DNA damage and structural changes in RBC membrane. *Food Chem. Toxicol.* **2012**, *50*, 2811–2818. [CrossRef]
96. Fisher-Wellman, K.; Bloomer, R.J. Acute exercise and oxidative stress: A 30 year history. *Dyn. Med.* **2009**, *8*, 1. [CrossRef]
97. Cai, D.; Frantz, J.D.; Tawa, N.E., Jr.; Melendez, P.A.; Oh, B.C.; Lidov, H.G.; Hasselgren, P.O.; Frontera, W.R.; Lee, J.; Glass, D.J.; et al. IKKbeta/NF-kappaB activation causes severe muscle wasting in mice. *Cell* **2004**, *119*, 285–298. [CrossRef]

98. Wang, Y.; Lin, Q.W.; Zheng, P.P.; Zhang, J.S.; Huang, F.R. DHA inhibits protein degradation more efficiently than EPA by regulating the PPARγ/NFκB pathway in C2C12 myotubes. *BioMed Res. Int.* **2013**, *2013*, 318981. [CrossRef]
99. Stark, A.H.; Crawford, M.A.; Reifen, R. Update on alpha-linolenic acid. *Nutr. Rev.* **2008**, *66*, 326–332. [CrossRef]
100. Innes, J.K.; Calder, P.C. Omega-6 fatty acids and inflammation. *Prostaglandins Leukot. Essent. Fat. Acids* **2018**, *132*, 41–48. [CrossRef]
101. Cornish, S.M.; Chilibeck, P.D. Alpha-linolenic acid supplementation and resistance training in older adults. *Appl. Physiol. Nutr. Metab.* **2009**, *34*, 49–59. [CrossRef]
102. Robinson, S.M.; Reginster, J.Y.; Rizzoli, R.; Shaw, S.C.; Kanis, J.A.; Bautmans, I.; Bischoff-Ferrari, H.; Bruyere, O.; Cesari, M.; Dawson-Hughes, B.; et al. Does nutrition play a role in the prevention and management of sarcopenia? *Clin. Nutr.* **2018**, *37*, 1121–1132. [CrossRef]
103. Dupont, J.; Dedeyne, L.; Dalle, S.; Koppo, K.; Gielen, E. The role of omega-3 in the prevention and treatment of sarcopenia. *Aging Clin. Exp. Res.* **2019**, *31*, 825–836. [CrossRef]
104. Storlien, L.H.; Pan, D.A.; Kriketos, A.D.; O'Connor, J.; Caterson, I.D.; Cooney, G.J.; Jenkins, A.B.; Baur, L.A. Skeletal Muscle Membrane Lipids and Insulin Resistance. *Lipids* **1996**, *31*, S261–S265. [CrossRef] [PubMed]
105. Imamura, F.; Micha, R.; Wu, J.H.; de Oliveira Otto, M.C.; Otite, F.O.; Abioye, A.I.; Mozaffarian, D. Effects of Saturated Fat, Polyunsaturated Fat, Monounsaturated Fat, and Carbohydrate on Glucose-Insulin Homeostasis: A Systematic Review and Meta-analysis of Randomised Controlled Feeding Trials. *PLoS Med.* **2016**, *13*, e1002087. [CrossRef] [PubMed]
106. Cabout, M.; Alssema, M.; Nijpels, G.; Stehouwer, C.D.A.; Zock, P.L.; Brouwer, I.A.; Elshorbagy, A.K.; Refsum, H.; Dekker, J.M. Circulating linoleic acid and alpha-linolenic acid and glucose metabolism: The Hoorn Study. *Eur. J. Nutr.* **2017**, *56*, 2171–2180. [CrossRef] [PubMed]
107. Lyudinina, A.Y.; Bushmanova, E.A.; Varlamova, N.G.; Bojko, E.R. Dietary and plasma blood alpha-linolenic acid as modulators of fat oxidation and predictors of aerobic performance. *J. Int. Soc. Sport. Nutr.* **2020**, *17*, 57. [CrossRef] [PubMed]
108. Kinsella, J.E. Alpha-linolenic acid: Functions and effects on linoleic acid metabolism and eicosanoid-mediated reactions. *Adv. Food Nutr. Res.* **1991**, *35*, 1–184. [CrossRef]
109. Pan, D.A.; Storlien, L.H. Dietary lipid profile is a determinant of tissue phospholipid fatty acid composition and rate of weight gain in rats. *J. Nutr.* **1993**, *123*, 512–519. [CrossRef]
110. Borkman, M.; Storlien, L.H.; Pan, D.A.; Jenkins, A.B.; Chisholm, D.J.; Campbell, L.V. The relation between insulin sensitivity and the fatty-acid composition of skeletal-muscle phospholipids. *N. Engl. J. Med.* **1993**, *328*, 238–244. [CrossRef]
111. Mickleborough, T.D. Omega-3 Polyunsaturated Fatty Acids in Physical Performance Optimization. *Int. J. Sport Nutr. Exerc. Metab.* **2013**, *23*, 83–96. [CrossRef]
112. Gurney, T.; Spendiff, O. Algae Supplementation for Exercise Performance: Current Perspectives and Future Directions for Spirulina and Chlorella. *Front. Nutr.* **2022**, *9*, 865741. [CrossRef]
113. Hosseini, A.M.; Keshavarz, S.A.; Nasli-Esfahani, E.; Amiri, F.; Janani, L. The effects of Chlorella supplementation on glycemic control, lipid profile and anthropometric measures on patients with type 2 diabetes mellitus. *Eur. J. Nutr.* **2021**, *60*, 3131–3141. [CrossRef]
114. Sales, K.M.; Reimer, R.A. Unlocking a novel determinant of athletic performance: The role of the gut microbiota, short-chain fatty acids, and "biotics" in exercise. *J. Sport Health Sci.* **2023**, *12*, 36–44. [CrossRef]

Disclaimer/Publisher's Note: The statements, opinions and data contained in all publications are solely those of the individual author(s) and contributor(s) and not of MDPI and/or the editor(s). MDPI and/or the editor(s) disclaim responsibility for any injury to people or property resulting from any ideas, methods, instructions or products referred to in the content.

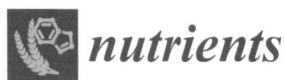

Review

Insights into the Chemical Compositions and Health Promoting Effects of Wild Edible Mushroom *Chroogomphus rutilus*

Bincheng Han [1,†], Jinhai Luo [1,2,†] and Baojun Xu [1,*]

[1] Food Science and Technology Program, Beijing Normal University-Hong Kong Baptist University United International College, Zhuhai 519087, China
[2] Centre for Cancer and Inflammation Research, School of Chinese Medicine, Hong Kong Baptist University, Hong Kong, China
* Correspondence: baojunxu@uic.edu.cn; Tel.: +86-756-3620636
[†] These authors contributed equally to this work.

Abstract: *Chroogomphus rutilus* is an edible mushroom that has been an important food source since ancient times. It is increasingly sought after for its unique flavor and medicinal value. It is one of the most important wild mushrooms for its medicinal and economic value. *C. rutilus* contains a variety of active ingredients such as vitamins, proteins, minerals, polysaccharides, and phenolics. *C. rutilus* and its active compounds have significant anti-oxidant, anti-tumor, immunomodulatory, anti-fatigue, hypoglycemic, gastroprotective, hypolipemic, and neuronal protective properties. This paper summarizes the fungal chemical compositions and health-promoting effects of *C. rutilus* by collecting the literature on the role of *C. rutilus* through its active ingredients from websites such as Google Scholar, Scopus, PubMed, and Web of Science. Current research on *C. rutilus* is limited to the cellular and animal levels, and further clinical trials are needed to conduct and provide theoretical support for further development.

Keywords: *Chroogomphus rutilus*; chemical compositions; health-promoting effects

Citation: Han, B.; Luo, J.; Xu, B. Insights into the Chemical Compositions and Health Promoting Effects of Wild Edible Mushroom *Chroogomphus rutilus*. *Nutrients* 2023, 15, 4030. https://doi.org/10.3390/nu15184030

Academic Editor: Jacqueline Isaura Alvarez-Leite

Received: 1 September 2023
Revised: 14 September 2023
Accepted: 15 September 2023
Published: 17 September 2023

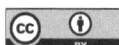

Copyright: © 2023 by the authors. Licensee MDPI, Basel, Switzerland. This article is an open access article distributed under the terms and conditions of the Creative Commons Attribution (CC BY) license (https://creativecommons.org/licenses/by/4.0/).

1. Introduction

Many health problems in today's society hurt people's quality of life and wellbeing. Some of these health problems include cardiovascular disease, obesity, diabetes, cancer, and immune system disorders. These problems are closely linked to modern lifestyles, dietary changes, and environmental factors [1]. Cardiovascular diseases, such as hypertension and hypercholesterolemia, have become major health problems worldwide [2]. Diets high in salt, sugar, and fat, physical inactivity, and stress can all contribute to the development of cardiovascular disease [3]. Obesity is also a growing problem that increases the risk of many non-communicable diseases not only related to cardiovascular disease, but also diabetes, joint disease, stroke, and other chronic diseases [4]. Cancer is one of the world's greatest health challenges. Environmental factors, unhealthy lifestyles (e.g., smoking, alcohol consumption, etc.), dietary patterns, and genetic mutations can all increase the risk of cancer [5]. The dysregulation of the immune system is also a key factor in the development of many diseases, including autoimmune and infectious diseases [6]. In the face of these health problems, there is an increasing emphasis on proactive health management measures, including improving diet, increasing physical activity, reducing stress, and boosting immunity [7]. Diet plays an important role in health management [8]. The consumption of nutrient-rich, functional foods is gradually increasing, as is the demand for natural, organic, low-fat, high-fiber, and antioxidant-rich foods [9].

Since ancient times, mushrooms have been a critical element in human life and culture as a kind of food source. It is an important part of the human diet to promote health and wellbeing [10]. Traditional Chinese medicine also often uses mushrooms as medicinal products [11]. China is a major country in mushroom cultivation and production [12].

Moreover, Heilongjiang Province, Jilin Province, and Liaoning Province in China have a forest coverage rate of 80%, abundant annual rainfall, abundant natural conditions, and abundant sunshine, which provide unique growth conditions for wild mushrooms and are the main mushroom-producing areas [13]. Mushroom mycelium is considered as a nutritional drug [14]. The fruiting body of the mushroom includes the cap and stalk [15]. In the past decades, the knowledge about the bioactive components and nutritional value of mushrooms has been increasing. Mushrooms are considered to be rich sources of many bioactive compounds.

Mushrooms are rich in high-quality carbohydrates [16]. Their high-quality protein [17], polysaccharides [18], unsaturated fatty acids [19], minerals [20], sterols and secondary metabolites [19], and vitamin D [21]. The important role of mushrooms in protecting and treating various health problems has always been appreciated, and mushrooms play a huge role in treating various degenerative diseases [22]. Mushrooms also play a significant role in the treatment of immunodeficiency, cancer, inflammation, hypertension, hyperlipidemia, hypercholesterolemia, and obesity [18]. The bioactive components of Agaricus campestris have the anti-oxidation effect [23] and anti-tumor [24] effect, which serves as antioxidants and anti-tumor drugs.

Chromogompuhus rutilus (*Gomphidius viscidus*, *Gomphidius rutilus*), abbreviated as *C. rutilus* and also known as the brown slime cap [25], red mushroom, pine umbrella, pine mushroom, and the copper spike, is a member of the genus *Chromogompus* in the family *Gomphidiaceae*. *C. rutilus* belongs to the *Basidiomycota*, *Agaricales*, and *Gomphidiaceae* families [26]. *Chromogompus* was originally a subgenus of *Gomphidius* [27] and was elevated to the genus status by Orson K in 1964 [28]. Molecular analyses have shown that *Gomphidius* is monophyletic [29,30]. As an ectomycorrhizal fungus, *Chroogomphus rutilus* is symbiotic with *Pinus densiflora* in Europe and is often found with *Lactobacillus* under Chinese pine forests in China [31].

Therefore, mushrooms have attracted wide attention in the research area of food nutrition, and this research may provide a way to prevent and treat some chronic diseases. In this case, we aim to provide an overview and summary of the nutritional value, fungal–chemical profile, and biological activity of *C. rutilus*, which will provide better knowledge of health improvement. With further progress in the related fields, it may be that *C. rutilus* can play a more important role in medicine. This paper aims to summarize the fungal chemistry, medicinal nutritional value, and biological activity of *C. rutilus* by collecting the literature on its active compounds from Google Scholar, Scopus, PubMed, and Web of Science. The keyword for collecting journal article includes *Chroogomphus rutilus*, *C. rutilus*, and antioxidant mushrooms. It is proven that *C. rutilus* is an edible mushroom with remarkable antioxidant, anti-tumor, immunomodulatory, anti-fatigue, hypoglycemia, gastric protective, hypolipidemic, and neuronal protective effects. However, research on *C. rutilus* is currently limited to the cellular and animal levels, and further clinical trials are needed to provide theoretical support for further development.

2. Description and Geographical Distribution of *C. rutilus*

The fruiting body of *C. rutilus* (Figure 1) is generally small. When it is first formed, it is generally bell-shaped or nearly cone-shaped. Later, it spreads out slowly, with a slight upward bulge in the middle and a light brown color. The flesh of the fungus is often a little red, and after drying, it is purplish-red. The fungus folds grow outwards along the base of the stipe. The stipe is 6–10 cm long and 1.5–2.5 cm thick, and the stipe tapers down and is solid [32] The growth conditions of *C. rutilus* are harsh, and it grows in the shady slopes with an altitude of 500–700 m. In summer and autumn, the solitary or gregarious *C. rutilus* can often be seen in the pine forest [33]. *C. rutilus*, as a precious understory resource, is common in the north temperate zone and mainly distributed in the pine forests northeast and southwest of China [34].

The pileus of *C. rutilus* is initially bell-shaped and gradually widens into a convex hemisphere. Later, it may become flat and slightly concave in the center, and its diameter is usually between 2 and 6 cm. The surface of the cap is smooth and glossy, there may be reddish-brown and pink fluff, and the edge may be slightly curled. The color of the cover is usually reddish-brown to orange-red, and sometimes it may be slightly orange-yellow [35]. The gill folds are widely spaced, and the common folds are attached to the lid and do not extend to the stem. The color of the pleats is similar to that of the cap but slightly lighter, usually reddish-brown to orange-red [36]. The stipe of *C. rutilus* is usually slender and erect, with a length of 4–10 cm and a diameter of about 0.5–1 cm. The surface of the stem has a rivet-like texture, hence the scientific name. The color of the stem is often red or orange-red, and sometimes it may gradually change to yellow towards the base [29]. The spores of *C. rutilus* are large, orange to brown, and oval in shape, and the color of the sporophores is usually brown [37].

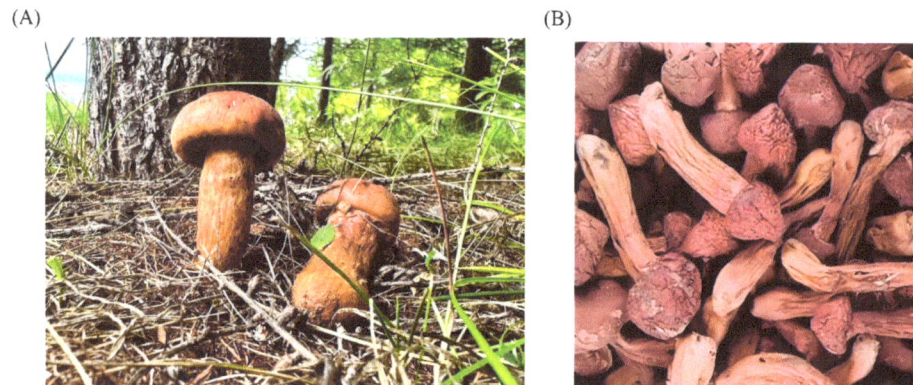

Figure 1. The fruiting body of *C. rutilus*: (**A**) the fresh fruiting body of *C. rutilus* collected from the Greater Khingan Mountains region of Heilongjiang Province, China; (**B**) the dry fruiting body of *C. rutilus*.

3. Fungal Chemical Characteristics of *C. rutilus*

3.1. Primary Metabolites of *C. rutilus*

C. rutilus is rich in primary metabolites, including proteins (12.3 g/100 g), eight essential amino acids, minerals (Ca, Fe, K, Na, etc.) [38], carbohydrates, fatty acids [39,40], polysaccharides (6–34 g/100 g), and riboflavin [41]. The silicified extract of *C. rutilus* contains 19 components. Xylitol (56.88%), glucitol (11.08%), fumaric acid (10.92%), and mannitol (6.79%) were identified as the major compounds [42]. The methylated extract contains 13 fatty acids, of which linoleic acid (41.61%) and oleic acid (35.87%) are the main fatty acids [42]. After extracting *C. rutilus* with different substances, it was concluded that hexane extract (IC$_{50}$, 2.22 ± 0.13 μg/mL) and ethyl acetate extract (IC$_{50}$, 2.28 ± 0.18 μg/mL) showed good lipid peroxidation inhibitory activity, while methanol extract showed good butyl cholinesterase inhibitory activity (IC$_{50}$, 45.5 ± 1.1 μg/mL). This biological activity is mainly attributed to polyols [42,43].

3.2. Secondary Metabolites of *C. rutilus*

C. rutilus contains different secondary metabolites (Table 1) including 5a, 8a-epidioxyergosta-6,22-dien-3b-ol, ergost-5, 24, (28)-diene-3b,7a,16b-triol, (24R)-ergost-5,7,22- triene-3b-ol, 3b,5a,9a-trihydroxy-(22E,24R)-ergosta-7,22-dien-6-one, 3b,5a-dihydroxy-(22E,24R)-ergosta-7,22-dien-6-one, 5a-ergosta-7,22-dien-3-one, ergosta-4,6,8(14),22tetraene-3-one, 5a-ergost-7-en-3b-ol, 4-hydroxybenzaldehyde, (4-hydroxyphenyl) acetic acid, methyl (4-hydroxyphenyl) acetate, butyl (4 hydroxyphenyl) acetate, butyl (4-hydroxyphenyl) acetate, 3-(3,4-dihydroxyphenyl)-2-propenoic acid, uracil, uridine, adenosine, a-methyl D- xyloside, D-ribonolactone, 6-hydroxy-5,7, dimethoxycoumarin, 7-hydroxycoumarin, esculetin, scopoletin, scoparone, fraxetin, 6,7,8- trimethoxycoumarin, phytodolor, 5,7-dimethoxycoumarin, fraxidin, and esculin [44]. Thus, it can be seen that *C. rutilus* is an important source of dietary fiber, natural anticancer, and antioxidant substances [45,46].

Table 1. The secondary metabolites of *C. rutilus*.

Components	Classification	Structure	Function	References
4-Hydroxybenzaldehyde	hydroxybenzaldehyde		Scavenged free radicals and promoted antioxidation	[47]
(4-hydroxyphenyl) acetic acid	monocarboxylic acid		Selectively inhibited tumor necrosis factor (TNF)-α-inducible levels of the redox-sensitive genes, vascular cell adhesion molecule-1, and monocyte chemoattractant protein-1	[48]
Methyl (4-hydroxyphenyl) acetate	methyl ester		Inhibited phenyl hydrazine-induced hemolysis of erythrocytes to scavenge most of the free radicals generated	[49]
3-(3,4-Dihydroxyphenyl)-2-propenoic acid	monocarboxylic acid		Scavenged free radicals and promoted antioxidation	[50]
Scopoletin	coumarin		Scavenged free radicals and promoted antioxidation. Activated some key antioxidant enzymes, such as superoxide dismutase (SOD), glutathione peroxidase (GPx), and glutathione -S- transferase (GST) to enhance the antioxidant defense system of cells	[51]
Fraxetin	coumarin		Scavenged free radicals and promoted antioxidation	[52]
Esculin	coumarin		Scavenged free radicals and promoted antioxidation	[53]
5a, 8a-Epidioxyergosta-6, 22-dien-3b-ol	ergosterol peroxide		Induced a cytotoxic effect on the OECM-1 cell strain and exerted an anti-tumor role	[54]
3b,5a-Dihydroxy-(22E, 24R)-ergosta-7,22-dien-6-one	ergostanoid		Exerted a cytotoxic effect on the MCF-7 cell strain and fulfilled an anti-tumor role	[55]

Table 1. Cont.

Components	Classification	Structure	Function	References
6-Hydroxy-5,7-dimethoxycoumarin	coumarins		Induced a cytotoxic effect on the L1210 cell strain and played an anti-tumor role	[56]
5,7-Dimethoxycoumarin	coumarins		Inhibited Mek 1/2 kinase activity and stimulated melanin production to inhibit melanoma	[57]
Adenosine	nucleoside		Inhibited the activities of T cells (proliferation, cytokine production, and cytotoxicity), NK cells (cytotoxicity), NKT cells (cytokine production and CD40L up-regulation), macrophages/dendritic cells (antigen presentation and cytokine production), and neutrophils (oxidative burst)	[58]
Scoparone	coumarins		Suppressed the responses of human mononuclear cells to phytohemagglutinin and mixed lymphocyte reaction for use against transplantation rejection and autoimmune disease	[59]
Uridine	nucleoside		Uridine is phosphorylated into nucleotides for the synthesis of DNA and RNA, as well as the synthesis of membrane components and glycosylation. Uridine nucleotides and UDP sugars may be released from neurons and glial cells. Used as neuroprotective agent for treating neurodegenerative diseases	[60]
5a-Ergosta-7,22-dien-3-one (Stellasterin)	lanostanoids		(External α-sialidase) inhibitors and antifungal agents, which play an immunomodulatory role. Hydroxyl groups can separate polar lipids and reduce blood fat and cholesterol	[61]
Ergosta-4,6,8(14),22tetraene-3-one	ergostanoid		Induced G2/M cell cycle arrest and apoptosis in human hepatocellular carcinoma HepG2 cells	[62]

Table 1. Cont.

Components	Classification	Structure	Function	References
6-Hydroxy-5,7-dimethoxycoumarin (Fraxinol)	coumarins		Inhibited the growth of Jurkat cell line tumor cells	[63]
6,7,8-Trimethoxycoumarin	coumarins		The gastric protective activity of GU induced by HCl/ethanol and indomethacin was improved, resulting in more than 90% reversal of GU	[64]
5,7-Dimethoxycoumarin (citropten)	coumarins		Inhibited the growth of A-375 melanoma cells	[65]
Fraxidin	coumarins		Exerted inhibitory effects towards aldose reductase activity and platelet aggregation	[66]
Scopoletin	coumarins		Scopoletin has obvious anti-inflammatory activity in inhibiting the overproduction of PGE2 and TNF-α and neutrophil infiltration	[67]
7-Hydroxycoumarin	coumarins		Inhibited [3H]thymidine, [3H]uridine, and [3H]leucine incorporation. Inhibited the intracellular production of prostate-specific antigen by LNCaP cells. Have direct antitumor (cytostatic) activity as well as immunomodulatory activity	[68]
Phytodolor	coumarins		The intracellular content of TNF-α and PTGS2 protein and the expression of TNF-α and PTGS2 gene were inhibited, and the induced apoptosis of LPS-activated human monocytes was inhibited in the absence of serum. In addition, phytodolor inhibited the translocation of p65 subunit of redox-regulated NF-κB in LPS-activated human macrophage nuclei. Played an anti-tumor role	[69]
Esculetin	coumarins		Exerted a cytotoxic effect on the Leukemia HL-60 cell strain and fulfilled an anti-tumor role	[70]

Table 1. Cont.

Components	Classification	Structure	Function	References
3b,5a,9a-Trihydroxy-(22E,24R)-ergosta-7,22-dien-6-one	ergostanoid		/	/
5a-Ergosta-7-en-3b-ol	ergostanoid		/	/

The main phytochemicals of *C. rutilus* are listed in Table 2, where these phytochemicals process diverse bioactivities, such as antioxidant, anti-fatigue, immunomodulatory, anti-tumor, anti-sugar, anti-hyperlipidemic, and gastric protective properties. *C. rutilus* can prevent lipid peroxidation and free radical damage due to its high antioxidant activity [71]. More specifically, the polysaccharides and phenolic compounds in *C. rutilus* have significant antioxidant activity [46], which can neutralize the free radicals and reduce the damage of oxidative stress to the body [72]. These compounds can scavenge the free radicals, enhance the activity of antioxidant enzymes, and adjust the redox balance [73,74]. The polysaccharides and phenolic compounds in *C. rutilus* showed certain anticancer activity [75]. These compounds can inhibit the growth and spread of tumor cells and induce programmed tumor death [76]. They can also regulate the function of the immune system and enhance the body's immune surveillance of tumors [77]. In addition, the triterpenoids in *C. rutilus* also have anti-angiogenesis effects [78] by blocking the blood supply to tumors. The polysaccharides and phenolic compounds in *C. rutilus* have certain anti-fatigue effects [79]. They can improve the body's energy metabolism, increase muscle endurance and adaptability, and reduce fatigue [80]. These compounds can also regulate the body's immune function, reduce the inflammatory response after exercise, and promote the body's recovery and repair [16].

Table 2. The major bioactive components from *C. rutilus* and their biological activities.

Compounds or Extracts	Biological Activity	Method	References
2-Methoxyadenine nucleoside, flavone	Antioxidant activity	Separating and purifying fruiting bodies and preparing macroporous resin	[39]
Polysaccharide	Antifatigue activity	Mice were given low (100 mg/kg/d), medium (250 mg/kg/d), and high (625 mg/kg/d) doses of Pleurotus eryngii polysaccharide	[75]
Polysaccharides (β-glucan and α-glucan)	Immunomodulatory activity	Organic extraction	[46]
Crude extract	Antitumor activity	Organic extraction (95% ethanol)	[45]

4. Biological Activity of *C. rutilus*

4.1. Formation and Function of Antioxidant Activity

Polyphenols have multiple hydroxyl structures, which makes them excellent free radical scavengers [81]. *C. rutilus* contains active compounds such as 4-hydroxybenzaldehyde, (4-hydroxyphenyl) acetic acid, methyl (4-hydroxyphenyl) acetate, 3-(3,4-dihydrohydroxyphenyl)-2-

propenoic acid, scopoletin, fraxetin, and esculin [44]. Among them, 4-hydroxybenzaldhyde and the coumarins scopoletin, fraxetin, and esculin can prevent oxidation by scavenging the free radicals [47,51–53]. At the same time, in other studies, (4-hydroxyphenyl) acetate was selectively inhibited by the tumor necrosis factor (TNF)-α-induced levels of the redox-sensitive genes, vascular cell adhesion molecule-1, and monocyte chemoattractant protein-1, inhibiting oxidation [48]. Methyl (4-hydroxyphenyl) acetate can reduce the degree of oxidation by inhibiting phenylhydrazine-induced hemolysis of radicals to scavenge most of the free radicals [49]. Currently, there is no literature to directly verify that the antioxidant activity of *C. rutilus* is produced by the above chemical components, but since these components can play an antioxidant role in fungi, *C. rutilus* may also have good antioxidant capacity, which requires further research to verify. Specifically, polyphenols react with free radicals via a redox reaction, thereby reducing the reactivity of free radicals and protecting the cells from oxidative damage [82].

In fungi, coumarins have a good antioxidant capacity [83], and *C. rutilus* also contains these substances, so *C. rutilus* is likely to have this ability. Polysaccharide compounds have a variety of biological activities, including antioxidant, anti-inflammatory, and immunomodulatory activities [84]. Scopoletin can activate some key antioxidant enzymes, such as superoxide dismutase (SOD), glutathione peroxide (GPX), and glutathione-*S*-transfer (GST), to enhance the antioxidant defense system of the cells [51]. This substance has also been found in *C. rutilus* [44], which may reduce the damage caused to the cells by oxidative stress.

C. rutilus is rich in vitamin C and vitamin E [85], which may also contribute to the antioxidant capacity of *C. rutilus*. As water-soluble and fat-soluble antioxidants, vitamin C and vitamin E can scavenge the free radicals, inhibit the generation of free radicals in the oxidation reaction chain, and protect the cells from oxidative damage [86]. In addition, *C. rutilus* is rich in some trace elements such as zinc, calcium, and iron [42,87]. As cofactors of antioxidant enzymes, these elements participate in the activity of antioxidant enzymes in the cells, thus enhancing the antioxidant defense capacity of the cells [88].

Moreover, the 2-methoxyadenine nucleoside was isolated and purified from the fruiting body of *C. rutilus* by Feng et al. in 2014 [39], which was determined to have a strong antioxidant capacity (EC_{50} is 0.06 mg/mL). In 2018, Sun et al. [31] found that the crude polysaccharide of *C. rutilus* has a good reducing ability, which was further separated and purified to obtain two polysaccharide components (GRMPW and GRMPS). The activity results showed that both of them had strong free radical scavenging ability. In the 2016 study, Zhang et al. [89] prepared the total flavonoids of *C. rutilus* via macroporous resin and determined its antioxidant effect. Its ability to scavenge DPPH and the hydroxyl radical (IC_{50} is 0.01 and 0.17 mg/mL) is stronger than that of positive medicine vitamin C. In conclusion, as a fungus rich in antioxidant compounds, the antioxidant properties of *C. rutilus* can be attributed to the synergistic effect of polyphenols, polysaccharides, vitamins, and trace elements.

In determining the redox state, we can evaluate its regulatory effect on the redox state in vivo by measuring the changes in the redox indices in the *C. rutilus* sample, such as the ratio of glutathione (GSH)/oxidized glutathione (GSSG) and the ratio of NADH/NAD^+ [90]. Using cellular models, such as the oxidative stress model in the cell culture, the protective effect of the *C. rutilus* sample on the cells was observed. Through the animal model, the influence of the *C. rutilus* sample on oxidative stress in animals was observed and the antioxidant activity of *C. rutilus* was comprehensively evaluated [91,92], revealing its antioxidant mechanism and effect.

Free radicals are highly active molecules produced by oxidation processes [93] that can cause cellular damage and oxidative stress [94]. The active components of *C. rutilus* can enhance the activities of antioxidant enzymes such as superoxide dismutase, glutathione peroxidase, and catalase in vivo [45,71]. These enzymes can further scavenge the free radicals in the body [95] and protect the cells from oxidative stress. Polysaccharides can enhance the activities of superoxide dismutase and glutathione peroxidase, reduce oxidative stress, improve mitochondrial function, and reduce the release of free radicals produced by mitochondria [96,97]. The polyphenolic compounds provide electron donors that help restore the reduced state and maintain redox balance [98]. Phenolic compounds also have anti-inflammatory effects and can reduce oxidative stress caused by inflammatory responses [99]. *C. rutilus* was also found to be rich in active compounds such as 4-hydroxybenzaldehyde, (4-hydroxyphenyl) acetic acid, methyl (4-hydroxyphenyl) acetate, 3-(3,4-dihydroxyphenyl)-2-propenoic acid, scopoletin, fraxetin, and esculin [44]. Further detailed experimental evidence is required to demonstrate the biological activity of *C. rutilus*.

Through these mechanisms, the antioxidant activity of *C. rutilus* helps prevent and alleviate the occurrence and development of many chronic diseases, including cardiovascular diseases, neurodegenerative diseases, and diabetes [45,100]. The generation and function of antioxidant activity make *C. rutilus* a potential natural antioxidant and health food [101]. The generation and function of antioxidant activity in *C. rutilus* can be studied using a few analytical methods, including free radical scavenging ability analysis, antioxidant enzyme activity analysis, redox state analysis, and cell and animal experiments [91,92,102,103].

4.2. Anti-Tumor Activity of C. rutilus

Abnormal cell proliferation caused by oxidative stress, inflammation, and immune response is related to the occurrence of many tumors [76]. Some fungi may contain compounds with antioxidant, anti-inflammatory, immunomodulatory, and anti-tumor activities, which can improve the immune system and reduce the risk of tumor occurrence [24].

C. rutilus has been extensively studied and is considered to have anti-tumor activity [40]. *C. rutilus* can inhibit the growth of tumor cells, and its extract can inhibit a variety of cancer cell lines, including lung cancer, liver cancer, and colon cancer [104]. The active compounds in *C. rutilus* can induce the apoptosis of tumor cells, which is an important cell self-destruction mechanism [105]. *C. rutilus* extract can increase the expression of apoptosis-related proteins such as Bax and caspase-3, while decreasing the expression of Bcl-2, thus promoting the apoptosis of cancer cells [106]. *C. rutilus* was found to have anti-angiogenic properties [107]. Tumor angiogenesis is a key process in tumor growth and metastasis [108]. *C. rutilus* contains 5a, 8a-epidioxyergosta-6,22-dien-3b-ol, 3b, 5a-dihydroxy-(22E,24R)-ergosta-7,22-dien-6-one, 6-hydroxy-5,7-dimethoxycoumarin, 5,7-dimethoxycoumarin, 7-dimethoxycoumarin, ergosta-4,6,8(14),22-tetraene-3-one, phytodolor, and esculetin [44]. Most of these chemical constituents are coumarin and ergostane, and these chemical constituents have been shown to have inhibitory effects on tumors through different mechanisms in other fungi. Among them, 5a, 8a-epidioxyergosta-6,22-dien-3b-ol, 3b, 5a-dihydroxy-(22E,24R)-ergosta-7,22-dien-6-one, and 6-hydroxy-5,7-dimethoxycoumarin have anti-OECM-1 tumor activity [55,56]. 5,7-Dimethoxycoumarin can stimulate melanogenesis and inhibit melanoma by inhibiting Mek 1/2 kinase activity [57]. Ergosta-4,6,8(14) and 22-tetraen-3-one induced G2/M cell cycle arrest and apoptosis in human hepatocellular carcinoma HepG2 cells, which reduced the incidence of liver cancer and the growth rate of liver cancer cells [62]. 6-Hydroxy-5,7-dimethoxycoumarin and 5,7-dimethoxycoumarin inhibited the growth of Jurkat tumor cells and A-375 tumor cells, respectively, and played an anti-tumor role [63,65]. Phytodolor inhibited the intracellular content of TNF-α and PTGS2 proteins and the expression of TNF-α and PTGS2 genes and inhibited the apoptosis of LPS-activated human monocytes in the absence of serum. In addition, phytodolor inhibited the translocation of the p65 subunit of redox-regulated NF-κB in the nucleus of LPS-activated human macrophages. It plays an anti-tumor role [69]. Esculetin has a cytotoxic effect on the leukemia cell line HL-60 and plays an anti-tumor role [70]. At present, there is no literature to directly verify that these chemical components in *C. rutilus* have the same effect, but since these components can play an anti-tumor role in fungi, *C. rutilus* may also have good anti-tumor ability, which needs further experimental research to verify. *C. rutilus* extract can promote the activation and proliferation of immune cells [80], These results confirmed that *C. rutilus* has anti-tumor activity.

4.3. Immunomodulatory Activity of C. rutilus

The immune system is an important part of maintaining the health of the body and acts as a line of defense against pathogens and abnormal cells [109]. Immunoregulation is a key process in the immune system that can balance the immune response, regulate the activity of immune cells, and maintain immune balance [110].

The active components in *C. rutilus* can regulate the activation and proliferation of immune cells (Figure 2). Adenosine and scoparone can inhibit T cell proliferation, cytokine production and cytotoxicity, and NK cell toxicity in other fungi), NKT cytokine production and CD40L upregulation, antigen presentation and cytokine production by macrophages or dendritic cells, and neutrophil oxidative burst activity. These cytokines play an important role in immune regulation and inflammation [111]. It also inhibits the human monocyte response to phytohaemagglutinin and mixed lymphocyte reaction and can be used to combat transplant rejection and autoimmune diseases [58,59]. *C. rutilus*, which plays an immunomodulatory role, also contains these two substances. At present, no experiment directly proves that the antioxidant activity of *C. rutilus* is produced by these two chemical components, but *C. rutilus* probably also has good immunomodulatory ability, which needs more research to verify.

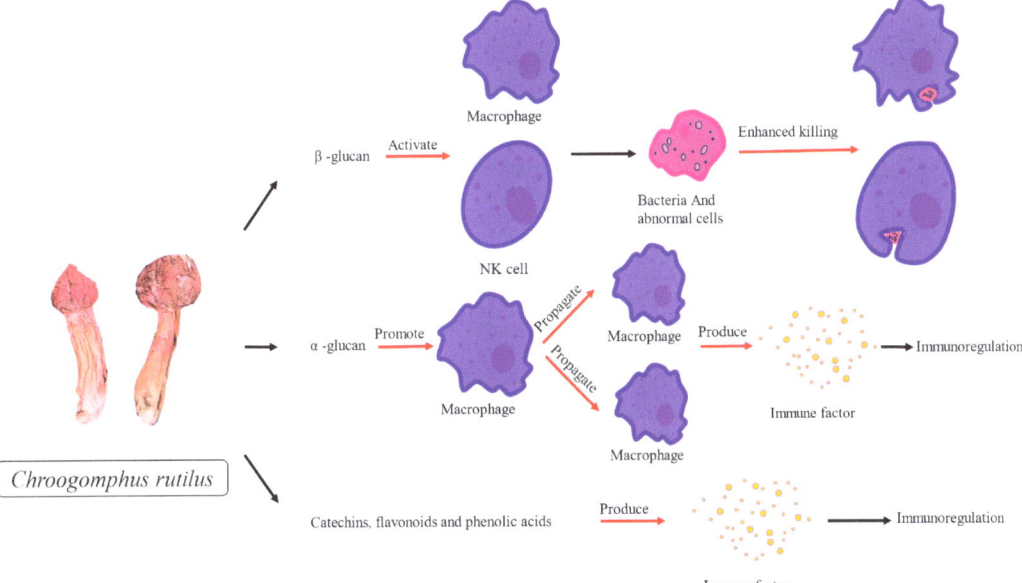

Figure 2. The summary of the mechanism of the immunomodulatory activity of *C. rutilus*.

The immunomodulatory activity of *C. rutilus* is closely related to the synergistic effects of polysaccharides (such as β-glucan and α-glucan), polyphenols (such as catechins, flavonoids, and phenolic acids), and antioxidants (such as vitamin C and vitamin E) [112–114]. Polysaccharides in *C. rutilus* are considered to be one of the important components of its immunomodulatory activity. It has been found that the polysaccharide compounds in *C. rutilus* mainly include β-glucan and α-glucan [46]. These polysaccharide compounds can stimulate the activation and proliferation of immune cells and enhance the ability of immune cells to produce cytokines [115]. For example, β-glucan can activate macrophages and natural killer cells and increase their killing effect on pathogens and abnormal cells [116]. In addition, α-glucan has an immunomodulatory effect, which can promote the proliferation of immune cells and the production of immune factors, thus enhancing the immune response [117]. The polyphenols in *C. rutilus* also play an important role in its immunomodulatory activity. The polyphenols found in *C. rutilus* are mainly catechins, flavonoids, and phenolic acids [42]. These compounds can regulate the balance of the immune response by regulating the activity of immune cells and the production of cytokines. For example, catechins have immunomodulatory effects that can regulate the function of immune cells and the production of cytokines [118].

In addition, antioxidants such as vitamin C and vitamin E are also involved in its immunomodulatory activity [119,120]. Vitamin C and vitamin E can reduce oxidative stress damage to immune cells and regulate the activity of immune cells and the immune response [121].

4.4. Anti-Fatigue Activity of C. rutilus

Fatigue is a common physical and psychological condition in modern society, which has a negative impact on individual health and the quality of life. As a natural herbal resource, *C. rutilus* has been extensively studied and shows potential anti-fatigue activity.

C. rutilus extract has an anti-fatigue effect and can delay the onset and development of fatigue. This activity is related to the synergistic effect of polysaccharides, polyphenols, and other bioactive substances in *C. rutilus* [122]. Polysaccharide compounds in *C. rutilus* are considered to be one of the important components of its anti-fatigue activity [122]. Crude polysaccharide compounds can provide energy supply and regulate energy metabolism, thus increasing the endurance and anti-fatigue ability of the body [79]. Polysaccharide compounds in *C. rutilus* have been found to improve the endurance of physical activity, reduce fatigue, and promote recovery [113,122].

Additionally, its anti-fatigue activity also includes the participation of polyphenols [113]. Polyphenols, such as the catechins and flavonoids abundant in *C. rutilus*, are believed to exhibit a beneficial anti-fatigue effect [123]. There are other bioactive substances in *C. rutilus*, such as vitamins, minerals, and amino acids [45], which may also play a role in anti-fatigue. Vitamins and minerals are involved in the regulation of energy metabolism and muscle function, which helps to improve the body's endurance and anti-fatigue ability [124]. Amino acids are the basic units of protein, which play an important role in maintaining normal muscle function and repairing damaged tissue [125]. In 2014, animal experiments were conducted to investigate the function of the *C. rutilus* polysaccharide in alleviating physical fatigue. Mice were given low (100 mg/kg/d), medium (250 mg/kg/d), and high (625 mg/kg/d) doses of the *C. rutilus* polysaccharide, and exhaustive swimming time, blood lactic acid, and blood urea were measured. The results showed that the effect of the mid-dose group was significant. Compared with the control group, the middle dose group of *C. rutilus* polysaccharide can significantly reduce the content of blood urea nitrogen and blood lactic acid and increase the glycogen storage in the body, indicating that the *C. rutilus* polysaccharide has a certain function of alleviating physical fatigue [75].

4.5. Hypoglycemia Activity of C. rutilus

Polysaccharide compounds have biological activities such as lowering blood glucose, improving islet function, and increasing insulin sensitivity [126]. These polysaccharide compounds may block the process of sugar digestion and absorption by interacting with glycosidase in the gut, thereby lowering the blood glucose levels [127].

In addition, fraxidin has been shown to inhibit aldose reductase activity and platelet aggregation, inhibit the rise of the blood sugar levels in the human body, and may play an anti-hyperglycemia role [52]. *C. rutilus* contains this chemical, which may play an anti-hyperglycemic role. However, there is no evidence that the anti-hyperglycemia effect of *C. rutilus* comes from fraxidin, which needs further research to prove. Further research has also shown that *C. rutilus* may exert its anti-sugar activity by regulating the insulin signaling pathway and improving insulin sensitivity [128]. These compounds may also affect the activities of key enzymes involved in glucose metabolism and promote glucose utilization and energy metabolism [128].

4.6. Gastric Protective Activity of C. rutilus

Studies have shown that *C. rutilus* has significant gastric protective activity (Figure 3), which has a positive effect on protecting the gastric mucosa, inhibiting gastric ulcers, and relieving gastric inflammation. The active constituents of *C. rutilus* are involved in its gastric protective activity. The polysaccharide compounds were found to be one of the important components of its gastric protective activity [129]. Polysaccharide compounds have a variety of biological activities, including anti-inflammatory, antioxidant, and mucosal protection [130]. *C. rutilus* contains 6,7,8-trimethoxycoumarin, and 6,7,8-trimethoxycoumarin can improve the gastric protective activity of GU induced by hydrochloric acid or ethanol and indomethacin, resulting in the reversal of GU by more than 90%. As a medicinal mushroom, *C. rutilus* probably also has gastric protective biological activity, which requires further studies to validate [44,64]. This improvement in gastric protective activity has been confirmed in other fungi. At the same time, the polysaccharide compounds in the plant can reduce the inflammatory response of the gastric mucosa and promote the repair and regeneration of the gastric mucosa [131].

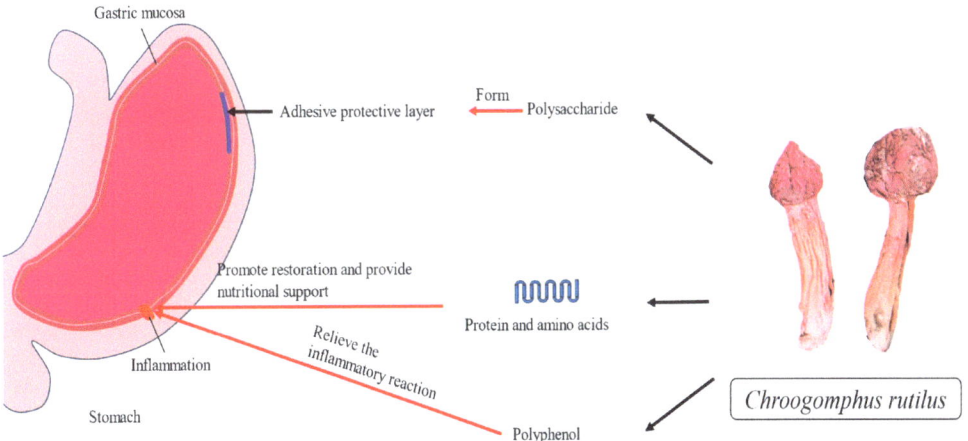

Figure 3. The summary of the mechanism of gastric protective activity of *Chroogomphus rutilus*.

In addition, the polyphenols also play an important role in its gastric protective activity. Polyphenols have antioxidant and anti-inflammatory effects, which can reduce the oxidative stress and inflammatory response of the gastric mucosa and protect the gastric mucosa from damage [99]. Moreover, protein, amino acids, vitamins, etc., are also involved in gastric protective activities. Protein and amino acids can provide nutrients needed for gastric mucosal repair and promote gastric mucosal recovery. Vitamins participate in the metabolism and repair of mucosal tissues and play an important role in gastric mucosal health [132,133]. *C. rutilus* may have good gastric protective activity because of the meaning of these substances, but this needs more follow-up experiments to verify.

4.7. Hypolipidemic Activity of C. rutilus

The active constituents of *C. rutilus* play an important role in its anti-hyperlipidemic activity. Polysaccharide compounds can regulate lipid metabolism and inhibit cholesterol synthesis [134]. Polysaccharide compounds can regulate blood lipid metabolism in many ways, including reducing the levels of total cholesterol, low-density lipoprotein cholesterol (LDL-C), and triacylglycerol, increasing the levels of high-density lipoprotein cholesterol (HDL-C) and promoting cholesterol excretion [135,136]. These effects help reduce the blood lipid levels and lipid accumulation in the blood, thus playing an anti-hyperlipidemic role.

Polyphenols have antioxidant activity, which can reduce lipid peroxidation and prevent the formation of lipid oxidation products, thus reducing the blood lipid levels [86]. Protein, amino acids, and dietary fiber can also regulate blood lipid metabolism and promote the balance of blood lipid metabolism [135]. Further studies have also shown that the anti-hyperlipidemic activity of C. rutilus is closely related to the regulation of relevant enzymes. For example, the active components can inhibit key enzymes in cholesterol synthesis, such as HMG-CoA reductase, resulting in reduced cholesterol synthesis [135]. In addition, the components of C. rutilus may also affect the expression of the genes involved in lipid metabolism, further regulating the balance of lipid metabolism [113,137]. The 5a-ergosta-7,22-dien-3-one contained in C. rutilus can be used as an (exo-α-sialidase) inhibitor and an antifungal agent, which plays an immunomodulatory role. Hydroxyl groups can separate polar lipids and reduce blood lipids and cholesterol. In other experimental studies, 5a-ergosta-7,22-dien-3-one has been proven to play a role in reducing blood lipids [44,61]. Another medicinal mushroom, C. rutilus, may also have good anti-hyperlipidaemic activity, which can be tested in subsequent experimental studies.

4.8. Neuroprotective Effects of C. rutilus

The crude polysaccharide has a protective effect against neuronal damage. Nervous system diseases such as Alzheimer's disease, Parkinson's disease, and stroke are usually associated with oxidative stress, inflammatory response, and neuronal damage [138,139] Polysaccharide compounds can regulate neuronal metabolic activity, improve nerve conduction and cell signaling, and promote neuronal survival and repair [140]. Studies have shown that C. rutilus and its extracts have significant activity in neuronal protection [46]. In addition, C. rutilus can also inhibit the inflammatory response and reduce cell death caused by neuronal inflammatory injury [46]. These protective effects may be related to the mechanism by which the active components of C. rutilus regulate the cell signaling pathways, reduce the release of inflammatory mediators, and promote the self-repair ability of the cells [114,135]. C. rutilus may have neuroprotective activity, and uridine can be phosphorylated to nucleotides for DNA and RNA synthesis and the synthesis and glycosylation of membrane components. Uridine nucleotides and UDP sugars can be released from the neurons and glial cells. It is used as a neuroprotective agent in the treatment of neurodegenerative diseases [60]. However, C. rutilus contains uridine, which may have a neuroprotective effect, but this has not been confirmed by any direct experiments and further research is needed to prove this.

5. Conclusions

Due to the taste and nutritional value of C. rutilus, people's demand for C. rutilus is increasing. C. rutilus is a fungus with potential medicinal value that has been extensively studied and found to have various biological activities. Due to its medicinal value, C. rutilus is also used in medicine to treat various diseases. As a species of medicinal mushroom, C. rutilus has shown a wide application prospect in clinical research. The properties of its active components, such as anti-tumor, cardiovascular protection, immunomodulation, anti-inflammation, anti-oxidation, and anti-aging, provide a basis for its further research and development in the fields of tumor treatment, cardiovascular diseases, immunomodulation, and anti-aging. However, further clinical research and practice are needed to verify its safety and efficacy and to promote its use in clinical practice. Due to its antioxidant, anti-tumor, immunomodulatory, anti-fatigue, anti-sugar, gastric protective, anti-hyperlipidaemic, and neuronal protective activities, C. rutilus has attracted a lot of attention in the fields of biochemistry and pharmacology. At the same time, the mechanism behind some of the medicinal activities has hardly been studied. Therefore, future research must pay attention to these potential mechanisms. Finally, despite the remarkable pharmacological effects of C. rutilus in vitro and in vivo, there is a lack of information on its safe use, therapeutic index, and risk–benefit ratio in humans. These data are very useful for the development of new pharmaceutical preparations based on the active principles of C. rutilus.

Author Contributions: B.H.: Literature investigation and Writing—Original draft preparation. J.L.: Literature investigation and Writing—Original draft preparation. B.X.: Conceptualization, Methodology, Software, Supervision, and Writing—Reviewing and Editing. All authors have read and agreed to the published version of the manuscript.

Funding: This project is supported by (Project code: UICR0200007-23) from BNU-HKBU United International College, China.

Data Availability Statement: Not applicable.

Conflicts of Interest: The authors declare no conflict of interest.

References

1. Habib, S.H.; Saha, S. Burden of non-communicable disease: Global overview. *Diabetesi. Metab. Synd.* **2010**, *4*, 41–47. [CrossRef]
2. Munzel, T.; Hahad, O.; Sørensen, M.; Lelieveld, J.; Duerr, G.D.; Nieuwenhuijsen, M.; Daiber, A. Environmental risk factors and cardiovascular diseases: A comprehensive expert review. *Cardiovasc. Res.* **2011**, *118*, 2880–2902. [CrossRef]
3. Buttar, H.S.; Li, T.; Ravi, N. Prevention of cardiovascular diseases: Role of exercise, dietary interventions, obesity and smoking cessation. *Exp. Clin. Cardiol.* **2005**, *10*, 229.
4. Bray, G.A.; Kim, K.K.; Wilding, J.P.; World Obesity Federation. Obesity: A chronic relapsing progressive disease process. A position statement of the World Obesity Federation. *Obes. Rev.* **2017**, *18*, 715–723. [CrossRef] [PubMed]
5. Wu, M.; Zhao, J.K.; Hu, X.S.; Wang, P.H.; Qin, Y.; Lu, Y.C.; Yang, J.; Liu, A.M.; Wu, D.L.; Zhang, Z.F.; et al. Association of smoking, alcohol drinking and dietary factors with esophageal cancer in high-and low-risk areas of Jiangsu Province, China. *World J. Gastroentero.* **2006**, *12*, 1686. [CrossRef] [PubMed]
6. Bach, J.F. Infections and autoimmune diseases. *J. Autoimmun.* **2005**, *25*, 74–80. [CrossRef]
7. Sharkey, B.J.; Gaskill, S.E. *Fitness & Health*; Human Kinetics: Champaign, IL, USA, 2013.
8. Dettmar, P.W.; Strugala, V.; Richardson, J.C. The key role alginates play in health. *Food Hydrocoll.* **2011**, *25*, 263–266. [CrossRef]
9. Mudgil, D.; Barak, S. *Functional Foods: Sources and Health Benefits*; Scientific Publishers: London, UK, 2011.
10. Kour, H.; Kour, D.; Kour, S.; Singh, S.; Hashmi, S.A.J.; Yadav, A.N.; Kumar, K.; Sharma, Y.P.; Ahluwalia, A.S. Bioactive compounds from mushrooms: An emerging bioresources of food and nutraceuticals. *Food Bonsci.* **2022**, *50*, 102124. [CrossRef]
11. Lee, K.H.; Morris-Natschke, S.L.; Yang, X.; Huang, R.; Zhou, T.; Wu, S.F.; Shi, Q.; Itokawa, H. Recent progress of research on medicinal mushrooms, foods, and other herbal products used in traditional Chinese medicine. *J. Tradit. Complement. Med.* **2012**, *2*, 1–12. [CrossRef]
12. Phan, C.W.; Tan, E.Y.Y.; Sabaratnam, V. Bioactive molecules in edible and medicinal mushrooms for human wellness. In *Bioactive Molecules in Food*; Springer: Cham, Switzerland, 2019; pp. 1597–1620.
13. Wang, S.; Yang, B.; Zhou, Q.; Li, Z.; Li, W.; Zhang, J.; Tuo, F. Radionuclide content and risk analysis of edible mushrooms in northeast China. *Radiat. Med. Prot.* **2021**, *2*, 165–170. [CrossRef]
14. Rathore, H.; Prasad, S.; Kapri, M.; Tiwari, A.; Sharma, S. Medicinal importance of mushroom mycelium: Mechanisms and applications. *J. Funct. Foods* **2019**, *56*, 182–193. [CrossRef]
15. Şen, A.; Acevedo-Fani, A.; Dave, A.; Ye, A.; Husny, J.; Singh, H. Plant oil bodies and their membrane components: New natural materials for food applications. *Crit. Rev. Food Sci.* **2022**, 1–24. [CrossRef] [PubMed]
16. Ma, G.; Yang, W.; Zhao, L.; Pei, F.; Fang, D.; Hu, Q. A critical review on the health promoting effects of mushrooms nutraceuticals. *Food Sci. Hum. Wellness* **2018**, *7*, 125–133. [CrossRef]
17. Goswami, B.; Majumdar, S.; Das, A.; Barui, A.; Bhowal, J. Evaluation of bioactive properties of Pleurotus ostreatus mushroom protein hydrolysate of different degree of hydrolysis. *LWT-Food Sci. Technol.* **2021**, *149*, 111768. [CrossRef]
18. Zhang, S.; Lei, L.; Zhou, Y.; Ye, F.Y.; Zhao, G.H. Roles of mushroom. polysaccharides in chronic disease management. *J. Integr. Agric.* **2022**, *21*, 1839–1866. [CrossRef]
19. Saini, R.K.; Rauf, A.; Khalil, A.A.; Ko, E.Y.; Keum, Y.S.; Anwar, S.; Alamri, A.; Rengasamy, K.R. Edible mushrooms show significant differences in sterols and fatty acid compositions. *S. Afr. J. Bot.* **2021**, *141*, 344–356. [CrossRef]
20. De Souza Lopes, L.; De Casssia Silva, M.; De Oliveira Faustino, A.; De Oliveira, L.L.; Kasuya, M.C.M. Bioaccessibility, oxidizing activity and co-accumulation of minerals in Li-enriched mushrooms. *LWT-Food Sci. Technol.* **2022**, *155*, 112989. [CrossRef]
21. Pedrali, D.; Gallotti, F.; Proserpio, C.; Pagliarini, E.; Lavelli, V. Kinetic study of vitamin D2 degradation in mushroom powder to improve its applications in fortified foods. *Lwt-Food Sci. Technol.* **2020**, *125*, 109248. [CrossRef]
22. Rathore, H.; Prasad, S.; Sharma, S. Mushroom nutraceuticals for improved nutrition and better human health: A review. *Pharma Nutr.* **2017**, *5*, 35–46. [CrossRef]
23. Mwangi, R.W.; Macharia, J.M.; Wagara, I.N.; Bence, R.L. The antioxidant potential of different edible and medicinal mushrooms. *Biomed. Pharmacother.* **2022**, *147*, 112621. [CrossRef]
24. Pathak, M.P.; Pathak, K.; Saikia, R.; Gogoi, U.; Ahmad, M.Z.; Patowary, P.; Das, A. Immunomodulatory effect of mushrooms and their bioactive compounds in cancer: A comprehensive review. *Biomed. Pharmacother.* **2022**, *149*, 112901. [CrossRef]
25. McKnight, K.H.; McKnight, V.B. *A Field Guide to Mushrooms: North America*; Houghton Mifflin Harcourt: Boston, MA, USA, 1987; Volume 34.

26. Sun, L.; He, W.; Xin, G.; Cai, P.; Zhang, Y.; Zhang, Z.; Wei, Y.; Sun, B.; Wen, X. Volatile components, total phenolic compounds, and antioxidant capacities of worm-infected *Gomphidius rutilus*. *Food Sci. Hum. Wellness* **2018**, *7*, 148–155. [CrossRef]
27. Singer, R. New and interesting species of *Basidiomycetes* III. *Sydowia* **1950**, *4*, 130–157.
28. Miller, O.K., Jr. Monograph of *Chroogomphus* (*Gomphidiaceae*). *Mycologia* **1964**, *56*, 526–549. [CrossRef]
29. Miller, O.K., Jr.; Aime, M.C. *Systematics, Ecology and World Distribution in the Genus Chroogomphus*; Trichomycetes Other Fungal Groups: Boca Raton, FL, USA, 2001; p. 315.
30. Miller, O.K., Jr. The Gomphidiaceae revisited: A worldwide perspective. *Mycologia* **2003**, *95*, 176–183. [CrossRef]
31. Jiang, X. Study on the special niche of the *Chroogomphus rutilus* and its undergrowth. *Liaoning Forest. Sci. Technol.* **2022**, *1*, 54–57.
32. Gao, C. *Chroogomphus rutilus* Polysaccharide Preparation and Bioactivity Analysis. Ph.D. Thesis, Liaoning Petrochemical University, Fushun, China, 2012.
33. Luan, Q.S. Research status, development and utilization of *Chroogomphus rutilus*. *Edible Fungi* **2002**, *24*, 2–3.
34. Jin, Z.M.; Chai, J.H.; He, T.T.; Peng, D. Study on antioxidant activity of polysaccharide from *Gomphidius rutilus*. *Hubei Agric. Sci.* **2020**, *59*, 123.
35. Scambler, R.; Niskanen, T.; Assyov, B.; Ainsworth, A.M.; Bellanger, J.M.; Loizides, M.; Moreau, P.A.; Kirk, P.M.; Liimatainen, K. Diversity of *Chroogomphus* (*Gomphidiaceae, Boletales*) in Europe, and typification of *C. rutilus*. *Ima. Fungus* **2018**, *9*, 271–290. [CrossRef] [PubMed]
36. Kuo, M. *The Genus Chroogomphus*; MushroomExpert. Com.: OH, USA, 2007. Available online: http://www.mushroomexpert.com/chroogomphus.html (accessed on 31 August 2023).
37. Martín, M.P.; Siquier, J.L.; Salom, J.C.; Telleria, M.T.; Finschow, G. Barcoding sequences clearly separate *Chroogomphus mediterraneus* (Gomphidiaceae, Boletales) from *C. rutilus*, and allied species. *Mycoscience* **2016**, *57*, 384–392. [CrossRef]
38. Mgbekem, M.A.; Lukpata, F.; Ndukaku, N.; Armon, M.; Uka, V.K.; Udosen, G.N.; Pricilla, A.B. Knowledge and utilization of mushroom as a food supplement among families in selected local government areas of Cross River State, Nigeria. *Food Sci. Nutr.* **2019**, *10*, 1287–1299. [CrossRef]
39. Feng, J.; Qin, S.L.; Hu, B.; Zhao, X.J.; Wang, L. Preliminary study on chemical constituents and biological activities of fruiting bodies of *Chroogomphus rutilus*. *Mycosystema* **2014**, *33*, 355–364.
40. Li, Z.; Bao, H. Overview of studies on chemical constituents and pharmacological activities of *Chroogomphus rutilus*. *J. Fungal Res.* **2015**, *13*, 181–186.
41. Fulgoni, V.L., III; Agarwal, S. Nutritional impact of adding a serving of mushrooms on usual intakes and nutrient adequacy using National Health and Nutrition Examination Survey 2011–2016 data. *Food Sci. Nutr.* **2021**, *9*, 1504–1511. [CrossRef]
42. Çayan, F.; Tel, G.; Duru, M.E.; Öztürk, M.; Türkoğlu, A.; Harmandar, M. Application of GC, GC-MSD, ICP-MS and spectrophotometric methods for the determination of chemical composition and in vitro bioactivities of *Chroogomphus rutilus*: The edible mushroom species. *Food Anal. Method* **2014**, *7*, 449–458. [CrossRef]
43. Cheung, P.C.K. The nutritional and health benefits of mushrooms. *Nutr. Bull.* **2010**, *35*, 292–299. [CrossRef]
44. Luo, J.; Zhou, W.; Cao, S.; Zhu, H.; Zhang, C.; Jin, M.; Li, G. Chemical constituents of *Chroogomphus rutilus* (Schaeff.) OK mill. *Biochem. Syst. Ecol.* **2015**, *61*, 203–207. [CrossRef]
45. Zhang, J.; Zhao, X.; Zhao, L.Q.; Zhao, J.; Qi, Z.; Wang, L.A. A primary study of the antioxidant, hypoglycemic, hypolipidemic, and antitumor activities of ethanol extract of brown slimecap mushroom, *Chroogomphus rutilus* (Agaricomycetes). *Int. J. Med. Mushrooms* **2017**, *19*, 905–913. [CrossRef]
46. Zhang, Y.; Lan, M.; Lü, J.P.; Li, J.F.; Zhang, K.Y.; Zhi, H.; Zhang, H.; Sun, J.M. Antioxidant, anti-inflammatory and cytotoxic activities of polyphenols extracted from *Chroogomphus rutilus*. *Chem. Biodivers.* **2020**, *17*, e1900479. [CrossRef]
47. Nobsathian, S.; Tuchinda, P.; Sobhon, P.; Tinikul, Y.; Poljaroen, J.; Tinikul, R.; Sroyraya, M.; Poomton, T.; Chaichotranunt, S. An antioxidant activity of the whole body of Holothuria scabra. *Chem. Biol. Technol. Agric.* **2017**, *4*, 4. [CrossRef]
48. Kunsch, C.; Luchoomun, J.; Chen, X.L.; Dodd, G.L.; Karu, K.S.; Meng, C.Q.; Marino, E.M.; Olliff, L.K.; Piper, J.D.; Qiu, F.H.; et al. AGIX-4207 [2-[4-[[1-[[3, 5-bis (1, 1-dimethylethyl)-4-hydroxyphenyl] thio]-1-methylethyl] thio]-2, 6-bis (1, 1-dimethylethyl) phenoxy] acetic acid], a novel antioxidant and anti-inflammatory compound: Cellular and biochemical characterization of antioxidant activity and inhibition of redox-sensitive inflammatory gene expression. *J. Pharmacol. Exp. Ther.* **2005**, *313*, 492–501.
49. Akbas, E.; Ekin, S.; Ergan, E.; Karakus, Y. Synthesis, DFT calculations, spectroscopy and in vitro antioxidant activity studies on 4-hydroxyphenyl substituted thiopyrimidine derivatives. *J. Mol. Struct.* **2018**, *1174*, 177–183. [CrossRef]
50. Choi, K.H.; Nam, K.C.; Lee, S.Y.; Cho, G.; Jung, J.S.; Kim, H.J.; Park, B.J. Antioxidant potential and antibacterial efficiency of caffeic acid-functionalized ZnO nanoparticles. *Nanomaterials* **2017**, *7*, 148. [CrossRef] [PubMed]
51. Jamuna, S.; Karthika, K.; Paulsamy, S.; Thenmozhi, K.; Kathiravan, S.; Venkatesh, R. Confertin and scopoletin from leaf and root extracts of Hypochaeris radicata have anti-inflammatory and antioxidant activities. *Ind. Crop. Prod.* **2015**, *70*, 221–230. [CrossRef]
52. Fernandez-Puntero, B.; Barroso, I.; Iglesias, I.; BENEDÍ, J.; VILLAR, A. Antioxidant activity of Fraxetin: In vivo and ex vivo parameters in normal situation versus induced stress. *Biol. Pharm. Bull.* **2001**, *24*, 777–784. [CrossRef]
53. Witaicenis, A.; Seito, L.N.; da Silveira Chagas, A.; de Almeida Junior, L.D.; Luchini, A.C.; Rodrigues-Orsi, P.; Helena Cestari, S.; Di Stasi, L.C. Antioxidant and intestinal anti-inflammatory effects of plant-derived coumarin derivatives. *Phytomedicine* **2014**, *21*, 240–246. [CrossRef]
54. Zhuang, Y.-S. Studies on the Chemical Constituents and Biological Activities of the Thermophilic Fungus, *Aspergillus terreus*. Master's Thesis, Taipei University of Technology, Taipei, Taiwan, 2011. [CrossRef]

55. Shylaja, G.; Sathiavelu, A. Cytotoxicity of endophytic fungus *Chaetomium cupreum* from the plant *Mussaenda luteola* against breast cancer cell line MCF-7. *Bangl. J. Pharmacol.* **2017**, *12*, 373–375. [CrossRef]
56. Rojas, J.O.H.N.; Londoño, C.E.S.A.R.; Ciro, Y. The health benefits of natural skin UVA photoprotective compounds found in botanical sources. *Int. J. Pharm. Pharm. Sci.* **2016**, *8*, 13–23.
57. Alesiani, D.; Cicconi, R.; Mattei, M.; Bei, R.; Canini, A. Inhibition of Mek 1/2 kinase activity and stimulation of melanogenesis by 5,7-dimethoxycoumarin treatment of melanoma cells. *Int. J. Oncol.* **2009**, *34*, 1727–1735.
58. Ohta, A. A metabolic immune checkpoint: Adenosine in tumor microenvironment. *Front. Immunol.* **2016**, *7*, 109. [CrossRef]
59. Huei-Chen, H.; Shu-Hsun, C.; Chao, P.D.L. Vasorelaxants from Chinese herbs, emodin and scoparone, possess immunosuppressive properties. *Eur. J. Pharmacol.* **1991**, *198*, 211–213. [CrossRef]
60. Dobolyi, A.; Juhász, G.; Kovács, Z.; Kardos, J. Uridine function in the central nervous system. *Curr. Top. Med. Chem.* **2011**, *11*, 1058–1067. [CrossRef]
61. Pallam, R.B.; Sarma, V.V. Metabolites of Ganoderma and their Applications in Medicine. In *Fungal Biotechnology: Prospects and Avenues*; CRC Press: Boca Raton, FL, USA, 2022; p. 175.
62. Zhao, Y.Y.; Shen, X.; Chao, X.; Ho, C.C.; Cheng, X.L.; Zhang, Y.; Lin, R.C.; Du, K.J.; Luo, W.J.; Chen, J.Y.; et al. Ergosta-4, 6, 8 (14), 22-tetraen-3-one induces G2/M cell cycle arrest and apoptosis in human hepatocellular carcinoma HepG2 cells. *Biochim. Biophys. Acta-Gen. Subj.* **2011**, *1810*, 384–390. [CrossRef]
63. Pereira, A.; Bester, M.; Soundy, P.; Apostolides, Z. Anti-proliferative properties of commercial *Pelargonium sidoides* tincture, with cell-cycle G0/G1 arrest and apoptosis in Jurkat leukaemia cells. *Pharm. Biol.* **2016**, *54*, 1831–1840. [CrossRef] [PubMed]
64. Son, D.J.; Lee, G.R.; Oh, S.; Lee, S.E.; Choi, W.S. Gastroprotective efficacy and safety evaluation of scoparone derivatives on experimentally induced gastric lesions in rodents. *Nutrients* **2015**, *7*, 1945–1964. [CrossRef] [PubMed]
65. Chodurek, E.; Orchel, A.; Orchel, J.; Kurkiewicz, S.; Gawlik, N.; Dzierżewicz, Z.; Stępień, K. Evaluation of melanogenesis in A-375 melanoma cells treated with 5,7-dimethoxycoumarin and valproic acid. *Cell Mol. Biol. Lett.* **2012**, *17*, 616–632. [CrossRef] [PubMed]
66. Fort, D.M.; Rao, K.; Jolad, S.D.; Luo, J.; Carlson, T.J.; King, S.R. Antihyperglycemic activity of *Teramnus labialis* (Fabaceae). *Phytomedicine* **2000**, *6*, 465–467. [CrossRef]
67. Ding, Z.; Dai, Y.; Hao, H.; Pan, R.; Yao, X.; Wang, Z. Anti-inflammatory effects of scopoletin and underlying mechanisms. *Pharm. Biol.* **2008**, *46*, 854–860. [CrossRef]
68. Marshall, M.E.; Kervin, K.; Benefield, C.; Umerani, A.; Albainy-Jenei, S.; Zhao, Q.; Khazaeli, M.B. Growth-inhibitory effects of coumarin (1, 2-benzopyrone) and 7-hydroxycoumarin on human malignant cell lines in vitro. *J. Cancer Res. Clin.* **1994**, *120*, S3–S10. [CrossRef]
69. Bonaterra, G.A.; Schwarzbach, H.; Kelber, O.; Weiser, D.; Kinscherf, R. Anti-inflammatory effects of Phytodolor®(STW 1) and components (poplar, ash and goldenrod) on human monocytes/macrophages. *Phytomedicine* **2019**, *58*, 152868. [CrossRef]
70. Chu, C.Y.; Tsai, Y.Y.; Wang, C.J.; Lin, W.L.; Tseng, T.H. Induction of apoptosis by esculetin in human leukemia cells. *Eur. J. Pharmacol.* **2001**, *416*, 25–32. [CrossRef] [PubMed]
71. Kalyoncu, F.; Oskay, M.; Kayalar, H. Antioxidant activity of the mycelium of 21 wild mushroom species. *Mycology* **2010**, *1*, 195–199. [CrossRef]
72. Wang, J.; Hu, S.; Nie, S.; Yu, Q.; Xie, M. Reviews on mechanisms of in vitro antioxidant activity of polysaccharides. *Oxid. Med. Cell Longev.* **2016**, *2016*, 5692852. [CrossRef]
73. López-Alarcón, C.; Denicola, A. Evaluating the antioxidant capacity of natural products: A review on chemical and cellular-based assays. *Anal. Chim. Acta.* **2013**, *763*, 1–10. [CrossRef]
74. Valko, M.; Rhodes, C.J.B.; Moncol, J.; Izakovic, M.M.; Mazur, M. Free radicals, metals and antioxidants in oxidative stress-induced cancer. *Chem-Biol. Interact.* **2006**, *160*, 1–40. [CrossRef] [PubMed]
75. Li, Z. Research on Chemical Constituents and Anti-Tumor Activity of *Chroogomphus rutilus*. Master's Thesis, Jilin Agricultural University, Changchun, China, 2014.
76. Mohamed, S.I.A.; Jantan, I.; Haque, M.A. Naturally occurring immunomodulators with antitumor activity: An insight on their mechanisms of action. *Int. Immunopharmacol.* **2017**, *50*, 291–304. [CrossRef]
77. Park, H.J. Current uses of mushrooms in cancer treatment and their anticancer mechanisms. *Int. J. Mol. Sci.* **2022**, *23*, 10502. [CrossRef]
78. Jana, P.; Acharya, K. Mushroom: A new resource for anti-angiogenic therapeutics. *Food Rev. Int.* **2022**, *38*, 88–109. [CrossRef]
79. Luo, C.; Xu, X.; Wei, X.; Feng, W.; Huang, H.; Liu, H.; Xu, R.; Lin, J.; Han, L.; Zhang, D. Natural medicines for the treatment of fatigue: Bioactive components, pharmacology, and mechanisms. *Pharmacol. Res.* **2019**, *148*, 104409. [CrossRef]
80. Zhou, Y.; El-Seedi, H.R.; Xu, B. Insights into health promoting effects and myochemical profiles of pine mushroom *Tricholoma matsutake*. *Crit. Rev. Food Sci.* **2021**, *63*, 5698–5723. [CrossRef] [PubMed]
81. Villaño, D.; Fernández-Pachón, M.S.; Moyá, M.L.; Troncoso, A.M.; García-Parrilla, M.C. Radical scavenging ability of polyphenolic compounds towards DPPH free radical. *Talanta* **2007**, *71*, 230–235. [CrossRef] [PubMed]
82. Losada-Barreiro, S.; Bravo-Diaz, C. Free radicals and polyphenols: The redox chemistry of neurodegenerative diseases. *Eur. J. Med. Chem.* **2017**, *133*, 379–402. [CrossRef] [PubMed]
83. Tsivileva, O.M.; Koftin, O.V.; Evseeva, N.V. Coumarins as fungal metabolites with potential medicinal properties. *Antibiotics* **2022**, *11*, 1156. [CrossRef] [PubMed]
84. Wang, L.; Li, J.Q.; Zhang, J.; Li, Z.M.; Liu, H.G.; Wang, Y.Z. Traditional uses, chemical components and pharmacological activities of the genus Ganoderma P. Karst.: A review. *Rsc. Adv.* **2020**, *10*, 42084–42097. [CrossRef] [PubMed]

85. Roosta, Z.; Hajimoradloo, A.; Ghorbani, R.; Hoseinifar, S.H. The effects of dietary vitamin C on mucosal immune responses and growth performance in *Caspian roach* (*Rutilus rutilus* caspicus) fry. *Fish Physiol. Biochem.* **2014**, *40*, 1601–1607. [CrossRef]
86. Kaur, C.; Kapoor, H.C. Antioxidants in fruits and vegetables–the millennium's health. *Int. J. Food Sci. Tech.* **2001**, *36*, 703–725. [CrossRef]
87. Vázquez, E.L.; García, F.P.; Canales, M.G. Major and trace minerals present in wild mushrooms. *Am.-Eurasian J. Agric. Environ. Sci.* **2016**, *16*, 1145–1158.
88. Aslani, B.A.; Ghobadi, S. Studies on oxidants and antioxidants with a brief glance at their relevance to the immune system. *Life Sci.* **2016**, *146*, 163–173. [CrossRef]
89. Zhang, H.; Yang, X.; Li, Z.; Yu, H. Study on antioxidant activity of *Chroogomphus rutilus* flavonoids in vitro. *Food Res. Dev.* **2016**, *37*, 109–113.
90. Petrushanko, I.; Bogdanov, N.; Bulygina, E.; Grenacher, B.; Leinsoo, T.; Boldyrev, A.; Gassmann, M.; Bogdanova, A. Na-K-ATPase in rat cerebellar granule cells is redox sensitive. *Am. J. Physiol-Reg. I* **2006**, *290*, R916–R925. [CrossRef]
91. Jayathilake, C.; Rizliya, V.; Liyanage, R. Antioxidant and free radical scavenging capacity of extensively used medicinal plants in Sri Lanka. *Procedia Food Sci.* **2016**, *6*, 123–126. [CrossRef]
92. Wolfe, K.L.; Liu, R.H. Cellular antioxidant activity (CAA) assay for assessing antioxidants, foods, and dietary supplements. *J. Agric. Food Chem.* **2007**, *55*, 8896–8907. [CrossRef] [PubMed]
93. Ifeanyi, O.E. A review on free radicals and antioxidants. *Int. J. Curr. Res. Med. Sci.* **2018**, *4*, 123–133.
94. Betteridge, D.J. What is oxidative stress? *Metabolism* **2000**, *49*, 3–8. [CrossRef]
95. Engwa, G.A. Free radicals and the role of plant phytochemicals as antioxidants against oxidative stress-related diseases. In *Phytochemicals: Source of Antioxidants and Role in Disease Prevention*; BoD–Books on Demand: Norderstedt, Germany, 2018; Volume 7, pp. 49–74.
96. Liu, Q.; Zhu, M.; Geng, X.; Wang, H.; Ng, T.B. Characterization of polysaccharides with antioxidant and hepatoprotective activities from the edible mushroom *Oudemansiella radicata*. *Molecules* **2017**, *22*, 234. [CrossRef]
97. Rajendran, K.; Karthikeyan, A.; Krishnan, U.M. Emerging trends in nano-bioactive-mediated mitochondria-targeted therapeutic stratagems using polysaccharides, proteins and lipidic carriers. *Int. J. Biol. Macromol.* **2022**, *208*, 627–641. [CrossRef]
98. Lv, J.; Han, R.; Huang, Z.; Luo, L.; Cao, D.; Zhang, S. Relationship between molecular components and reducing capacities of humic substances. *Acs. Earth Space Chem.* **2018**, *2*, 330–339. [CrossRef]
99. Zhang, H.; Tsao, R. Dietary polyphenols, oxidative stress and antioxidant and anti-inflammatory effects. *Curr. Opin. Food Sci.* **2016**, *8*, 33–42. [CrossRef]
100. Zhang, X.; Sun, H.; Wang, L.; Wang, Y.; Liu, C.; Bai, Y.; Li, J.; Guan, Z. Protective effect of crude polysaccharide from *Chroogomphus rutilus* on MPTP injury in mouse DA neurons. *Mycosystema* **2011**, *30*, 77–84.
101. Zhao, B.; Zhao, J.; Lv, M.; Li, X.; Wang, J.; Yue, Z.; Shi, J.; Zhang, G.; Sui, G. Comparative study of structural properties and biological activities of polysaccharides extracted from *Chroogomphus rutilus* by four different approaches. *Int. J. Biol. Macromol.* **2021**, *188*, 215–225. [CrossRef]
102. Ghiselli, A.; Serafini, M.; Natella, F.; Scaccini, C. Total antioxidant capacity as a tool to assess redox status: Critical view and experimental data. *Free Radical Bio. Med.* **2000**, *29*, 1106–1114. [CrossRef] [PubMed]
103. Lee, S.E.; Hwang, H.J.; Ha, J.S.; Jeong, H.S.; Kim, J.H. Screening of medicinal plant extracts for antioxidant activity. *Life Sci.* **2003**, *73*, 167–179. [CrossRef]
104. Du, J.; Zhang, H.; Chen, P. GC-MS analysis of chemical constituents of fruiting body of *Chroogomphus rutilus* and screening of anti-tumor active components of petroleum ether extract. *Jiangsu Agric. Sci.* **2019**, *10*, 197–201.
105. Ouyang, F.; Wang, G.; Guo, W.; Zhang, Y.; Xiang, W.; Zhao, M. AKT signalling and mitochondrial pathways are involved in mushroom polysaccharide-induced apoptosis and G1 or S phase arrest in human hepatoma cells. *Food Chem.* **2013**, *138*, 2130–2139. [CrossRef]
106. Chen, J.H.; Cao, J.L.; Chu, Y.L.; Wang, Z.L.; Yang, Z.T.; Wang, H.L. T-2 toxin-induced apoptosis involving Fas, p53, Bcl-xL, Bcl-2, Bax and caspase-3 signaling pathways in human chondrocytes. *J. Zhejiang Univ. Sci. B* **2008**, *9*, 455–463. [CrossRef]
107. SEVİNDİK, M. Antioxidant and oxidant potantials and element contents of *Chroogomphus rutilus* (Agaricomycetes). *Mantar Dergisi* **2021**, *12*, 29–32.
108. Hicklin, D.J.; Ellis, L.M. Role of the vascular endothelial growth factor pathway in tumor growth and angiogenesis. *J. Clin. Oncol.* **2005**, *23*, 1011–1027. [CrossRef]
109. Pickard, J.M.; Zeng, M.Y.; Caruso, R.; Núñez, G. Gut microbiota: Role in pathogen colonization, immune responses, and inflammatory disease. *Immunol. Rev.* **2017**, *279*, 70–89. [CrossRef]
110. Sun, M.; He, C.; Cong, Y.; Liu, Z. Regulatory immune cells in regulation of intestinal inflammatory response to microbiota. *Mucosal Immunol.* **2015**, *8*, 969–978. [CrossRef] [PubMed]
111. Asadullah, K.; Sterry, W.; Trefzer, U. Cytokines: Interleukin and interferon therapy in dermatology. *Clin. Exp. Dermatol.* **2002**, *27*, 578–584. [CrossRef] [PubMed]
112. Akpi, U.K. In Vitro Antimicrobial Activities of Some Selected Edible and Non-Edible Mushrooms. Ph.D. Thesis, Universiti Kebangsaan Malaysia, Bangi, Malaysia, 2017.
113. Geng, P.; Siu, K.C.; Wang, Z.; Wu, J.Y. Antifatigue functions and mechanisms of edible and medicinal mushrooms. *Biomed. Res. Int.* **2017**, *2017*, 9648496. [CrossRef]
114. Zhao, S.; Gao, Q.; Rong, C.; Wang, S.; Zhao, Z.; Liu, Y.; Xu, J. Immunomodulatory effects of edible and medicinal mushrooms and their bioactive immunoregulatory products. *J. Fungus* **2020**, *6*, 269. [CrossRef]

115. Jiang, W.; Xu, J. Immune modulation by mesenchymal stem cells. *Cell Proliferat.* **2020**, *53*, e12712. [CrossRef]
116. Cifaldi, L.; Prencipe, G.; Caiello, I.; Bracaglia, C.; Locatelli, F.; De Benedetti, F.; Strippoli, R. Inhibition of natural killer cell cytotoxicity by interleukin-6: Implications for the pathogenesis of macrophage activation syndrome. *Arthritis Rheumatol.* **2015**, *67*, 3037–3046. [CrossRef]
117. Rizza, P.; Moretti, F.; Belardelli, F. Recent advances on the immunomodulatory effects of IFN-α: Implications for cancer immunotherapy and autoimmunity. *Autoimmunity* **2010**, *43*, 204–209. [CrossRef]
118. Ganeshpurkar, A.; Saluja, A. Immunomodulatory effect of rutin, catechin, and hesperidin on macrophage function. *Indian J. Biochem. Bio.* **2020**, *57*, 58–63.
119. Lewis, E.D.; Meydani, S.N.; Wu, D. Regulatory role of vitamin E in the immune system and inflammation. *Iubmb. Life* **2019**, *71*, 487–494. [CrossRef]
120. Mousavi, S.; Bereswill, S.; Heimesaat, M.M. Immunomodulatory and antimicrobial effects of vitamin C. *Eur. J. Microbiol. Immunol.* **2019**, *9*, 73–79. [CrossRef] [PubMed]
121. El-Senousey, H.K.; Chen, B.; Wang, J.Y.; Atta, A.M.; Mohamed, F.R.; Nie, Q.H. Effects of dietary vitamin C, vitamin E, and alpha-lipoic acid supplementation on the antioxidant defense system and immune-related gene expression in broilers exposed to oxidative stress by dexamethasone. *Poultry Sci.* **2018**, *97*, 30–38. [CrossRef] [PubMed]
122. Li, Z. Extraction and Alleviate Physical Fatigue of Polysaccharides from *Gomphidius rutilus*. Master's Thesis, Changchun University of Technology, Changchun, China, 2016.
123. Malaguti, M.; Angeloni, C.; Hrelia, S. Polyphenols in exercise performance and prevention of exercise-induced muscle damage. *Oxid. Med. Cell. Longev.* **2013**, *2013*, 825928. [CrossRef] [PubMed]
124. Xu, C.; Lv, J.; Lo, Y.M.; Cui, S.W.; Hu, X.; Fan, M. Effects of oat β-glucan on endurance exercise and its anti-fatigue properties in trained rats. *Carbohyd. Polym.* **2013**, *92*, 1159–1165. [CrossRef] [PubMed]
125. Filippin, L.I.; Moreira, A.J.; Marroni, N.P.; Xavier, R.M. Nitric oxide and repair of skeletal muscle injury. *Nitric Oxide-Biol. Ch.* **2009**, *21*, 157–163. [CrossRef]
126. Yu, W.; Zeng, D.; Xiong, Y.; Shan, S.; Yang, X.; Zhao, H.; Lu, W. Health benefits of functional plant polysaccharides in metabolic syndrome: An overview. *J. Funct. Foods* **2022**, *95*, 105154. [CrossRef]
127. Gong, L.; Feng, D.; Wang, T.; Ren, Y.; Liu, Y.; Wang, J. Inhibitors of α-amylase and α-glucosidase: Potential linkage for whole cereal foods on prevention of hyperglycemia. *Food Sci. Nutr.* **2020**, *8*, 6320–6337. [CrossRef]
128. Deveci, E.; Çayan, F.; Tel-Çayan, G.; Duru, M.E. Inhibitory activities of medicinal mushrooms on α-amylase and α-glucosidase-enzymes related to type 2 diabetes. *S. Afr. J. Bot.* **2021**, *137*, 19–23. [CrossRef]
129. Lv, M.S. Structure Characterization and Biological Activities of Polysaccharide from *Chroogomphis rutilus*. Master's Thesis, Northeast Forestry University, Harbin, China, 2021.
130. He, X.; Wang, X.; Fang, J.; Chang, Y.; Ning, N.; Guo, H.; Huang, L.; Huang, X.; Zhao, Z. Structures, biological activities, and industrial applications of the polysaccharides from *Hericium erinaceus* (Lion's Mane) mushroom: A review. *Int. J. Biol. Macromol.* **2017**, *97*, 228–237. [CrossRef]
131. Chen, W.; Wu, D.; Jin, Y.; Li, Q.; Liu, Y.; Qiao, X.; Zhang, J.; Dong, G.; Li, Z.; Li, T.; et al. Pre-protective effect of polysaccharides purified from *Hericium erinaceus* against ethanol-induced gastric mucosal injury in rats. *Int. J. Biol. Macromol.* **2020**, *159*, 948–956. [CrossRef] [PubMed]
132. Bequette, B.J. Amino acid metabolism in animals: An overview. *Amino Acids Anim. Nutr.* **2003**, *2*, 103–124.
133. Sirisinha, S. The pleiotropic role of vitamin A in regulating mucosal immunity. *Asian Pac. J. Allergy Immunol.* **2015**, *33*, 71–89.
134. Wu, Q.; Wang, Q.; Fu, J.; Ren, R. Polysaccharides derived from natural sources regulate triglyceride and cholesterol metabolism: A review of the mechanisms. *Food Funct.* **2019**, *10*, 2330–2339. [CrossRef] [PubMed]
135. Ganesan, K.; Xu, B. Anti-diabetic effects and mechanisms of dietary polysaccharides. *Molecules* **2019**, *24*, 2556. [CrossRef] [PubMed]
136. Pérez-Moreno, J.; Martínez-Reyes, M. Edible ectomycorrhizal mushrooms: Biofactories for sustainable development. In *Biosystems Engineering: Biofactories for Food Production in the Century XXI*; Springer International Publishing: Cham, Switzerland, 2014; pp. 151–233.
137. Ghorbanpour, M.; Omidvari, M.; Abbaszadeh-Dahaji, P.; Omidvar, R.; Kariman, K. Mechanisms underlying the protective effects of beneficial fungi against plant diseases. *Biol. Control* **2018**, *117*, 147–157. [CrossRef]
138. Amor, S.; Puentes, F.; Baker, D.; Van Der Valk, P. Inflammation in neurodegenerative diseases. *Immunology* **2010**, *129*, 154–169. [CrossRef]
139. Leszek, J.; E Barreto, G.; Gasiorowski, K.; Koutsouraki, E.; Aliev, G. Inflammatory mechanisms and oxidative stress as key factors responsible for progression of neurodegeneration: Role of brain innate immune system. *Cns. Neurol. Disord-Drug* **2016**, *15*, 329–336. [CrossRef] [PubMed]
140. Chen, S.L.; Chen, Z.G.; Dai, H.L.; Ding, J.X.; Guo, J.S.; Han, N.; Jiang, B.G.; Jiang, H.J.; Li, J.; Li, S.P.; et al. Repair, protection and regeneration of peripheral nerve injury. *Neural. Regen. Res.* **2015**, *10*, 1777. [CrossRef] [PubMed]

Disclaimer/Publisher's Note: The statements, opinions and data contained in all publications are solely those of the individual author(s) and contributor(s) and not of MDPI and/or the editor(s). MDPI and/or the editor(s) disclaim responsibility for any injury to people or property resulting from any ideas, methods, instructions or products referred to in the content.

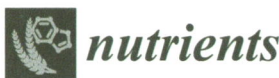 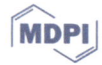

Review

Vaccinium uliginosum and *Vaccinium myrtillus*—Two Species—One Used as a Functional Food

Agnieszka Kopystecka [1], Ilona Kozioł [1], Dominika Radomska [2], Krzysztof Bielawski [2,*], Anna Bielawska [3] and Monika Wujec [4,*

[1] Students' Scientific Circle on Medical Law at the Department of Humanities and Social Medicine, Medical University of Lublin, 20-093 Lublin, Poland; aga.kop@interia.eu (A.K.); ilona.koziol9@gmail.com (I.K.)
[2] Department of Synthesis and Technology of Drugs, Faculty of Pharmacy, Medical University of Bialystok, Kilinskiego 1 Street, 15-089 Bialystok, Poland; dominika.radomska@sd.umb.edu.pl
[3] Department of Biotechnology, Faculty of Pharmacy, Medical University of Bialystok, Kilinskiego 1 Street, 15-089 Bialystok, Poland; anna.bielawska@umb.edu.pl
[4] Department of Organic Chemistry, Faculty of Pharmacy, Medical University of Lublin, 4a Chodzki Str., 20-093 Lublin, Poland
* Correspondence: krzysztof.bielawski@umb.edu.pl (K.B.); monika.wujec@umlub.pl (M.W.)

Abstract: *Vaccinium uliginosum* L. (commonly known as bog bilberry) and *Vaccinium myrtillus* L. (commonly known as bilberry) are species of the genus *Vaccinium* (family *Ericaceae*). The red–purple–blue coloration of blueberries is attributed largely to the anthocyanins found in bilberries. Anthocyanins, known for their potent biological activity as antioxidants, have a significant involvement in the prophylaxis of cancer or other diseases, including those of metabolic origin. Bilberry is the most important economically wild berry in Northern Europe, and it is also extensively used in juice and food production. A review of the latest literature was performed to assess the composition and biological activity of *V. uliginosum* and *V. myrtillus*. Clinical studies confirm the benefits of *V. uliginosum* and *V. myrtillus* supplementation as part of a healthy diet. Because of their antioxidant, anti-inflammatory, anti-cancer, and apoptosis-reducing activity, both bog bilberries and bilberries can be used interchangeably as a dietary supplement with anti-free radical actions in the prevention of cancer diseases and cataracts, or as a component of sunscreen preparations.

Keywords: bog bilberry; *Vaccinium uliginosum*; *Vaccinium myrtillus*; bilberry; bioactive compounds; bioactive natural products; dietary supplement

Citation: Kopystecka, A.; Kozioł, I.; Radomska, D.; Bielawski, K.; Bielawska, A.; Wujec, M. *Vaccinium uliginosum* and *Vaccinium myrtillus*—Two Species—One Used as a Functional Food. *Nutrients* **2023**, *15*, 4119. https://doi.org/10.3390/nu15194119

Academic Editor: Jacqueline Isaura Alvarez-Leite

Received: 18 August 2023
Revised: 20 September 2023
Accepted: 22 September 2023
Published: 23 September 2023

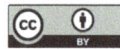

Copyright: © 2023 by the authors. Licensee MDPI, Basel, Switzerland. This article is an open access article distributed under the terms and conditions of the Creative Commons Attribution (CC BY) license (https://creativecommons.org/licenses/by/4.0/).

1. Introduction

Vaccinium uliginosum L. (bog bilberry) and *Vaccinium myrtillus* L. (bilberry) are species of the genus *Vaccinium* (family *Ericaceae*). They are low-growing deciduous shrubs that produce dark purple fruits (berries) which are edible (Figure 1). Commonly called bilberries, their fruits are highly valued as a rich source of anthocyanins, which are naturally occurring compounds. In fresh berries, their content is about 0.5% [1–4]. In addition to fresh fruit, berries can also be consumed as frozen, dried, juices, jams, and food supplements [5]. It has recently become more popular to consume fermented products made from bilberries [6,7]. In vitro studies have shown that bilberry extracts have an impact on the effects of, among other things, anti-glycation and the scavenging of external radicals. Strong antioxidant properties were also found because of the occurrence of abundant bioactive substances, such as anthocyanins and flavanols [1,8,9]. Thanks to these properties, the supplementation of bilberries can have an impact on health in many cases of diseases. Its known pharmacological effects include vascular regulation, dysentery, antigens, diabetic retinopathy, and potential anti-cancer effects [10–14].

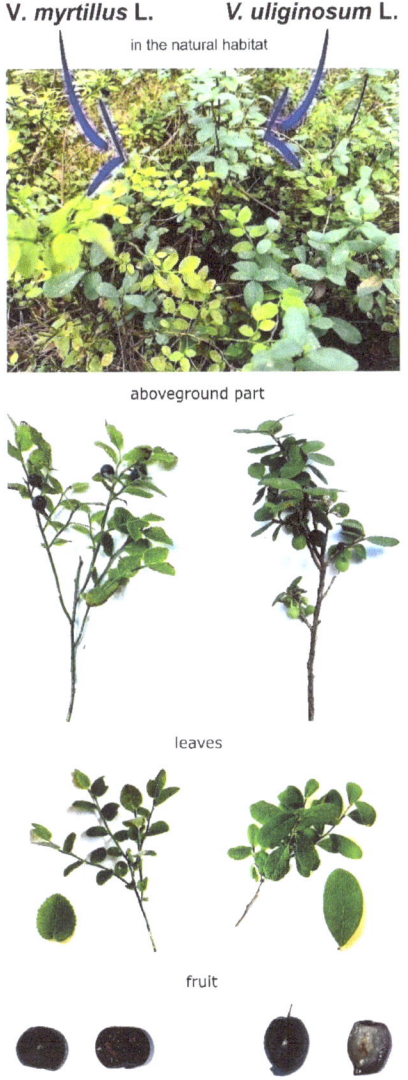

Figure 1. *V. myrtillus* and *V. uliginosum* in their natural habitat and the external appearance of their parts (leaves and fruit).

There are many studies on *Vaccinium* species, but so far there is no comparison of both species, *V. uliginosum* and *V. myrtillus*, especially in terms of their biological activity and possible use as functional food. The biological effect of the fruit extract of *V. uliginosum* is known primarily from both Chinese and European folk medicine. In the presented review, we want to present the similarities and differences between two species growing side by side in their natural habitat.

2. Occurrence

Most *V. myrtillus* and *V. uliginosum* are mainly acquired from their native habitats [15,16]. These members of the *Ericaceae* family grow best in humid and moderate climates. Mountains and high mountains are the most common habitats in their southernmost distribution [17]. *V. myrtillus* is found in European mountains and forests, while *V. uliginosum* grows in areas of Asia, Europe, and North America [18]. *V. uliginosum, V. myrtillus,* and *V. vitis-idaea* are the species that grow on the Iberian Peninsula. Observations of *V. uliginosum* on Portugal's mainland suggest fragmented populations and uncertain survival in the uppermost parts of Serra da Estrela. Serra da Estrela as well as Serra da Freita both have fragmented populations of *V. myrtillus*, but the latter is more plentiful in northern Portugal's mountains [19]. Bilberry (*Vaccinium myrtillus* L.) is the most important economically wild berry in Northern Europe, and it is also extensively used in juice and food production. The bog bilberry is used to a lesser extent, but it is widespread in northern areas [20]. Compared to cultivated species, wild berries have a more complex chemical composition [18]. A very important aspect is also climate and weather conditions, which determine the content of the various bioactive substances (phenolic acids, anthocyanins, etc.) in blueberries [21]. In turn, the qualitative–quantitative composition of phenolic compounds in bilberries depends on the plant parts used, growth stage, and genetic factors [22,23]. For this reason, buyers are interested in the origin of the berries, as those from specific areas or countries often have a higher price. As spectrophotometers are quick and easy to use, they are highly suitable for commercial purposes, especially for evaluating berry quality [24–26].

A study by Urbanaviciene and Dalia et al. determined the physicochemical properties, as well as the levels of total anthocyanins (TAC) and polyphenols (TPC) present in *V. myrtillus* populations, which occur in areas of Northern Europe (Lithuania, Latvia, Finland, and Norway), along with their ability to scavenge free radicals. In the investigation, *V. myrtillus* had pH values ranging from 2.94 to 3.47. Approximately 232.7 to 475.5 mg/100 g of fresh weight (FW) were obtained from the investigated *V. myrtillus* samples. The content of TPC was the highest in Norway and the lowest in Lithuania and varied between 452–902 mg/100 g FW. According to the study, the antioxidant capacity of *V. myrtillus* oscillated between 60.9 and 106.0 mol TE/g FW, with the lowest value in populations from Lithuania and the highest from Norway [27]. The main ingredients that make up more than 50% of the Lithuanian bilberry water extract are cyanidin-3-O-glucoside, cyanidin-3-O-arabinoside, delphinidin-3-O-galactoside, peonidin-3-O-glucoside, petunidin-3-O-glucoside, delphinidin glycosides, and cyanidin [28]. According to Szakiel et al., the content of triterpenoids in the leaves of *V. myrtillus* from wild habitats varies significantly depending on its location in Poland and Finland. Polish leaves were significantly richer in lupeol, and friedelin was only found on Finnish leaves, while taraxasterol was only found on leaves of plants from Poland. Polish leaves contained more than three times as much 2α-hydroxyursolic and 2α-hydroxyoleanolic acids as Finnish leaves, but they had similar levels of oleanolic and ursolic acids [29].

3. *V. uliginosum* and *V. myrtillus* Composition

Blueberry composition depends on the genotype of the plant [30–32]. *V. uliginosum* berries contain many anthocyanins and flavonols. *V. uliginosum* has a characteristic profile of flavonols and anthocyanins compared to other berries of the *Vaccinium* family, which can be used to distinguish bog bilberry from *V. myrtillus* [33]. *V. myrtillus* seeds and oils contain natural antioxidants, anti-inflammatory, anti-atherosclerotic, and anticancer compounds, such as tocochromanols, carotenoids, flavonoids, phytosterols, and phenolic acids [34,35]. The caloric energy intake of fresh bilberries is approximately 45 kcal/100 g. They consist of water (84%), carbohydrates (9.6%), proteins (0.7%), fats (0.4%), and fibers (about 3.5%) [36]. This is compared to dry bilberry, which has 395 kcal/100 g and contains 94% carbohydrates, 3% proteins, and 1.5% fats [37]. The pH value of the bog bilberry's berry (*V. uliginosum* L.) was relatively high (pH = 3.5), and their titratable acidity, in turn, was moderate (1 g of citric acid/100 g). The main identified soluble sugar was fructose (concentration of 2138 ± 149 mg/100 g FW), while glucose was the second in amount (concentration of 1664 ± 121 mg/100 g FW) [38].

3.1. Polyphenols

Polyphenols are a group of naturally occurring compounds found in various plant foods, including berries from the *Vaccinium* genus (Figure 2).

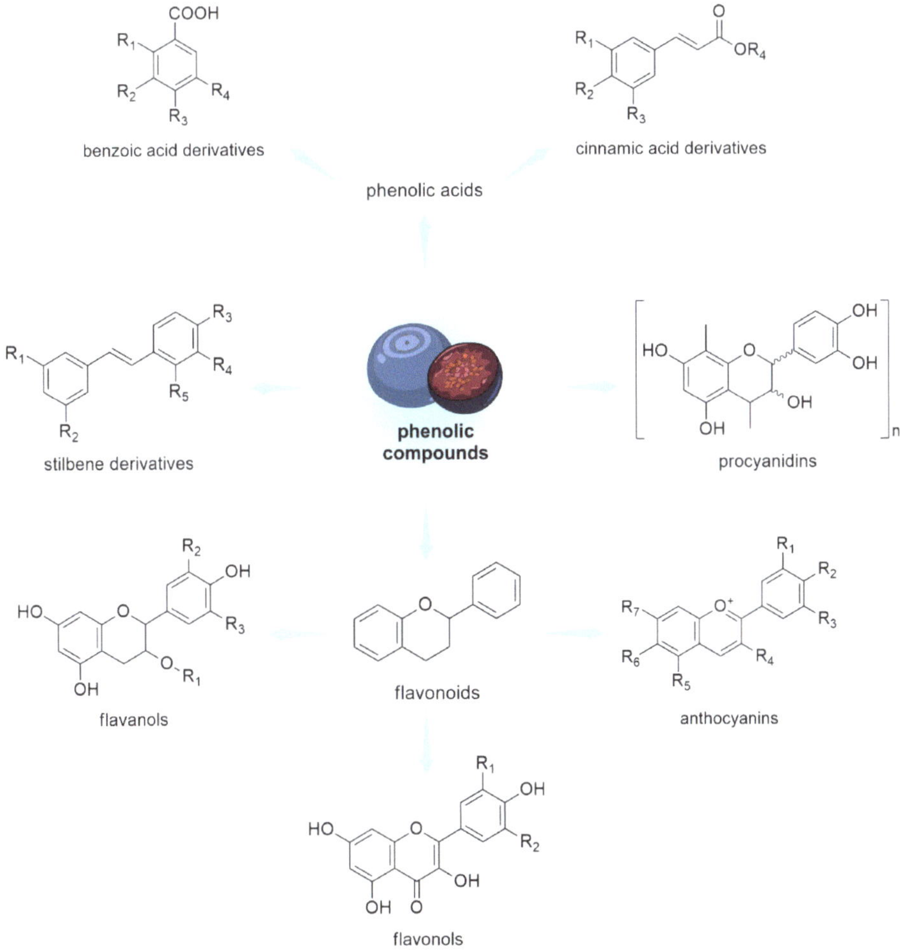

Figure 2. Phenolic compounds in *V. uliginosum* and *V. myrtillus*.

The content and availability of polyphenols in blueberries can be affected by various factors, including agricultural practices, storage, and processing technologies. Organic farming practices, which avoid synthetic pesticides and fertilizers, may promote higher polyphenol content in blueberries. This is because plants often produce more phytochemicals, including polyphenols, as a defense mechanism against pests and diseases. Harvesting techniques are very important too. Picking blueberries at the right ripeness can affect their polyphenol content. Polyphenol levels may increase as the berries ripen [39]. Using gentle harvesting methods to avoid damaging the berries can help preserve their polyphenol content. Proper temperature, pressure, and humidity control during storage are crucial to prevent polyphenol degradation [40]. Cold storage can help maintain polyphenol levels in fresh blueberries. Modified Atmosphere Packaging (MAP) involves adjusting the gas composition inside the packaging to extend the shelf life of blueberries while preserving their polyphenols [41]. Processing technology conditions are the most important factors influencing the content of polyphenols in products made from berries. Freeze drying is a method that can preserve the polyphenol content in blueberries by removing moisture without significant heat exposure, which can degrade polyphenols [42]. Drying blueberries at lower temperatures can help retain their polyphenol content compared to high-temperature drying methods. Processing blueberries into purees or juices can concentrate polyphenols. However, some heat exposure during processing may cause a slight reduction in polyphenol levels. Changes in the phenolic composition of berries may be related to various treatments, including ozone pretreatment using ultrasound [43] or using cold plasma [44].

Conventional methods for polyphenol extraction have limitations and drawbacks, which can include the use of harsh solvents, high energy consumption, and potential degradation of the polyphenols. These drawbacks have led to a growing demand for more sustainable and eco-friendly extraction techniques. To maximize the efficiency of polyphenol extraction while maintaining the total polyphenol content (TPC) and antioxidant capacity of the extract, it is essential to assess and compare different extraction conditions. Some novel technologies such as an ultrasound, microwave, cold plasma, pulsed electric field, and pressurized liquid were used as alternatives assisting the extraction process [45]. Factors such as temperature, pressure, and processing time can significantly influence the outcome.

It is important to note that while these technologies and practices can influence polyphenol content, the specific impact may vary depending on factors such as the blueberry variety and environmental conditions.

Polyphenol compounds in berries of *Vaccinium* spp. were determined by different methods (Table 2).

Table 1. Method of characterization of some polyphenol compounds in berries of *Vaccinium* genus.

Polyphenol Compounds	Method of Characterization	References
delphinidin-3-*O*-galactoside malvidin-3-*O*-galactoside malvidin-3-*O*-arabinoside delphinidin-3-*O*-arabinoside	CIELAB HPLC-DAD	[46]
delphinidin 3-glucoside cyanidin 3-glucoside petunidin 3-glucoside delphinidin 3-glucoside	HPLC-DAD	[47]
chlorogenic acid quercetin-3-*O*-galactoside quercetin-3-*O*-glucuronide delphinidin-3-*O*-galactoside delphinidin-3-*O*-glucoside cyanidin-3-*O*-galactoside petunidin-3-*O*-glucoside	HPLC-UV/DAD HPLC-ESI-MS MS	[48]
delphinidin 3-*O*-glucoside malvidin 3-*O*-glucoside myricetin 3-*O*-hexoside quercetin 3-*O*-galactoside	HPLC-DAD HPLC-ESI-MS	[49]
cyanidin-3-*O*-glucoside cyanidin-3-*O*-rutinoside catechin quercetin-3-*O*-galactoside quercetin-3-*O*-arabinoside myricetin 3-*O*-hexose	HPLC-FT-ICR MS/MS	[50]

Table 2. Method of characterization of some polyphenol compounds in berries of *Vaccinium* genus.

Polyphenol Compounds	Method of Characterization	References
gallic acid vanillic acid ferulic acid caffeic acid *p*-coumaric acid quercetin	HPLC	[51]
(–)-epicatechin kaempferol derivative chlorogenic acid ellagic acid	HPLC	[52]
glycosides of quercetin myricetin kaempferol isorhamnetin syringetin laricitrin	HPLC–MS	[53]

The colors used in Table 2: red—phenolic acids, green—flavonols, and violet—anthocyanins.

Quercetin, kaempferol, phenolic acid, and gentisic acid were the largest fraction of polyphenols identified in *V. myrtillus* extracts [54]. In one of the studies on *V. uliginosum gaultherioides* and *V. myrtillus* berries, differences in terms of relative percentages of total monomeric anthocyanins (TMA) concerning total soluble polyphenols (TSP) were shown, which was the predominant polyphenolic class in blueberry, but this was not observed in bog bilberry [55]. The bog bilberry juice was abundant in myricetin-3-*O*-galactoside and quercetin-3-*O*-galactoside [56]. The ferric reducing antioxidant power (FRAP) test yielded the highest antioxidant capacity values (117 μmol TE/g FW), followed by the oxygen radical absorbance capacity (ORAC) test (84 μmol TE/g FW) [38]. In a study by Wang Yu et al. in 10 different populations of *V. uliginosum* from the Changbai Mountains (China), the content of TF (total flavonoids), TA (total anthocyanins), and TP (total phenols) was assessed, and the spatial distribution and correlation between these components were examined. Fifteen anthocyanins were identified and described, and the amount of malvidin-glucoside, petunidin-glucoside, and delphinidin-glucoside was the highest in this phytochemical group. TF, TA, and TP values were the highest in the Dongfanghong forest farm (DFHI) and the Lanjia forest farm (LJII) populations, respectively. As compared to the other samples, the TF content of the DFHI-8 sample was higher, as was the TA content of the LJIII-1 and the TP content of the LJIII-4. At an altitude from 740 to 838 m, TA and TP content exhibited a positive correlation. In turn, at altitudes >838 m, their dependence showed negative values [57].

Antioxidant properties of juices of bog blueberry (*Vaccinium uliginosum*) were evaluated by ABTS scavenging capacity (RSC), FRAP, ORAC, TPC (total phenolic content), and TAC (total anthocyanin content) assays. The TPC values ranged from 0.85 to 2.81 mg gallic acid equivalent/mL; ORAC, FRAP, and RSC values were 4.21–45.68, 3.07–17.8, and 6.38–20.9 μmol Trolox equivalent/g, respectively. Bog blueberry had a very high TAC, 14.19 mg/100 mL. In the ABTS decolorization test, blueberry juices showed the highest RSC (20.9 μmol TE/g), FRAP (31.99 μmol Fe^{2+}/g and 17.80 μmol TE/g), and ORAC (45.68 μmol TE/g). Bog bilberry, even though it contained moderate amounts of quantified compounds, showed a very high antioxidant capacity; it had a slightly different chromatographic profile. It was found that there was a moderate negative correlation between berry weight and both FRAP and ORAC assays. Berries with a larger mass probably accumulate more macronutrients, e.g., carbohydrates. The values obtained in the FRAP and ORAC assays also correlated with quinic and chlorogenic acid concentrations ($p \leq 0.01$). According to the results of this study, new cultivars exhibiting higher antioxidant capacity can potentially be created through the use of the germplasm of half-highbush blueberry and *V. uliginosum* [58].

The team of Bayazid AB et al. conducted in vitro studies evaluating the antioxidant and anti-inflammatory properties of 70% ethanolic extracts of bilberry. Antioxidant activity was measured by total phenols, flavonoids, and ascorbic acid. Bilberry extract dose-dependently inhibited linoleic acid oxidation and showed free radical elimination activity. This extract reversed pro-inflammatory cytokines such as inducible nitric oxide synthase (iNOS), cyclooxygenase 2 (COX-2), tumor necrosis factor α (TNF-α), and interleukin-6 (IL-6) in LPS (lipopolysaccharide)-induced RAW 264.7 cells and suppressed NO (nitric oxide) generation. It was suggested that *V. myrtillus* blueberry extract is a natural preparation with strong antioxidant properties and acts as an anti-inflammatory agent due to its high concentration of anthocyanins [59].

3.1.1. Flavonols and Flavanols

Latti et al., in their studies, were the first to show the presence of kaempferol and isorhamnetin aglycones in *V. uliginosum*. In their study, about 1/4 of bog blueberry samples contained more flavonols than anthocyanins [33].

One study found that EC (epicatechin) and EGC (epigallocatechin) were the major flavanols in blueberry juice [56]. *V. uliginosum* also contains flavonols such as laricitrin, syringetin, myricetin, and quercetin. Based on the findings of myricetin and quercetin arabinosides, the minor laricitrin, isorhamnetin, and syringing pentosides were further named arabinosides. Both laricitrin and isorhamnetin were also detected in *V. myrtillus* [33]. Laricithrin, isorhamnetin, myricetin, kaempferol, syringetinhexosides, pentosides, and glucuronides, as well as glucuronide and pentosides QUE (quercetin), were identified in bilberry and bog bilberry in various amounts, and flavonol predominance in bog bilberry [55]. Figure 3 shows the chemical structures of flavonols and flavanols (and the sugars to which they are linked) that are contained in *V. uliginosum* and *V. myrtillus*.

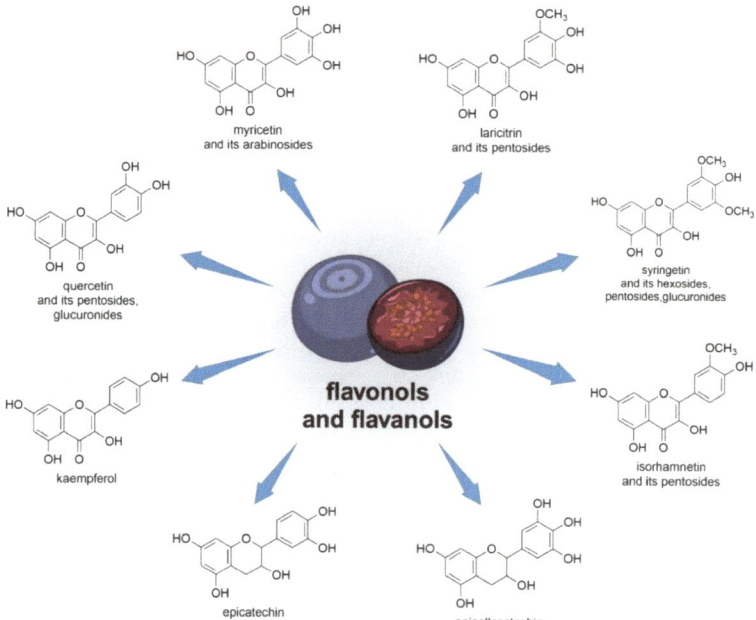

Figure 3. Chemical structures of flavonols and flavanols (and the sugars to which they are linked) that are contained in *V. uliginosum* and *V. myrtillus*.

Due to the very high concentration of quercetin-3-galactoside, the prevalence of quercetin-3-rhamnoside in blueberries contrasts with QUE and its derivatives in *V. uliginosum* subsp. *gaultheroides*. Blueberries contained about ten times more QUE-3-RHA than bog blueberries [55].

3.1.2. Anthocyanins

Compared with some common edible berries, bog bilberries contain more complex anthocyanins [60]. It was found that the TAC in blueberries is about 6 g/kg of fruit [61]. Holkem et al. researched *V. myrtillus* extracts. It was proven that the best antiproliferative effect was shown by an anthocyanin-rich extract due to the abundance of bioactive substances occurring in it; for this extract, there was an elevation in the antioxidative effect after the introduction of bacteria [62]. In one study conducted on *V. myrtillus* juice, results indicated that blueberry juice and cyanidin increased mitochondrial activity and reduced intracellular reactive oxygen species (ROS) generation and hydrogen peroxide-induced lipid peroxidation. In addition, the juice caused an increase in the activity of antiradical enzymes—superoxide dismutase (SOD) and catalase (CAT) [63]. It has been proven that they have antioxidant, anti-cancer, and anti-inflammatory effects and that these compounds can alleviate chronic and acute colitis [64,65]. Bog bilberries were the subject of one study that identified five key anthocyanidins, among which malvidin 3-glucoside was the main compound. It was observed that the TAC fraction showed particularly high variability in antioxidant capacity, which was mainly influenced by the type of phenolic structure that was eluted by solid-phase extraction (SPE) [38].

V. uliginosum, in their structure, have an aglycone part and a glycosyl part. Malvidin, delphinidin, cyanidin, peonidin, and petunidin constitute the aglycone part (Figure 4), while arabinoside, glucoside, xyloside and galactoside belong to the glycosyl part of the compound. In the course of the research, it was observed that specific habitats conditioned noticeable differences in the quantitative composition of anthocyanidin glycosides [33]. Most anthocyanins in *V. uliginosum* derived from B-ring tri-substituted anthocyanidins ($80 \pm 3\%$); the most important was the malvidin-type ($46 \pm 6\%$), followed by cyanidin ($21 \pm 3\%$), delphinidin ($13 \pm 3\%$), petunidin ($13 \pm 0\%$), and peonidin ($7 \pm 1\%$) [38].

V. myrtillus anthocyanin extracts contain at least 16 anthocyanin monomers [66]. In its extract composition were cyanidin-3-O-rutinoside, delphinidin-3-galactoside, delphinidin-3-glucoside, cyanidin-3-galactoside, and chlorogenic acid as the main native phenolic compounds. They were also contained in the extract in smaller amounts of petunidin-3-glucoside, malvidin-3-glucoside, and cyanidin-3-glucoside. Cyanidin-3-O-rutinoside was higher in *V. uliginosum* compared to *V. myrtillus*, accounting for 136.8909 mg/g $\pm$ 11.48 (36.63%) and 43.5743 mg/g $\pm$ 4.01 (26.40%) of total anthocyanins, respectively [50]. The comparative analysis shows that the two *Vaccinium* species have different quantitative compositions of the 15 tested anthocyanins, all at different concentrations ($p < 0.001$). It was found that in bilberry there is a predominance of all target anthocyanins, except for malvidin-3-glucoside (its concentration was 471 mg and 230 mg/100 d.w. for *V. uliginosum* subsp. *gaultherioides* and *V. myrtillus*, respectively). Malvidin derivatives represented a major percentage of the anthocyanins found in bog bilberry—approximately 50% of the total concentration of target anthocyanins. The other anthocyanins identified in *V. uliginosum* occurred as follows (from lowest to highest concentration): peonidin < cyanidin = petunidin < delphinidin. As with *V. myrtillus*, glycoside abundance was also different (70% of the total), with glucosides accounting for 70% of the total, while galactosides and arabinosides were found at very similar percentages (16% and 14%, respectively) [55].

It is known that polyphenols and anthocyanins have a strong impact on antioxidant activity—the higher their content, the more potent their free-radical-eliminating action [67–71]. The team of Kusznierewicz et al. analyzed the content of bioactive substances in samples of wild and bog bilberry from Poland. They determined the content of anthocyanins and polyphenols in dry and fresh samples (Table 3) [72].

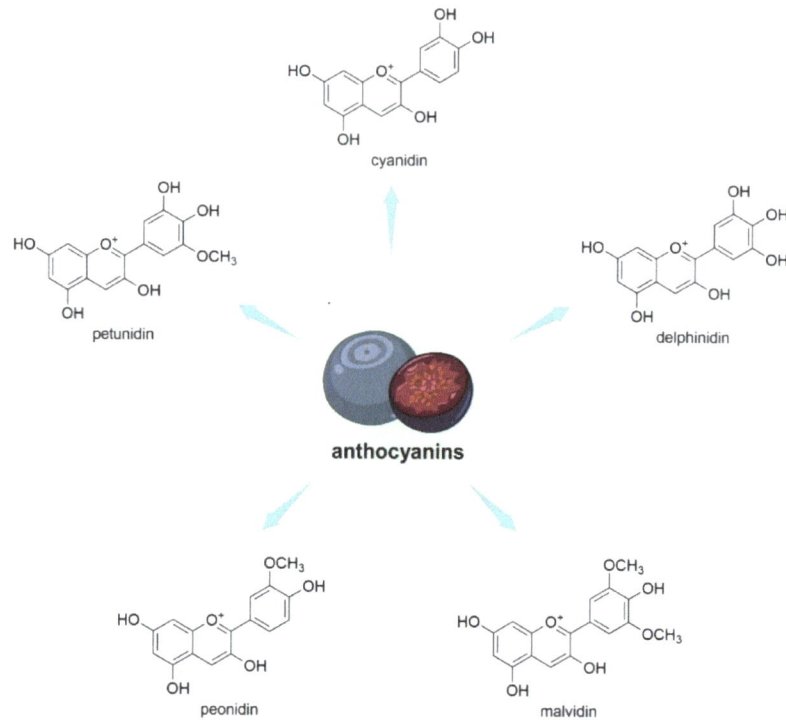

Figure 4. Chemical structures of aglycone parts of anthocyanins (so-called anthocyanidins) that are contained in *V. uliginosum* and *V. myrtillus*.

Table 3. The total content of anthocyanins and other polyphenolic compounds in dry and fresh weight of Polish *V. myrtillus* and *V. uliginosum*.

	Dry Samples		Fresh Samples	
	Total Anthocyanins Content (mg/g)	Total Phenolics Content (mg/g)	Total Anthocyanins Content (mg/g)	Total Phenolics Content (mg/g)
V. myrtillus	21.8 ± 0.1	26.6 ± 0.1	19.4 ± 0.1	23.7 ± 0.1
V. uliginosum	14.3 ± 0.3	21.1 ± 0.3	12.4 ± 0.2	18.2 ± 0.2

The polyphenolic compounds had comparable contents. Furthermore, the antioxidant activity of *V. myrtillus* and *V. uliginosum* was also essentially similar. The obtained results suggested that both berries are a good dietary source of anthocyanins.

3.1.3. Proanthocyanidins

In the dry weight (DW) of *V. uliginosum*, the main monomers and dimers of proanthocyanidins, i.e., procyanidin B2 (Figure 5), EC, phlorizin, taxifolin, gallocatechin, and EGC, were determined using a validated quantitative method. In total, the total procyanidin content was 159.4 µg/g DW, and the main monomers and dimers were EC and procyanidin B2. The content of phlorizin was 2.942 µg/g DW, and that of taxifolin was 2.807 µg/g DW. In turn, gallocatechin and EGC were identified in the tested fruits only in trace amounts [73].

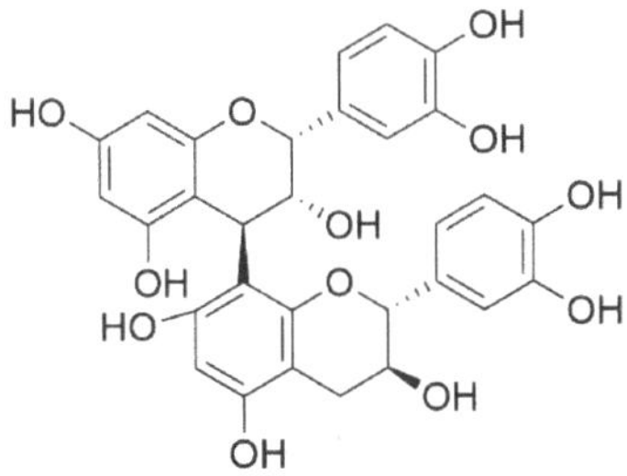

Figure 5. Chemical structures of procyanidin B2 contained in *V. uliginosum*.

3.1.4. Phenolic Acids

The antioxidant effects of *V. myrtillus* fruit were shown to depend on its phenolic content. Researchers found that even very low doses of the compound produced intracellular antioxidant activity [74]. Researchers have also proven that leaves contain more phenolic compounds compared to fruits [75].

It was determined that the main phenolic acids of bog bilberry juice are protocatechuic and chlorogenic acids [56]. The total content of phenolic acids in the dry matter of bilberries is approximately 2 mg/g [73]. Similar contents of flavonoids (EC and quercetin-3-glucoside) and *p*-coumaric acid were found in *V. uliginosum* and *V. myrtillus*. It was reported that *V. uliginosum* subsp. *gaultherioides* contains twenty-fold chlorogenic acid than *V. myrtillus*. Blueberries contained about ten times more cryptochlorogenic acid (Figure 5) than bog bilberries [55]. Ellagic, gallic, *p*-coumaric, ferulic, and syringic acids constitute a higher percentage of phenolic and hydroxycinnamic acids in *V. myrtillus* fruits. Moreover, the fruit of *V. myrtillus* also contains small quantities of vanillic acid, salicylic acid, and hydroxybenzoic acid [75].

In one study, the quantitative composition of eleven phenolic acids (Figure 6) and seventeen anthocyanin 3-glycosides in *V. uliginosum* was identified and determined. Caffeic acid (351 and 1076 µg/100 g in free and glycoside form, respectively) and syringic acid (in ester form 3524 µg/100 g FW) were the main phenolic acids of bog bilberry. It is also worth mentioning that the content of major phenolic acids in *Vaccinium* berries seems to suggest intra- and interspecies differences [38].

3.2. Other Organic Acids

Bilberry fruits also contain simple organic acids (citric/shikimic/malic/quinic acid; Figure 7) [75]. Among the main organic acids, in terms of concentration, in *V. uliginosum* are citric acid, malic acid, and ascorbic acid, with concentrations of 172 ± 11, 21 ± 4, and 12 ± 1 mg/100 g FW, respectively [34].

3.3. PUFAs (Polyunsaturated Fatty Acids)

PUFAs (polyunsaturated fatty acids) are a group of exogenous fatty acids that have to be supplemented through food. This is because the human organism lacks the enzymes needed to form double bonds in the chain of fatty acids outside C-9; thus, they cannot be synthesized in our body. Fatty acids *n*-3 and *n*-6 are part of phospholipids, which are important building components of cell membranes. Importantly, the proportion of these acids in tissues depends on their dietary intake. In addition to the above, they are also essential compounds during the synthesis of many biologically active molecules, for example, prostaglandins [34].

One study evaluated the chemical properties of cold-extracted native oils from *V. myrtillus* seeds to identify the qualitative composition of the fatty acids they contain and their positional distribution. It has been proven that seeds of *V. myrtillus* are abundant in PUFAs. The analysis conducted in this study showed a high α-linolenic acid (*n*-3) content in *V. myrtillus* oil, which was 28.99%. Additionally, oleic acid was detected as the predominant one in bilberry—21.02%. A very important and particularly desirable aspect of human nutrition is that vegetable oils in people's diets should be characterized by a low n-6/n-3 acid ratio. *V. myrtillus* oils have been shown to have an n-3/n-6 ratio of 1–2, indicating that they may be beneficial in people after heart attacks and cardiac surgery [34]. Figure 8 contains the chemical formulas of the fatty acids detected in *V. myrtillus* seed oil.

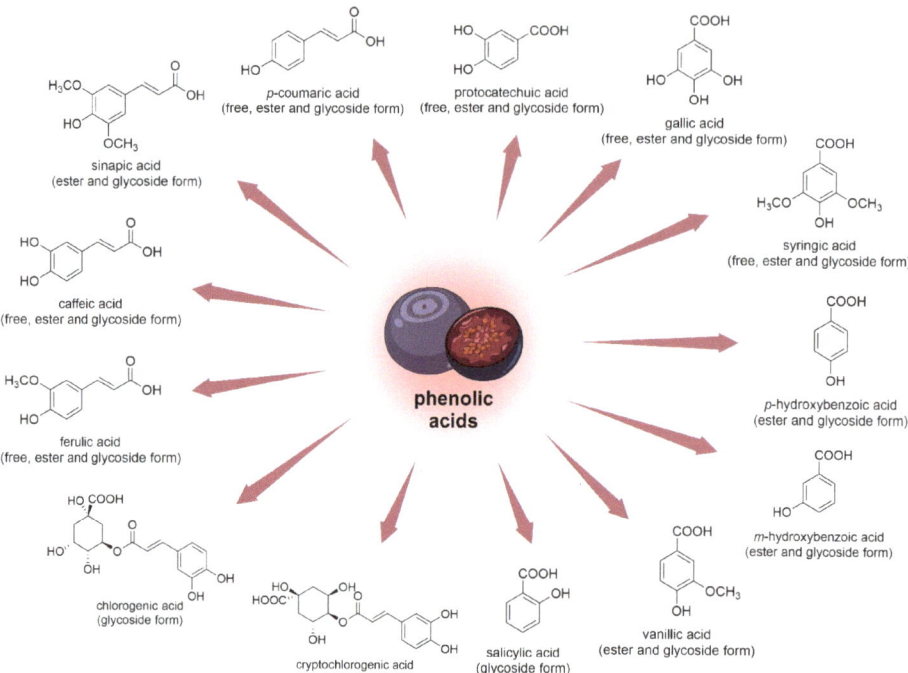

Figure 6. Chemical structures of phenolic acids (and their forms) that are contained in the fruits of *V. uliginosum* and *V. myrtillus* [38,55].

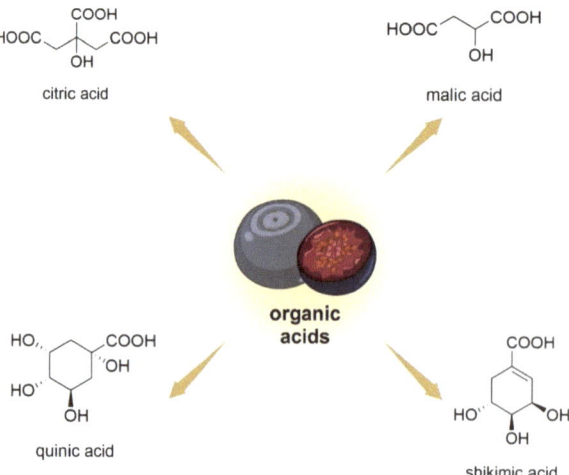

Figure 7. Chemical structures of organic acids that are contained in *V. uliginosum* and *V. myrtillus* fruits.

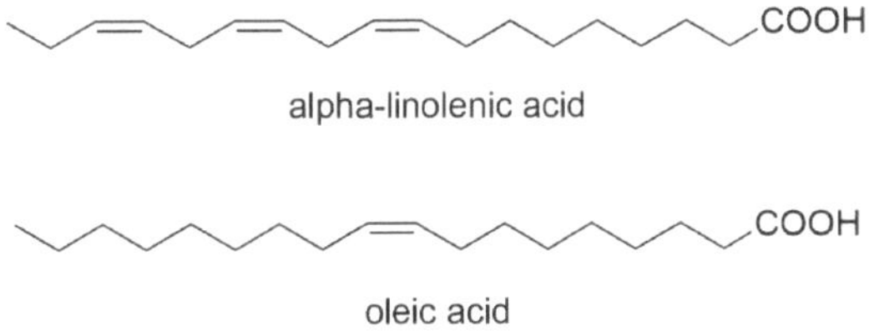

Figure 8. Chemical structures of fatty acids that are contained in *V. myrtillus* seed oil.

3.4. α-Tocopherol

Bederska-Łojewska D. et al. found that *V. myrtillus* seed oils have higher levels of α-tocopherol (Figure 9) than commercial tocopherol-rich oils (made from soybean and corn), and 4.84 mg of vitamin E were found per 100 g of blueberry [34].

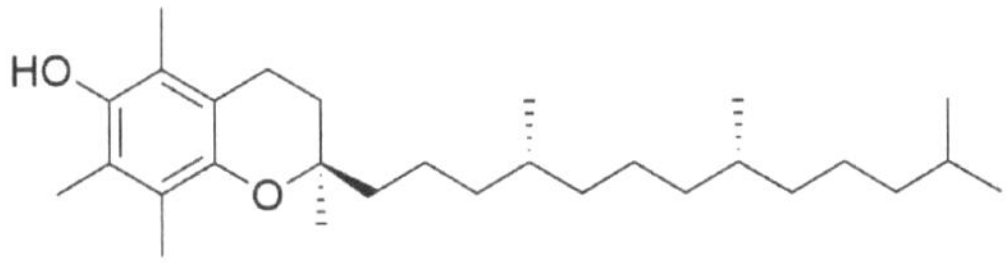

Figure 9. Chemical structure of α-tocopherol.

4. Composition and Potential of Wax

The surfaces of the berries are covered by a specific waxy epidermis. Its main purpose is to protect against harmful UV radiation and prevent excessive water loss. The composition and morphology of bilberry and bog bilberry epidermal waxes were investigated. The study found that the composition of bog bilberry wax was characterized by a predominance of fatty acids, while bilberry was abundant in triterpenoids. In bilberry wax, it was discovered triterpene compounds (alcohols, i.e., lupeol, α- and β-amyrin, and acids, i.e., ursolic acid, oleanolic acid), while bog bilberry contained only triterpene acids—oleanolic acid and ursolic acid (3.1% and 1.8%, respectively) [20]. Wax content per berry increased throughout fruit development, reaching 367.6 g. Based on GC-MS analysis, triterpenoids, primary alcohols, fatty acids, compounds containing a carbonyl group (aldehydes, ketones), and alkanes predominate in the cuticular wax of fruit. Cuticular wax is generally composed of oleanolic acid as its dominant triterpenoid. As bilberry fruits develop, their wax composition changes. The proportion of triterpenoids in bilberries decreased during fruit development and the proportion of total aliphatic compounds increased [76]. The epidermal wax of bog bilberry was characterized by a predominance of fatty acids (54.8% of the total), among which arachidic acid was found in the highest amount. In bilberry, fatty acids accounted for 31.7% of the quantitative composition, and montanic acid and cerotic acid were dominant. Alkanes represented a minor part of the cuticular wax of both bilberry (2.4%) and bog bilberry (1.4%). The wax contained 10.3% aldehydes in bilberry and 7.2% bog bilberry, respectively, and octacosanal was the dominant aldehyde in both species. In turn, the fraction containing ketones was the second most quantitative component of bilberry wax (22.5% of the total), of which 2-heneicosanone was the most abundant ketone. Minor quantities of ketones were also detected in blueberry fruit wax (3.6%) [20]. The identified compounds that are the dominant part of the wax of *V. uliginosum* and *V. myrtillus* are shown in Figure 10.

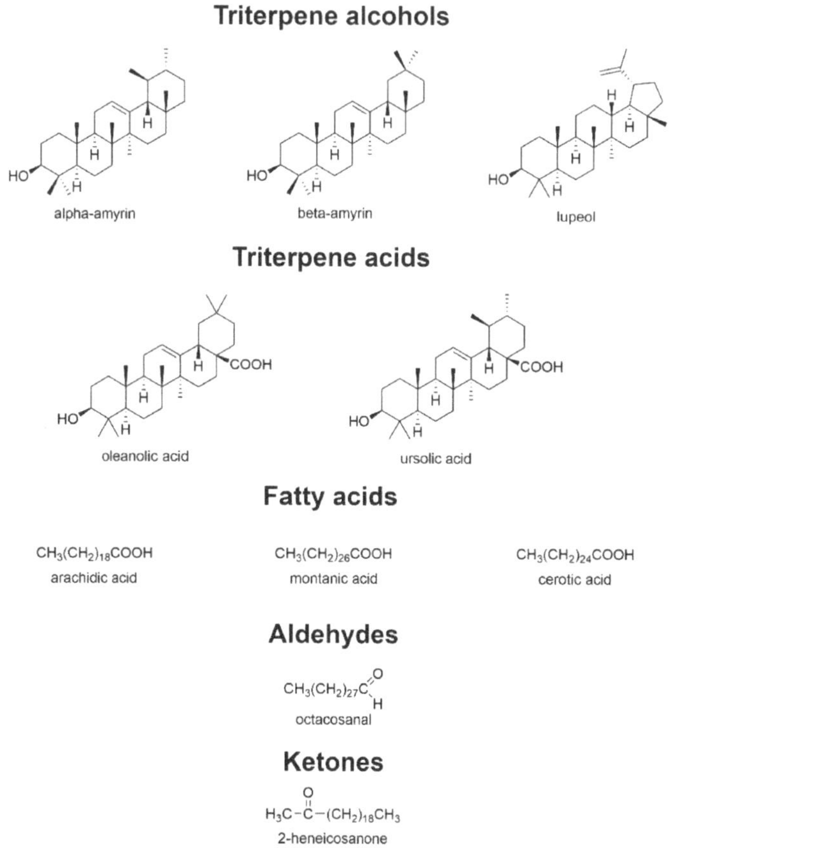

Triterpene alcohols

alpha-amyrin   beta-amyrin   lupeol

Triterpene acids

oleanolic acid   ursolic acid

Fatty acids

$CH_3(CH_2)_{18}COOH$
arachidic acid

$CH_3(CH_2)_{26}COOH$
montanic acid

$CH_3(CH_2)_{24}COOH$
cerotic acid

Aldehydes

$CH_3(CH_2)_{27}CHO$
octacosanal

Ketones

$H_3C-CO-(CH_2)_{18}CH_3$
2-heneicosanone

Figure 10. Chemical structures of compounds that are the dominant part of the wax of *V. uliginosum* and *V. myrtillus*.

5. The Use of Berries

5.1. Dermatology

Kyungae et al. investigated the photoprotective properties of the *V. uliginosum* dietary extract in hairless mice irradiated with ultraviolet B (UVB) radiation. In their study, *V. uliginosum* induced significant alterations in the water retention ability of the skin, TEWL (transepidermal water loss), and parameters related to wrinkles and skin thickness. Oral administration of *V. uliginosum* induced the upregulation of TIMP (tissue inhibitor of metalloproteinase) and antioxidant-related genes, and simultaneously reduced MMP (matrix metalloproteinase) expression. In addition, it was also responsible for a decrease in the levels of p38 protein, JNK (c-Jun N-terminal kinase), inflammation-activated cytokines, and UVB-induced ERK (extracellular signal-regulated kinase) phosphorylation. Additionally, *V. uliginosum* extract enriched in anthocyanins after the oral application had a positive effect on the condition and appearance of the skin after exposure to UV radiation [77]. One study investigated the potential of berry wax to block UV-B radiation. The highest SPF (sun protection factor) showed bog bilberry fruit cuticle wax. The presence of cinnamic acid and vitamin E is probably responsible for high SPF levels. Compared to lingonberry wax (supercritical fluid extraction), bilberry wax has higher levels of α-tocopherol and cinnamic acid, while bog bilberry cuticular wax is rich in cinnamic acid [20].

V. uliginosum extract has also been proven to be excellent for use in dietary supplements designed to take care of skin conditions, due to its abundant anthocyanin content and its anti-free radical activity [77]. One study tested the ability of anthocyanins from *V. myrtillus* to pass through the outer layer of the epidermis and prevent damage caused by the sun. A nanoberry (approximately 100 nm in diameter) exhibiting various elastic properties passed through the outer layer of the epidermis without causing harm. HaCaT cells (normal epidermal cells) in the nanoberry-containing environment remained further viable, despite being exposed to UV radiation. It was found that nanoberries can be actively taken up by cells, and the substances transported by them exhibit health-promoting effects for the skin, protect against UV radiation and facilitate wound healing [78].

Another study evaluated a topical formulation of *V. myrtillus* bilberry leaf extract and bilberry seed oil, which is a by-product of food production. In the leaf extract, the presence of chlorogenic acid was revealed as the most numerous among the phenolic acids, flavonoids—in the largest amount of isoquercetin and resveratrol—while in seed oil, the essential unsaturated fatty acids ω-3 and ω-6 were identified in a preferred proportion, close to 1. The anti-free radical potency was also assessed by wild blueberry extract and seed oil. In a study involving healthy volunteers, the impact of topically applied oil-in-water (o/w) creams containing these wild bilberry isolates was studied. Using wild bilberry isolates as active ingredients, o/w cream was found to improve the skin barrier function and tolerability, as well as retain the pH value of the skin and significantly increase stratum corneum hydration. A cream formulated with wild bilberry isolates as biologically active compounds may be used to treat skin disorders associated with oxidative stress and/or dry skin in addition to their good sensory properties [79].

5.2. Ophthalmology

V. uliginosum extract contains numerous antioxidant compounds, the supplementation of which has a proven effect in alleviating the symptoms of dry eye [80–82]. In a randomized, double-blind study, participants were divided into two groups—the study group (29 subjects) and the control group (30 subjects). The study group received oral tablets with *V. uliginosum* extract (1000 mg/day, total polyphenol content 9.1 mg/g) and the control group took a placebo (lactose). The duration of the trial was 4 weeks. The study proved that taking *V. uliginosum* extract significantly alleviated the visual discomfort caused by working in front of a computer and tablet screen. In the study group, they suggested significant improvement, including questions about "tired eyes" ($p = 0.001$), "irritated eyes" ($p = 0.010$), "eye pain" ($p = 0.038$), "watery eyes" ($p = 0.005$), "dry eyes" ($p = 0.003$), "visual discomfort" ($p = 0.018$), and "blurred vision" ($p = 0.035$). The control group showed improvement only for "tired eyes" ($p = 0.002$) and "irritated eyes" ($p = 0.033$) [83].

Researchers demonstrated that *V. uliginosum* extracts protected retinal cells from light-induced damage [84]. One study investigated the protective action of anthocyanins isolated from *V. uliginosum* on retinal cells against damage caused by microwave radiation. The study determined the cell apoptosis index (AI), malondialdehyde (MDA), glutathione (GSH), and SOD activity. The mRNA expression levels of HO-1 (heme oxygenase-1) and Nrf2 (nuclear factor 2-related factor 2) proteins were also investigated. The rate of cell apoptosis was reported to be notably elevated in the control group in comparison to the *V. uliginosum* treatment group, and the decrease in AI was correlated with dose. MDA and GSH in the study group were also lower and SOD activity was significantly higher. The expression of mRNA Nrf2 and HO-1 proteins increased marginally after irradiation and rose in the treated group. Based on this study, it was revealed that anthocyanins extracted from *V. uliginosum* have a stabilizing effect on the cell membrane, reduce apoptosis, and alleviate oxidative stress-induced damage to mouse retinal photoreceptor cells. Activation of the Nrf2/HO-1 signaling pathway and induction of HO-1 enzyme expression may be responsible for the above mechanism [85].

In a study carried out by Choi et al., the effect of *V. uliginosum* L. on cataract formation in Sprague–Dawley (SD) rat pups was assessed. The morphological analysis of the lens showed that the use of extract inhibits m-calpain-mediated proteolysis, PARP (Poly (ADP)-ribose polymerase) cleavage, and oxidative stress in the lens. *V. uliginosum* suppressed cataract development in a dose-dependent manner by preserving the expression of Nrf-2/HO-1 pathway proteins, maintaining cellular antioxidant protection, and inhibiting the insolubility of soluble proteins, including crystallins [86].

The team of Yoon SM et al. evaluated the effectiveness of *V. uliginosum* L. (VU) and its fractions in the prevention of AMD (age-related macular degeneration) development in human RPE (retinal pigment epithelium) cells exposed to blue light (ARPE-19 cells). During the viability assay, ARPE-19 cells were treated simultaneously with A2E (*N*-retinyl-*N*-retinylidene ethanolamine) and VU (or a fraction thereof). It was observed that after the exposure of ARPE-19 cells to A2E and blue light, the total protein level declined by 55%, which implies a reduced cell survival by blue light-induced A2E photooxidation. In turn, the treatment of the tested cells with VU (concentration of 500 µg/mL) resulted in a 28.7% reduction in the percentage of dead cells (in comparison with the A2E-BL group) after exposure to blue light. A fast atom bombardment mass spectrometry (FAB-MS; cell-free system) analysis revealed that anthocyanin and polyphenol decreased the A2E oxidation peak. The results of this study show that anthocyanin and polyphenol efficiently suppress the A2E oxidation induced by blue light exposure. VU extract, as well as its fractions, have a prophylactic action on RPE cell damage and AMD induced by blue light exposure [87–89]. FH (fraction of *Vaccinium uliginosum* L.) suppressed PMA-induced activity of AP1 and NF-κB proteins in a dose-dependent manner in A549 cells. In the course of the study, it was found that treatment using FH induced a reduction in *CXCL2* and *RASD1* gene expression and exerted antioxidant activity ($\downarrow$ROS) in comparison with A2E-laden RPE cells illuminated with blue light [89].

The team of Lee BL et al. conducted a study in which RPEs were tested for their resistance to damage from blue light using polyphenol-containing extracts. According to their findings, *V. uliginosum* extract and eluted fractions may be possibly used as a therapy strategy for age-related macular degeneration [88].

Additionally, for studies using *V. myrtillus* and/or *V. uliginosum*, we highlight two clinical trials in the field of ophthalmology investigating the impact of extracts from these plants on the organ of vision. The first of them (NCT number: NCT04063644) was designed to study the efficacy of eye drops containing *V. myrtillus* in their composition in the course of dry eye syndrome and their effect on improving visual acuity [90]. Meanwhile, the second trial (NCT number: NCT02641470) evaluated the preventive action of *V. uliginosum* extract against asthenopia induced by spending time in front of a computer monitor. Pills containing 1000 mg/day of *V. uliginosum* extract (DA9301) or a placebo were given orally to participants for 4 weeks, and then the results were assessed using an appropriate questionnaire [91].

5.3. Gynecology

In the study, Ozlem et al. *V. myrtillus* prevented I/R (ischemia-reperfusion) injury in ovarian tissue. In the control group (without receiving medication) that underwent 1-h ischemia and 2-h reperfusion ovary, malondialdehyde (MDA) levels were notably elevated, and enzymatic activities of CAT and SOD were markedly decreased compared to groups with the same damage but receiving a single dose of 200 mg/kg *V. myrtillus*. Moreover, in a histopathologic examination, the damage to ovarian tissues was significantly greater and had a significantly higher DNA damage and apoptosis in the group without a dose of *V. myrtillus*. As part of a gynecology practice, ovarian torsion is diagnosed and subsequently treated medically. This treatment, unfortunately, has limited protective effects if ovarian torsion occurs [92].

The treatment of ovarian cancer is a tremendous challenge for clinicians because it is often chemoresistant. In one study, the antiproliferative activity of 36% anthocyanin-enriched *V. myrtillus* extract in ovarian cancer cells that were sensitive and resistant to conventional chemotherapeutic treatment was studied. The tested mixture consisted of delphinidin, cyanidin, malvidin, peonidin and petunidin (in the proportion 33:28:16:16:7, respectively), which were in glycosylated forms. The above results lead to the conclusion that this mixture can sensitize chemotherapy-resistant ovarian cancer cells and reduce, in a dose-dependent manner, the effective dose of cisplatin required for a therapeutic response. Additionally, this study provides some evidence suggesting the possible benefits of combining conventionally used paclitaxel with a naturally derived product such as berry anthocyanidins in the treatment of chemo-resistant ovarian tumors [93].

5.4. Diabetology

Bilberry polyphenols have been shown to positively impact metabolic health in several animal studies, but studies are often conducted with pharmacological doses that have little nutritional relevance [94–96].

Recent studies show that protein tyrosine phosphatase 1B (PTP1B) and α-glycosidase have demonstrated effectiveness in controlling type 2 diabetes. Alternative treatment methods for this disease may include combined therapeutic strategies. By inhibiting these enzymes, polysaccharides may be absorbed and disintegrated more slowly, and blood glucose levels may rise more quickly post-prandial. In the insulin signaling pathway, the overexpression of PTP1B can inhibit insulin expression as a negative regulator [97]. The anthocyanins from *V. uliginosum* are the most potent inhibitors of PTP1B (IC_{50}= 3.06 ± 0.02 μg/mL). Based on the molecular docking research, cyanidin-3-O-glucoside had the lowest affinity for inhibiting PTP1B versus any other skeleton, whereas cyanidin-3-O-glucoside exhibited the highest affinity for inhibiting PTP1B (binding energy (E_B) = −7.8 kcal/mol), interacting with its two binding sites [98].

A randomized, double-blind, placebo-controlled crossover study was conducted on 20 patients. The treatment lasted 4 weeks. The study design involved receiving two capsules twice a day and was divided into two arms—the placebo group (starch) and the intervention group (*V. myrtillus*; 1.4 g/day of anthocyanin extract). After the treatment period, there was a 6-week procedure for the washout of the drug from the body, after which the patients' treatment regimen was switched. The study enrolled patients diagnosed with type 2 diabetes treated with hypoglycemic drugs with a BMI (body mass index) > 23 kg/m^2 and no evidence of cardiovascular disease. In the group that supplemented with bilberry, there was a tendency to reduce fasting glucose and HBA1c levels; in the placebo group, this relationship was not noticed. This may indicate that higher doses or longer duration of treatment may favor glycemic control [99]. In another study, aqueous and methanol extracts were proven to be effective α-glucosidase inhibitors. Through the inhibition of α-glucosidase by *V. myrtillus* extracts, patients with type 2 diabetes can control their glycemic level through diet [100].

In a study by Xingguo Li et al., a new polysaccharide fraction (VUP-1) from *V. uliginosum* L. was obtained using pressurized water extraction, and purified using a polyamide resin column and column chromatography. VUP-1, from the fruits of *V. uliginosum* L., is a heteropolysaccharide consisting of galacturonic acid, galactose, glucose, mannose, and arabinose, with an MW (molecular weight) of 4.98×10^4 kDa. The inhibition of α-amylase by VUP-1 is moderate and characterized by high antioxidant activities. Furthermore, VUP-1 inhibits dicarbonyl compound formation. The results indicate that VUP-1 had an uptake effect on free radicals (OH and DPPH) in a dose-dependent manner ($p < 0.05$). The results of this study indicate that polysaccharides from *V. uliginosum* L. could potentially be used as oral hypoglycemic agents [101].

Kim J et al. conducted a study to determine whether *V. myrtillus* bilberry helps prevent diabetes-induced retinal vascular dysfunction in vivo. Streptozotocin-induced diabetic rats were orally fed *V. myrtillus* extract (VME; 100 mg/kg) for 6 weeks. Diabetic rats undergoing treatment with VME exhibited a notable decline in fluorescein leakage in fluorescein-dextran angiography. VME treatment reduced specific indicators of diabetic retinopathy, such as the degradation of OCLN (occludin), ZO-1 (zonula occludens-1), CLDN5 (claudin-5), and VEGF (retinal vascular endothelial growth factor) expression in diabetic rats. It has been proven that VME can prevent or retard the development of early diabetic retinopathy [102].

In a study by Pemmari T et al. conducted in obese mice induced by a high-fat diet, the effects of dried blueberry powder on parameters such as body weight increase, systemic inflammation, glucose/lipid metabolism, and changes in gene expression in liver and adipose tissue were investigated. Blueberry supplementation prevented the rise of alanine transaminase (ALT; a marker of liver damage) and many proteins involved in the inflammatory response, such as serum amyloid A (SAA), CXC chemokine ligand 14 (CXCL14) and monocyte chemoattractant protein-1 (MCP1) induced by the high-fat diet. As a result of blueberry supplementation, serum insulin, glucose, and cholesterol concentrations were partly reduced, systemic and hepatic inflammation was suppressed, and undesirable changes in glucose/lipid metabolism were retarded. Consequently, blueberry supplementation appeared to support a healthier metabolic phenotype during obesity development [103].

Type 2 diabetes is very often not a single disease entity in the people suffering from it. Most patients are diagnosed with multiple coexisting factors associated with the development of this disease, among others, including impaired glucose tolerance or dyslipidemia and associated further atherosclerosis [104]. Table 4 shows clinical trials investigating the effects of *V. myrtillus*, not only on type 2 diabetes but also in the above-mentioned metabolic disorders.

Table 4. Clinical trials evaluating the effects of *V. myrtillus* on metabolic disorders. This table is compiled from the information available at https://www.clinicaltrials.gov/, accessed on 9 August 2023.

NCT Number	Study Title	Clinical Trial Status	Study Design	Condition	References
NCT01860547	The Effect of the Bioactives of Sea Buckthorn and Bilberry on the Risk of Metabolic Diseases	Not applicable	Randomized, open-label, crossover assignment	• Type 2 Diabetes • Atherosclerosis	[105]
NCT01414647	The Effect of Diet Rich in Nordic Berries on Gut Microbiota, Glucose and Lipid Metabolism and Metabolism on Fenolic Compounds	Not applicable	Randomized, open-label, crossover assignment	• Metabolic Syndrome • Impaired Glucose Tolerance • Low-grade Inflammation • Dyslipidemia	[106]
NCT03415503	Anthocyanin Supplementation Improves Blood Lipids in a Dose-response Manner in Subjects with Dyslipidemia	Phase 3	Randomized, double-blind (participant, investigator), parallel assignment	• Dyslipidemia	[107]
NCT04054284	Safety and Efficacy of a Complex Herbal Tea Mixture in Type 2 Diabetics	Not applicable	Randomized, quadruple-blind (participant, care provider, investigator, outcomes assessor), parallel assignment	• Type 2 Diabetes	[108]

5.5. Cardiology

In the clinical picture of cardiovascular disease, high levels of circulating microvesicles (MVs) and an increased risk of atherosclerosis can be distinguished. A study available in the literature evaluated the effect of bilberry extract (BE) on participants' MV levels and its impact on endothelial vesicles in vitro. Patients with myocardial infarction were supplemented with BE for eight weeks. The findings showed that BE supplementation positively affected the MV profile in participants' blood and decreased extracellular vesicle release via a P2X7 receptor-dependent mechanism. The cardioprotective effect of blueberries has been proven [109]. The antioxidant properties of *V. myrtillus* may partly explain its ability to protect rats from doxorubicin (DOX)-induced cardiotoxicity. DOX-induced elevations of lactate dehydrogenase (LDH), creatine phosphokinase (CPK), creatine kinase-myocardial band (CK-MB), and troponin I (TNI) activity in serum were significantly inhibited by bilberries. The treatment with *V. myrtillus* reduced the severity of histological lesions in rat tissue sections (Figure 11) [110].

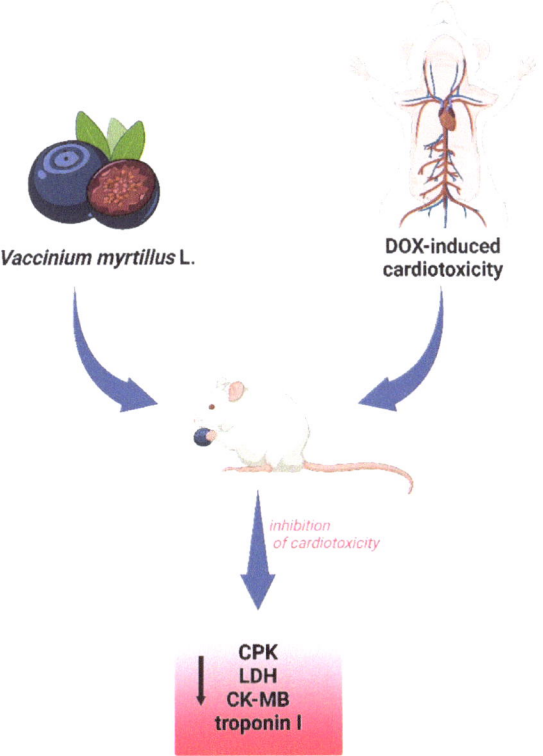

Figure 11. Cardioprotective effect of *V. myrtillus* against doxorubicin toxicity. DOX—doxorubicin, CPK—creatine phosphokinase, CK-MB—creatine kinase-myocardial band, and LDH—lactate dehydrogenase.

Habanova M et al. conducted a study of 25 women and 11 men who ate frozen blueberries (3 times a week, 150 g each) for 6 weeks. The consumption of blueberries resulted in decreased parameters of glucose ($p = 0.005$), γ-glutamyltransferase ($p = 0.046$), albumin ($p = 0.001$), TG (triglyceride; $p = 0.001$), total cholesterol (TC; $p = 0.017$), LDL-C (low-density lipoprotein cholesterol; $p = 0.0347$), and elevated HDL-C (high-density lipoprotein cholesterol; $p = 0.044$). Additionally, in the male population, a positive influence of bilberry consumption on albumin ($p = 0.028$), γ-glutamyltransferase ($p = 0.013$), aspartate aminotransferase ($p = 0.012$), glucose ($p = 0.015$), TC ($p = 0.004$), and HDL-C ($p = 0.009$) was observed, with a rise in LDL-C ($p = 0.007$) also noted. The study showed that the systematic consumption of blueberries may reduce the risk of cardiovascular disease by lowering the levels of TG and LDL-C with a simultaneous increase in HDL-C [111]. In another study of 32 adult rats supplemented with *V. myrtillus* powder (2 g/day) for four weeks, a significant improvement in diabetic dyslipidemia was observed by lowering TC, TG, LDL-C, and

VLDL-C in plasma [112]. The studies show that regularly consuming frozen bilberries for even a short period can improve humans' lipid profile [111].

In one study conducted on rats, it was proven that *V. myrtillus* bilberry anthocyanin (BA) notably enhanced total antioxidant ability, total CAT and SOD activity, leading to reduced levels of glycated serum protein (GSP), MDA, TG, TC LDL-C and lower Castelli Index I and II values (TC/HDL-C and LDL-C/HDL-C, respectively) [113].

5.6. Antimicrobial Activity

The team of Benassai E et al., during green synthesis and using aqueous extracts of bilberry (*Vaccinium myrtillus* L.) and bog bilberry fruit (*Vaccinium uliginosum* L. subsp. *gaultherioides*), obtained mixtures that contained copper nanoparticles (Cu-NPs) in their composition and then underwent microbiological investigation. The obtained mixtures were characterized by potent and extensive antimicrobial activity (fungi, Gram-negative and positive bacteria), and their activity was stronger in most cases compared to equivalent concentrations of copper salts [114]. In one study, the authors focused on evaluating the antibacterial activity of *V. uliginosum* extract and its fractions against Gram-negative (*Vibrio parahaemolyticus, Salmonella enteritidis*) and Gram-positive (*Staphylococcus aureus, Listeria monocytogenes*) bacteria. The crude extract (BBE) of wild blueberry (*Vaccinium uliginosum*) was achieved by extraction with methanol, and the F1, F2, and F3 fractions (sugars/acids, phenols, and anthocyanins/proanthocyanidins, respectively) were isolated. The F3 strain exhibited the most potent antibacterial effect compared to the other examined strains, and then the F2, F1 and BBE strains. Gram-negative bacteria, compared to Gram-positive bacteria, exhibited greater sensitivity to all fractions, with the sensitivity of the tested species, as follows (least→most sensitive): *S. aureus*→*L. monocytogenes*→*S. enteritidis* →*V. parahaemolyticus*. The received results indicate that the investigated blueberry fractions (in particular, F3) suppress the growth of bacteria, whose route of infection is food, as a consequence of damage to their cytoplasmic membrane. This information could be used to create new natural preservatives to protect food from pathogenic microorganisms in the future [115].

Different concentrations of anthocyanins from *V. uliginosum* were applied to four types of pathogens to test their antibacterial properties. A positive correlation was found between anthocyanin concentration and antimicrobial activity. Overall, significant antimicrobial activity against *S. enteritidis, V. parahaemolyticus, L. monocytogenes*, and *St. aureus* was observed when anthocyanins were used at 0.53 mg/mL. Anthocyanins at 0.26 mg/mL completely suppressed *S. aureus*, and reduced *L. monocytogenes* by 3.27 log and *S. enteritidis* by 1.07 log. The presence of anthocyanins also increased protein efflux from *L. monocytogenes, S. enteritidis, S. aureus*, and *V. parahaemolyticus* across damaged membranes [101].

The study by Satoh, Yutaroh, and Kazuyuki Ishihara aimed to identify the antibacterial compounds present in *V. myrtillus* that inhibited periodontopathic bacteria. Oil/water separation was used to extract the acetone-soluble fraction of *V. myrtillus*. In the following step, the extract was purified by chromatography using silica gel. The total extract had an MIC (minimum inhibitory concentration) of 500 g/mL against *Porphyromonas gingivalis*. An antibacterial fraction called NU4-TDC was found to be effective against *P. gingivalis*. This product had MICs above 62.5 µg/mL for *Streptococcus mutans*, 26.0 µg/mL for *P. gingivalis*, 59.1 µg/mL for *Fusobacterium nucleatum*, and 45.1 µg/mL for *Prevotella intermedia*. Based on the above-mentioned research, it can be concluded that bilberry extract has antimicrobial properties. The semi-purified fraction (NU4-TDC) also demonstrated antimicrobial activity when tested against *P. intermedia, P. gingivalis*, and *F. nucleatum* [116].

In another investigation, a team of researchers undertook to determine the antifungal effects and content of particular compounds in essential oils from *Vaccinium myrtillus*. It was found that the essential oil extracted from this plant consists of 41.07% 1,8-cineole, 12.72% β-linalool, 12.17% α-pinene, and 6.48% myrtenol. *V. myrtillus* essential oil suppressed mycelial growth in *Alternaria solani, Verticillium dahlia* Kleb, *Sclerotinia sclerotiorum* (Lib.), and *Fusarium oxysporumf.* sp. *radicis-lycopersici* (Sacc.) W.C. Synder & H.N. Hans (FORL) by

100%, 57.91%, 61.38%, and 80.36% respectively. The findings of this research revealed that *V. myrtillus* essential oil exhibits potent antifungal properties [117].

5.7. Oncology

Colorectal cancer is a malignant process that develops in the final part of the gastrointestinal tract and is one of the most lethal types of cancer globally. Lippert E et al. assessed the influence of an anthocyanin-rich blueberry extract on colorectal tumor progression and growth after administration of azoxymethane (AOM)/sodium dextran sulfate (DSS) using an in vivo mouse model. Mice fed 10% anthocyanins exhibited markedly ($p < 0.004$) less reduction in colon length compared to the control group, providing evidence of reduced inflammation. Moreover, mice in the control group and those receiving 1% anthocyanins showed a higher average number of tumors when compared to individuals receiving 10% anthocyanin-rich extract. Anthocyanins prevented the initiation and progression of colorectal cancer in Balb/c mice exposed to AOM/DSS [118].

In another study, the impact of a standardized *V. myrtillus* extract on human colorectal adenocarcinoma cells (Caco-2) was investigated. The tested extract contained anthocyanins 237.9 ± 17.1 mg CGE (cyanidin-3-glucoside equivalent)/g, phenols 338.5 ± 28.0 mg GAE (gallic acid equivalent)/g, and flavonoids 735.4 ± 18.2 mg QE (quercetin equivalent)/g. It was measured whether *V. myrtillus* may modify the expression of genes related to cholesterol biosynthesis. One of the main transcription factors for cholesterol uptake and biosynthesis is SREBP2 (sterol regulatory element-binding protein 2). It regulates LDLR (LDL receptor) and HMGR (3-hydroxy-3-methylglutaryl coenzyme A reductase). After treatment with blueberries, the abundance of SREBP2 and HMGR mRNA decreased in a statistically significant way. In contrast, LDLR expression in Caco-2 cells increased 2-fold. In conclusion, the *V. myrtillus* extract modulated genes that are involved in cholesterol metabolism in the intestine [119].

Mauramo M. et al. performed a study to investigate the influence of bilberry powder on OSCC (oral squamous cell carcinoma) cells using in vitro/in vivo assays. In a study comparing 0.01 mg/mL cetuximab with 0, 1, 10, and 25 mg/mL powder obtained from whole berries, invasion, proliferation, migration, and viability were assessed in OSCC cells (HSC-3). The in vitro study revealed that bilberry powder exhibited antiproliferative activity and inhibited the migration and invasion process, while the suppression of tumor progression was observed in the in vivo investigation. The inhibitory activity of the tested powder intensified with rising concentrations and was more pronounced in cancer cells when compared to normal cells. When compared with cetuximab, bilberry powder exhibited comparable or even more potent activity in a dose-dependent manner [120].

It was tested whether the exosomal *V. myrtillus* bilberry's anthocyanins and their aglycones anthocyanidins (ExoAnthos) would increase the therapeutic effectiveness over free Anthos against A549 lung cancer cells. The antiproliferative activity of Anthos and ExoAnthos was determined using subcutaneous lung cancer xenografts in athymic nude mice, and then it was compared with exosomes alone. Regardless of the tumor cell type, ExoAnthos exerted a notably stronger dose-dependent antiproliferative effect compared to free Anthos. The greater efficacy of exosomal Anthos is partly due to their intrinsic activity, which is an 'add-on' effect not observed with traditional systems [121].

Li J et al. studied the effect of BA on healthy ageing in 12-month-old ageing female rats. The findings suggest that the intake of a medium dose of BA (MBA) markedly elevated relative the liver weight by 7.34% compared to an ageing control group. In feces, MBA decreased bacterial enzyme activity and increased short-chain fatty acids. The results of the Western blot analysis indicated an increased expression of ZO-1, OCLN, and autophagy-related proteins (ATP6 V0C (bafilomycin A1-binding subunit of vacuolar ATPase), ATG4D (autophagy-related 4D cysteine peptidase), and CTSB (cathepsin B)) in ageing rats. MBA induced AMPK (5′AMP-activated protein kinase) and FOXO3a (forkhead box O3) phosphorylation and inhibited mTOR (mammalian target of rapamycin) phosphorylation, indicating that blueberry anthocyanin induced autophagy through the

AMPK/mTOR signaling pathway. Furthermore, the activation of autophagy additionally promoted the ability to counteract the effects of oxidative stress and enhanced the intestinal epithelial barrier function in ageing female rats [113].

Kausar H. et al. carried out a study in which they found that combining suboptimal equimolar concentrations of anthocyanidins from *V. myrtillus* with marginal effects on the viability of normal cells synergistically suppressed the proliferation of two aggressive NSCLC (non-small cell lung cancer) cell lines. A mixture of anthocyanidins significantly induced the apoptotic process and cell cycle arrest in the G_2/M phase and suppressed the cancer cell migration and invasion process compared to a single anthocyanidin. The improved efficacy of the combinatorial treatment was probably a result of the enhanced cleavage of the apoptosis mediators Bcl2 and PARP, its effect on the oncogenic Wnt/Notch pathway and its downstream signaling molecules (β-catenin, c-myc, cyclin B1 and D1, MMP9, pERK, and VEGF), and elevated suppression of NF-κB activation via the TNF-α-dependent pathway. H1299 xenografts were significantly inhibited in nude mice by both the native mixture of anthocyanidins in bilberries (0.5 mg per subject) and delphinidin (1.5 per subject) [122].

Besides in vitro and in vivo animal research, one clinical trial can be found (NCT number: NCT01674374, phase 2) which focused on the treatment of mucositis induced by radiotherapy and chemotherapy for HNSCC (head and neck squamous cell carcinoma). Immediately after the appearance of symptoms of inflammation and ulceration present in the oral cavity, patients were given granules, which in their composition contained, among other things, *V. myrtillus* extract or a placebo. The intake of the preparation lasted up to 4 weeks after the end of radiotherapy, with the duration of therapy not to exceed 11 weeks. After this period, participants were asked to assess their quality of life and fill out an appropriate questionnaire [123].

6. Side Effects

According to the American Herbal Products Association, bilberries have been recognized as a class 1 herb, and are therefore considered safe to consume when used in appropriate amounts [124]. In clinical trials, no disturbing side effects were noted. Interactions with other drugs have also not been demonstrated [97,125–127]. It is important to monitor patients for bleeding disorders, due to the antiplatelet effect of *V. myrtillus*; this applies to patients who take antiplatelet drugs and additionally supplement with blueberry extract for a longer period.

7. Conclusions

Health benefits, biological activity, and the composition of blueberry and bog bilberry were reviewed. Blueberries contain large amounts of anthocyanins, which are known for their potent biological activity as antioxidants and, according to studies, may be involved in the prophylaxis of cancer or other diseases, including those of metabolic origin—these reports indicate the incredible health potential of blueberries. Because of their antioxidant, anti-inflammatory, anti-cancer, and apoptosis-reducing activity, both bog bilberries and bilberries can be used interchangeably as a dietary supplement with anti-free radical action, in the prevention of cancer diseases and cataracts, or as a component of sunscreen preparations. The composition of both blueberries was analyzed, and they contain many bioactive compounds (including antioxidants and flavonols) with a beneficial effect on health.

Vaccinium uliginosum has not yet been as well researched in terms of both the content of metabolites and its biological activity as other *Vaccinium* species. There are many studies indicating the prevention and possible treatment of cancer with products derived from *V. uliginosum* blueberries, but they are still little confirmed.

Author Contributions: Conceptualization, A.K. and M.W.; methodology, I.K. and A.K.; software, M.W. and A.K.; formal analysis, A.K., I.K. and D.R.; investigation, A.K.; resources, M.W. and I.K.; writing—original draft preparation, A.K., I.K., D.R., A.B., K.B. and M.W.; writing—review and editing, all authors; visualization, A.K., D.R. and M.W. All authors have read and agreed to the published version of the manuscript.

Funding: This research received no external funding.

Institutional Review Board Statement: Not applicable.

Informed Consent Statement: Not applicable.

Data Availability Statement: No new data were created or analyzed in this study. Data sharing is not applicable to this article.

Acknowledgments: All figures (except Figures 1, 5 and 8–10) and the graphical abstract were created with BioRender.com (accessed on 9–10 August 2023).

Conflicts of Interest: The authors declare no conflict of interest.

References

1. Han, E.-K.; Kwon, H.-S.; Shin, S.-G.; Choi, Y.-H.; Kang, I.-J.; Chung, C.-K. Biological Effect of *Vaccinium uliginosum* L. on STZ-Induced Diabetes and Lipid Metabolism in Rats. *J. Korean Soc. Food Sci. Nutr.* **2012**, *41*, 1727–1733. [CrossRef]
2. Fraisse, D.; Bred, A.; Felgines, C.; Senejoux, F. Stability and Antiglycoxidant Potential of Bilberry Anthocyanins in Simulated Gastrointestinal Tract Model. *Foods* **2020**, *9*, 1695. [CrossRef] [PubMed]
3. Popović, D.; Đukić, D.; Katić, V.; Jović, Z.; Jović, M.; Lalić, J.; Golubović, I.; Stojanović, S.; Ulrih, N.P.; Stanković, M.; et al. Antioxidant and Proapoptotic Effects of Anthocyanins from Bilberry Extract in Rats Exposed to Hepatotoxic Effects of Carbon Tetrachloride. *Life Sci.* **2016**, *157*, 168–177. [CrossRef] [PubMed]
4. Karppinen, K.; Zoratti, L.; Nguyenquynh, N.; Häggman, H.; Jaakola, L. On the Developmental and Environmental Regulation of Secondary Metabolism in *Vaccinium* spp. Berries. *Front. Plant Sci.* **2016**, *7*, 655. [CrossRef] [PubMed]
5. Benzie, I.F.; Wachtel-Galor, S. *Herbal Medicine: Biomolecular and Clinical Aspects*, 2nd ed.; CRC Press/Taylor & Francis: Boca Raton, FL, USA, 2011.
6. Liu, S.; Laaksonen, O.; Yang, W.; Zhang, B.; Yang, B. Pyranoanthocyanins in Bilberry (*Vaccinium myrtillus* L.) Wines Fermented with Schizosaccharomyces Pombe and Their Evolution during Aging. *Food Chem.* **2020**, *305*, 125438. [CrossRef] [PubMed]
7. Behrends, A.; Weber, F. Influence of Different Fermentation Strategies on the Phenolic Profile of Bilberry Wine (*Vaccinium myrtillus* L.). *J. Agric. Food Chem.* **2017**, *65*, 7483–7490. [CrossRef]
8. Chen, L.; Zhang, X.; Wang, Q.; Li, W.; Liu, L. Effect of *Vaccinium myrtillus* Extract Supplement on Advanced Glycation End-Products: A Pilot Study (P06-098-19). *Curr. Dev. Nutr.* **2019**, *3*, 616. [CrossRef]
9. Fraisse, D.; Bred, A.; Felgines, C.; Senejoux, F. Screening and Characterization of Antiglycoxidant Anthocyanins from *Vaccinium myrtillus* Fruit Using DPPH and Methylglyoxal Pre-Column HPLC Assays. *Antioxidants* **2020**, *9*, 512. [CrossRef]
10. Maulik, M.; Mitra, S.; Sweeney, M.; Lu, B.; Taylor, B.E.; Bult-Ito, A. Complex Interaction of Dietary Fat and Alaskan Bog Blueberry Supplementation Influences Manganese Mediated Neurotoxicity and Behavioral Impairments. *J. Funct. Foods* **2019**, *53*, 306–317. [CrossRef]
11. Lesjak, M.; Beara, I.; Simin, N.; Pintać, D.; Majkić, T.; Bekvalac, K.; Orčić, D.; Mimica-Dukić, N. Antioxidant and Anti-Inflammatory Activities of Quercetin and Its Derivatives. *J. Funct. Foods* **2018**, *40*, 68–75. [CrossRef]
12. Chan, S.W.; Tomlinson, B. Effects of Bilberry Supplementation on Metabolic and Cardiovascular Disease Risk. *Molecules* **2020**, *25*, 1653. [CrossRef]
13. Bujor, O.C.; Tanase, C.; Popa, M.E. Phenolic Antioxidants in Aerial Parts of Wild *Vaccinium* Species: Towards Pharmaceutical and Biological Properties. *Antioxidants* **2019**, *8*, 649. [CrossRef] [PubMed]
14. Pires, T.C.S.P.; Caleja, C.; Santos-Buelga, C.; Barros, L.; Ferreira, I.C.F.R. *Vaccinium myrtillus* L. Fruits as a Novel Source of Phenolic Compounds with Health Benefits and Industrial Applications—A Review. *Curr. Pharm. Des.* **2020**, *26*, 1917–1928. [CrossRef] [PubMed]
15. Szakiel, A.; Pączkowski, C.; Huttunen, S. Triterpenoid Content of Berries and Leaves of Bilberry *Vaccinium myrtillus* from Finland and Poland. *J. Agric. Food Chem.* **2012**, *60*, 11839–11849. [CrossRef] [PubMed]
16. Vrancheva, R.; Ivanov, I.; Dincheva, I.; Badjakov, I.; Pavlov, A. Triterpenoids and Other Non-Polar Compounds in Leaves of Wild and Cultivated *Vaccinium* Species. *Plants* **2021**, *10*, 94. [CrossRef] [PubMed]
17. Anadon-Rosell, A.; Palacio, S.; Nogués, S.; Ninot, J.M. *Vaccinium myrtillus* Stands Show Similar Structure and Functioning under Different Scenarios of Coexistence at the Pyrenean Treeline. *Plant Ecol.* **2016**, *217*, 1115–1128. [CrossRef]
18. Ștefanescu, B.E.; Szabo, K.; Mocan, A.; Crisan, G. Phenolic Compounds from Five *Ericaceae* Species Leaves and Their Related Bioavailability and Health Benefits. *Molecules* **2019**, *24*, 2046. [CrossRef] [PubMed]

19. Gonçalves, A.C.; Sánchez-Juanes, F.; Meirinho, S.; Silva, L.R.; Alves, G.; Flores-Félix, J.D. Insight into the Taxonomic and Functional Diversity of Bacterial Communities Inhabiting Blueberries in Portugal. *Microorganisms* **2022**, *10*, 2193. [CrossRef] [PubMed]
20. Trivedi, P.; Karppinen, K.; Klavins, L.; Kviesis, J.; Sundqvist, P.; Nguyen, N.; Heinonen, E.; Klavins, M.; Jaakola, L.; Väänänen, J.; et al. Compositional and Morphological Analyses of Wax in Northern Wild Berry Species. *Food Chem.* **2019**, *295*, 441–448. [CrossRef] [PubMed]
21. Diaconeasa, Z. Time-Dependent Degradation of Polyphenols from Thermally-Processed Berries and Their In Vitro Antiproliferative Effects against Melanoma. *Molecules* **2018**, *23*, 2534. [CrossRef]
22. Bujor, O.C.; Le Bourvellec, C.; Volf, I.; Popa, V.I.; Dufour, C. Seasonal Variations of the Phenolic Constituents in Bilberry (*Vaccinium myrtillus* L.) Leaves, Stems and Fruits, and Their Antioxidant Activity. *Food Chem.* **2016**, *213*, 58–68. [CrossRef] [PubMed]
23. Mikulic-Petkovsek, M.; Schmitzer, V.; Slatnar, A.; Stampar, F.; Veberic, R. A Comparison of Fruit Quality Parameters of Wild Bilberry (*Vaccinium myrtillus* L.) Growing at Different Locations. *J. Sci. Food Agric.* **2015**, *95*, 776–785. [CrossRef]
24. Skrovankova, S.; Sumczynski, D.; Mlcek, J.; Jurikova, T.; Sochor, J. Bioactive Compounds and Antioxidant Activity in Different Types of Berries. *Int. J. Mol. Sci.* **2015**, *16*, 24673–24706. [CrossRef] [PubMed]
25. Bobinaitė, R.; Pataro, G.; Lamanauskas, N.; Šatkauskas, S.; Viškelis, P.; Ferrari, G. Application of Pulsed Electric Field in the Production of Juice and Extraction of Bioactive Compounds from Blueberry Fruits and Their By-Products. *J. Food Sci. Technol.* **2015**, *52*, 5898. [CrossRef] [PubMed]
26. Raudonė, L.; Liaudanskas, M.; Vilkickytė, G.; Kviklys, D.; Žvikas, V.; Viškelis, J.; Viškelis, P. Phenolic Profiles, Antioxidant Activity and Phenotypic Characterization of *Lonicera caerulea* L. Berries, Cultivated in Lithuania. *Antioxidants* **2021**, *10*, 115. [CrossRef] [PubMed]
27. Urbonaviciene, D.; Bobinaite, R.; Viskelis, P.; Bobinas, C.; Petruskevicius, A.; Klavins, L.; Viskelis, J. Geographic Variability of Biologically Active Compounds, Antioxidant Activity and Physico-Chemical Properties in Wild Bilberries (*Vaccinium myrtillus* L.). *Antioxidants* **2022**, *11*, 588. [CrossRef]
28. Liudvinaviciute, D.; Rutkaite, R.; Bendoraitiene, J.; Klimaviciute, R.; Dagys, L. Formation and Characteristics of Alginate and Anthocyanin Complexes. *Int. J. Biol. Macromol.* **2020**, *164*, 726–734. [CrossRef]
29. Szakiel, A.; Pączkowski, C.; Koivuniemi, H.; Huttunen, S. Comparison of the Triterpenoid Content of Berries and Leaves of Lingonberry *Vaccinium vitis-Idaea* from Finland and Poland. *J. Agric. Food Chem.* **2012**, *60*, 4994–5002. [CrossRef]
30. Mi, J.C.; Howard, L.R.; Prior, R.L.; Clark, J.R. Flavonoid Glycosides and Antioxidant Capacity of Various Blackberry, Blueberry and Red Grape Genotypes Determined by High-Performance Liquid Chromatography/Mass Spectrometry. *J. Sci. Food Agric.* **2004**, *84*, 1771–1782. [CrossRef]
31. Može, Š.; Polak, T.; Gašperlin, L.; Koron, D.; Vanzo, A.; Poklar Ulrih, N.; Abram, V. Phenolics in Slovenian Bilberries (*Vaccinium myrtillus* L.) and Blueberries (*Vaccinium corymbosum* L.). *J. Agric. Food Chem.* **2011**, *59*, 6998–7004. [CrossRef]
32. Wu, X.; Prior, R.L. Systematic Identification and Characterization of Anthocyanins by HPLC-ESI-MS/MS in Common Foods in the United States: Fruits and Berries. *J. Agric. Food Chem.* **2005**, *53*, 2589–2599. [CrossRef] [PubMed]
33. Lätti, A.K.; Jaakola, L.; Riihinen, K.; Kainulainen, P.S. Anthocyanin and Flavonol Variation in Bog Bilberries (*Vaccinium uliginosum* L.) in Finland. *J. Agric. Food Chem.* **2010**, *58*, 427–433. [CrossRef] [PubMed]
34. Bederska-Łojewska, D.; Pieszka, M.; Marzec, A.; Rudzińska, M.; Grygier, A.; Siger, A.; Cieślik-Boczula, K.; Orczewska-Dudek, S.; Migdał, W. Physicochemical Properties, Fatty Acid Composition, Volatile Compounds of Blueberries, Cranberries, Raspberries, and Cuckooflower Seeds Obtained Using Sonication Method. *Molecules* **2021**, *26*, 7446. [CrossRef] [PubMed]
35. Alves, E.; Simoes, A.; Domingues, M.R. Fruit Seeds and Their Oils as Promising Sources of Value-Added Lipids from Agro-Industrial Byproducts: Oil Content, Lipid Composition, Lipid Analysis, Biological Activity and Potential Biotechnological Applications. *Crit. Rev. Food Sci. Nutr.* **2021**, *61*, 1305–1339. [CrossRef]
36. Michalska, A.; Łysiak, G. Bioactive Compounds of Blueberries: Post-Harvest Factors Influencing the Nutritional Value of Products. *Int. J. Mol. Sci.* **2015**, *16*, 18642–18663. [CrossRef] [PubMed]
37. Frum, A.; Dobrea, C.M.; Rus, L.L.; Virchea, L.I.; Morgovan, C.; Chis, A.A.; Arseniu, A.M.; Butuca, A.; Gligor, F.G.; Vicas, L.G.; et al. Valorization of Grape Pomace and Berries as a New and Sustainable Dietary Supplement: Development, Characterization, and Antioxidant Activity Testing. *Nutrients* **2022**, *14*, 3065. [CrossRef] [PubMed]
38. Colak, N.; Torun, H.; Gruz, J.; Strnad, M.; Hermosín-Gutiérrez, I.; Hayirlioglu-Ayaz, S.; Ayaz, F.A. Bog Bilberry Phenolics, Antioxidant Capacity and Nutrient Profile. *Food Chem.* **2016**, *201*, 339–349. [CrossRef]
39. Kalt, W.; Forney, C.F.; Martin, A.; Prior, R.L. Antioxidant Capacity, Vitamin C, Phenolics, and Anthocyanins after Fresh Storage of Small Fruits. *J. Agric. Food Chem.* **1999**, *47*, 4638–4644. [CrossRef]
40. Zhang, W.; Shen, Y.; Li, Z.; Xie, X.; Gong, E.S.; Tian, J.; Si, X.; Wang, Y.; Gao, N.; Shu, C.; et al. Effects of High Hydrostatic Pressure and Thermal Processing on Anthocyanin Content, Polyphenol Oxidase and β-Glucosidase Activities, Color, and Antioxidant Activities of Blueberry (*Vaccinium* spp.) Puree. *Food Chem.* **2021**, *342*, 128564. [CrossRef] [PubMed]
41. Pinto, L.; Palma, A.; Cefola, M.; Pace, B.; D'Aquino, S.; Carboni, C.; Baruzzi, F. Effect of Modified Atmosphere Packaging (MAP) and Gaseous Ozone Pre-Packaging Treatment on the Physico-Chemical, Microbiological and Sensory Quality of Small Berry Fruit. *Food Packag. Shelf Life* **2020**, *26*, 100573. [CrossRef]

42. Muñoz-Fariña, O.; López-Casanova, V.; García-Figueroa, O.; Roman-Benn, A.; Ah-Hen, K.; Bastias-Montes, J.M.; Quevedo-León, R.; Ravanal-Espinosa, M.C. Bioaccessibility of Phenolic Compounds in Fresh and Dehydrated Blueberries (*Vaccinium corymbosum* L.). *Food Chem. Adv.* **2023**, *2*, 100171. [CrossRef]
43. Maryam, A.; Anwar, R.; Malik, A.U.; Raheem, M.I.U.; Khan, A.S.; Hasan, M.U.; Hussain, Z.; Siddique, Z. Combined Aqueous Ozone and Ultrasound Application Inhibits Microbial Spoilage, Reduces Pesticide Residues and Maintains Storage Quality of Strawberry Fruits. *J. Food Meas. Charact.* **2021**, *15*, 1437–1451. [CrossRef]
44. Hou, Y.; Wang, R.; Gan, Z.; Shao, T.; Zhang, X.; He, M.; Sun, A. Effect of Cold Plasma on Blueberry Juice Quality. *Food Chem.* **2019**, *290*, 79–86. [CrossRef] [PubMed]
45. Ebrahimi, P.; Lante, A. Environmentally Friendly Techniques for the Recovery of Polyphenols from Food By-Products and Their Impact on Polyphenol Oxidase: A Critical Review. *Appl. Sci.* **2022**, *12*, 1923. [CrossRef]
46. Cesa, S.; Carradori, S.; Bellagamba, G.; Locatelli, M.; Casadei, M.A.; Masci, A.; Paolicelli, P. Evaluation of Processing Effects on Anthocyanin Content and Colour Modifications of Blueberry (*Vaccinium* spp.) Extracts: Comparison between HPLC-DAD and CIELAB Analyses. *Food Chem.* **2017**, *232*, 114–123. [CrossRef] [PubMed]
47. Marhuenda, J.; Alemán, M.D.; Gironés-Vilaplana, A.; Pérez, A.; Caravaca, G.; Figueroa, F.; Mulero, J.; Zafrilla, P. Phenolic Composition, Antioxidant Activity, and in Vitro Availability of Four Different Berries. *J. Chem.* **2016**, *2016*, 5194901. [CrossRef]
48. Prencipe, F.P.; Bruni, R.; Guerrini, A.; Rossi, D.; Benvenuti, S.; Pellati, F. Metabolite Profiling of Polyphenols in Vaccinium Berries and Determination of Their Chemopreventive Properties. *J. Pharm. Biomed. Anal.* **2014**, *89*, 257–267. [CrossRef] [PubMed]
49. Wang, L.J.; Su, S.; Wu, J.; Du, H.; Li, S.S.; Huo, J.W.; Zhang, Y.; Wang, L.S. Variation of Anthocyanins and Flavonols in *Vaccinium uliginosum* Berry in Lesser Khingan Mountains and Its Antioxidant Activity. *Food Chem.* **2014**, *160*, 357–364. [CrossRef] [PubMed]
50. Xiao, T.; Guo, Z.; Sun, B.; Zhao, Y. Identification of Anthocyanins from Four Kinds of Berries and Their Inhibition Activity to α-Glycosidase and Protein Tyrosine Phosphatase 1B by HPLC-FT-ICR MS/MS. *J. Agric. Food Chem.* **2017**, *65*, 6211–6221. [CrossRef] [PubMed]
51. Hajazimi, E.; Landberg, R.; Zamaratskaia, G. Simultaneous Determination of Flavonols and Phenolic Acids by HPLC-CoulArray in Berries Common in the Nordic Diet. *LWT* **2016**, *74*, 128–134. [CrossRef]
52. Levaj, B.; Dragović-Uzelac, V.; Delonga, K.; Kovačević Ganić, K.; Banović, M.; Bursać Kovačević, D. Polyphenols and Volatiles in Fruits of Two Sour Cherry Cultivars, Some Berry Fruits and Their Jams. *Food Technol. Biotechnol.* **2010**, *48*, 538–547.
53. Mikulic-Petkovsek, M.; Slatnar, A.; Stampar, F.; Veberic, R. HPLC-MSn Identification and Quantification of Flavonol Glycosides in 28 Wild and Cultivated Berry Species. *Food Chem.* **2012**, *135*, 2138–2146. [CrossRef]
54. Sezer, E.D.; Oktay, L.M.; Karadadaş, E.; Memmedov, H.; Selvi Gunel, N.; Sözmen, E. Assessing Anticancer Potential of Blueberry Flavonoids, Quercetin, Kaempferol, and Gentisic Acid, Through Oxidative Stress and Apoptosis Parameters on HCT-116 Cells. *J. Med. Food* **2019**, *22*, 1118–1126. [CrossRef] [PubMed]
55. Ancillotti, C.; Ciofi, L.; Pucci, D.; Sagona, E.; Giordani, E.; Biricolti, S.; Gori, M.; Petrucci, W.A.; Giardi, F.; Bartoletti, R.; et al. Polyphenolic Profiles and Antioxidant and Antiradical Activity of Italian Berries from *Vaccinium myrtillus* L. and *Vaccinium uliginosum* L. Subsp. Gaultherioides (Bigelow) S.B. Young. *Food Chem.* **2016**, *204*, 176–184. [CrossRef] [PubMed]
56. Wei, M.; Wang, S.; Gu, P.; Ouyang, X.; Liu, S.; Li, Y.; Zhang, B.; Zhu, B. Comparison of Physicochemical Indexes, Amino Acids, Phenolic Compounds and Volatile Compounds in Bog Bilberry Juice Fermented by *Lactobacillus plantarum* under Different PH Conditions. *J. Food Sci. Technol.* **2018**, *55*, 2240. [CrossRef] [PubMed]
57. Wang, Y.; Liu, X.; Chen, J.Z.; Tian, X.; Zheng, Y.H.; Hao, J.; Xue, Y.J.; Ding, S.Y.; Zong, C.W. The Variation of Total Flavonoids, Anthocyanins and Total Phenols in *Vaccinium uliginosum* Fruits in Changbai Mountain of China Is Closely Related to Spatial Distribution. *J. Berry Res.* **2022**, *12*, 463–481. [CrossRef]
58. Kraujalyte, V.; Venskutonis, P.R.; Pukalskas, A.; Česoniene, L.; Daubaras, R. Antioxidant Properties, Phenolic Composition and Potentiometric Sensor Array Evaluation of Commercial and New Blueberry (*Vaccinium corymbosum*) and Bog Blueberry (*Vaccinium uliginosum*) Genotypes. *Food Chem.* **2015**, *188*, 583–590. [CrossRef] [PubMed]
59. Bayazid, A.B.; Chun, E.M.; Al Mijan, M.; Park, S.H.; Moon, S.K.; Lim, B.O. Anthocyanins Profiling of Bilberry (*Vaccinium myrtillus* L.) Extract That Elucidates Antioxidant and Anti-Inflammatory Effects. *Food Agric. Immunol.* **2021**, *32*, 713–726. [CrossRef]
60. Jin, Y.; Zhang, Y.; Liu, D.; Liu, D.; Zhang, C.; Qi, H.; Gu, W.; Yang, L.; Zhou, Z. Efficient Homogenization-Ultrasound-Assisted Extraction of Anthocyanins and Flavonols from Bog Bilberry (*Vaccinium uliginosum* L.) Marc with Carnosic Acid as an Antioxidant Additive. *Molecules* **2019**, *24*, 2537. [CrossRef] [PubMed]
61. Seeram, N.P. Berry Fruits: Compositional Elements, Biochemical Activities, and the Impact of Their Intake on Human Health, Performance, and Disease. *J. Agric. Food Chem.* **2008**, *56*, 627–629. [CrossRef]
62. Holkem, A.T.; Robichaud, V.; Favaro-Trindade, C.S.; Lacroix, M. Chemopreventive Properties of Extracts Obtained from Blueberry (*Vaccinium myrtillus* L.) and Jabuticaba (*Myrciaria cauliflora* Berg.) in Combination with Probiotics. *Nutr. Cancer* **2021**, *73*, 671–685. [CrossRef] [PubMed]
63. Cásedas, G.; González-Burgos, E.; Smith, C.; López, V.; Gómez-Serranillos, M.P. Regulation of Redox Status in Neuronal SH-SY5Y Cells by Blueberry (*Vaccinium myrtillus* L.) Juice, Cranberry (*Vaccinium macrocarpon* A.) Juice and Cyanidin. *Food Chem. Toxicol.* **2018**, *118*, 572–580. [CrossRef] [PubMed]
64. Sharma, A.; Lee, H.J. Anti-Inflammatory Activity of Bilberry (*Vaccinium myrtillus* L.). *Curr. Issues Mol. Biol.* **2022**, *44*, 4570–4583. [CrossRef]

65. Piberger, H.; Oehme, A.; Hofmann, C.; Dreiseitel, A.; Sand, P.G.; Obermeier, F.; Schoelmerich, J.; Schreier, P.; Krammer, G.; Rogler, G. Bilberries and Their Anthocyanins Ameliorate Experimental Colitis. *Mol. Nutr. Food Res.* **2011**, *55*, 1724–1729. [CrossRef] [PubMed]
66. Pan, F.; Liu, Y.; Liu, J.; Wang, E. Stability of Blueberry Anthocyanin, Anthocyanidin and Pyranoanthocyanidin Pigments and Their Inhibitory Effects and Mechanisms in Human Cervical Cancer HeLa Cells. *RSC Adv.* **2019**, *9*, 10842. [CrossRef] [PubMed]
67. Scalzo, J.; Politi, A.; Pellegrini, N.; Mezzetti, B.; Battino, M. Plant Genotype Affects Total Antioxidant Capacity and Phenolic Contents in Fruit. *Nutrition* **2005**, *21*, 207–213. [CrossRef] [PubMed]
68. Prior, R.L.; Cao, G.; Martin, A.; Sofic, E.; McEwen, J.; O'Brien, C.; Lischner, N.; Ehlenfeldt, M.; Kalt, W.; Krewer, G.; et al. Antioxidant Capacity as Influenced by Total Phenolic and Anthocyanin Content, Maturity, and Variety of *Vaccinium* Species. *J. Agric. Food Chem.* **1998**, *46*, 2686–2693. [CrossRef]
69. Wang, S.Y.; Lin, H.S. Antioxidant Activity in Fruits and Leaves of Blackberry, Raspberry, and Strawberry Varies with Cultivar and Developmental Stage. *J. Agric. Food Chem.* **2000**, *48*, 140–146. [CrossRef]
70. Sellappan, S.; Akoh, C.C.; Krewer, G. Phenolic Compounds and Antioxidant Capacity of Georgia-Grown Blueberries and Blackberries. *J. Agric. Food Chem.* **2002**, *50*, 2432–2438. [CrossRef] [PubMed]
71. Moyer, R.A.; Hummer, K.E.; Finn, C.E.; Frei, B.; Wrolstad, R.E. Anthocyanins, Phenolics, and Antioxidant Capacity in Diverse Small Fruits: *Vaccinium*, *Rubus*, and *Ribes*. *J. Agric. Food Chem.* **2002**, *50*, 519–525. [CrossRef]
72. Kusznierewicz, B.; Piekarska, A.; Mrugalska, B.; Konieczka, P.; Namieśnik, J.; Bartoszek, A. Phenolic Composition and Antioxidant Properties of Polish Blue-Berried Honeysuckle Genotypes by HPLC-DAD-MS, HPLC Postcolumn Derivatization with ABTS or FC, and TLC with DPPH Visualization. *J. Agric. Food Chem.* **2012**, *60*, 1755–1763. [CrossRef]
73. Wang, C.; Zhang, M.; Wu, L.; Wang, F.; Li, L.; Zhang, S.; Sun, B. Qualitative and Quantitative Analysis of Phenolic Compounds in Blueberries and Protective Effects on Hydrogen Peroxide-Induced Cell Injury. *J. Sep. Sci.* **2021**, *44*, 2837–2855. [CrossRef] [PubMed]
74. Bornsek, S.M.; Ziberna, L.; Polak, T.; Vanzo, A.; Ulrih, N.P.; Abram, V.; Tramer, F.; Passamonti, S. Bilberry and Blueberry Anthocyanins Act as Powerful Intracellular Antioxidants in Mammalian Cells. *Food Chem.* **2012**, *134*, 1878–1884. [CrossRef] [PubMed]
75. Vaneková, Z.; Rollinger, J.M. Bilberries: Curative and Miraculous—A Review on Bioactive Constituents and Clinical Research. *Front. Pharmacol.* **2022**, *13*, 909914. [CrossRef] [PubMed]
76. Trivedi, P.; Nguyen, N.; Klavins, L.; Kviesis, J.; Heinonen, E.; Remes, J.; Jokipii-Lukkari, S.; Klavins, M.; Karppinen, K.; Jaakola, L.; et al. Analysis of Composition, Morphology, and Biosynthesis of Cuticular Wax in Wild Type Bilberry (*Vaccinium myrtillus* L.) and Its Glossy Mutant. *Food Chem.* **2021**, *354*, 129517. [CrossRef] [PubMed]
77. Jo, K.; Bae, G.Y.; Cho, K.; Park, S.S.; Suh, H.J.; Hong, K.B. An Anthocyanin-Enriched Extract from *Vaccinium uliginosum* Improves Signs of Skin Aging in UVB-Induced Photodamage. *Antioxidants* **2020**, *9*, 844. [CrossRef] [PubMed]
78. Bucci, P.; Prieto, M.J.; Milla, L.; Calienni, M.N.; Martinez, L.; Rivarola, V.; Alonso, S.; Montanari, J. Skin Penetration and UV-Damage Prevention by Nanoberries. *J. Cosmet. Dermatol.* **2018**, *17*, 889–899. [CrossRef]
79. Tadić, V.M.; Nešić, I.; Martinović, M.; Rój, E.; Brašanac-Vukanović, S.; Maksimović, S.; Žugić, A. Old Plant, New Possibilities: Wild Bilberry (*Vaccinium myrtillus* L., Ericaceae) in Topical Skin Preparation. *Antioxidants* **2021**, *10*, 465. [CrossRef]
80. Pastori, V.; Tavazzi, S.; Lecchi, M. Lactoferrin-Loaded Contact Lenses: Eye Protection against Oxidative Stress. *Cornea* **2015**, *34*, 693–697. [CrossRef]
81. Choi, W.; Kim, J.C.; Kim, W.S.; Oh, H.J.; Yang, J.M.; Lee, J.B.; Yoon, K.C. Clinical Effect of Antioxidant Glasses Containing Extracts of Medicinal Plants in Patients with Dry Eye Disease: A Multi-Center, Prospective, Randomized, Double-Blind, Placebo-Controlled Trial. *PLoS ONE* **2015**, *10*, e0139761. [CrossRef]
82. Galbis-Estrada, C.; Pinazo-Durán, M.D.; Martínez-Castillo, S.; Morales, J.M.; Monleón, D.; Zanon-Moreno, V. A Metabolomic Approach to Dry Eye Disorders. The Role of Oral Supplements with Antioxidants and Omega 3 Fatty Acids. *Mol. Vis.* **2015**, *21*, 555.
83. Park, C.Y.; Gu, N.; Lim, C.Y.; Oh, J.H.; Chang, M.; Kim, M.; Rhee, M.Y. The Effect of *Vaccinium uliginosum* Extract on Tablet Computer-Induced Asthenopia: Randomized Placebo-Controlled Study. *BMC Complement. Altern. Med.* **2016**, *16*, 296. [CrossRef]
84. Yin, L.; Pi, Y.L.; Zhang, M.N. The Effect of *Vaccinium uliginosum* on Rabbit Retinal Structure and Light-Induced Function Damage. *Chin. J. Integr. Med.* **2012**, *18*, 299–303. [CrossRef] [PubMed]
85. Yin, L.; Fan, S.J.; Zhang, M. nian Protective Effects of Anthocyanins Extracted from *Vaccinium uliginosum* on 661W Cells Against Microwave-Induced Retinal Damage. *Chin. J. Integr. Med.* **2022**, *28*, 620–626. [CrossRef] [PubMed]
86. Choi, J.I.; Kim, J.; Choung, S.Y. Polyphenol-Enriched Fraction of *Vaccinium uliginosum* L. Protects Selenite-Induced Cataract Formation in the Lens of Sprague-Dawley Rat Pups. *Mol. Vis.* **2019**, *25*, 118. [PubMed]
87. Yoon, S.M.; Lee, B.L.; Guo, Y.R.; Choung, S.Y. Preventive Effect of *Vaccinium uliginosum* L. Extract and Its Fractions on Age-Related Macular Degeneration and Its Action Mechanisms. *Arch. Pharm. Res.* **2016**, *39*, 21–32. [CrossRef]
88. Lee, B.L.; Kang, J.H.; Kim, H.M.; Jeong, S.H.; Jang, D.S.; Jang, Y.P.; Choung, S.Y. Polyphenol-Enriched *Vaccinium uliginosum* L. Fractions Reduce Retinal Damage Induced by Blue Light in A2E-Laden ARPE19 Cell Cultures and Mice. *Nutr. Res.* **2016**, *36*, 1402–1414. [CrossRef] [PubMed]
89. Jin, H.L.; Choung, S.Y.; Jeong, K.W. Protective Mechanisms of Polyphenol-Enriched Fraction of *Vaccinium uliginosum* L. Against Blue Light-Induced Cell Death of Human Retinal Pigmented Epithelial Cells. *J. Funct. Foods* **2017**, *39*, 28–36. [CrossRef]

90. ClinicalTrials.gov. Quality of Life and Visual Acuity of Visglyc Eye Drops on Dry Eye Patients. Available online: https://www.clinicaltrials.gov/study/NCT04063644 (accessed on 9 August 2023).
91. ClinicalTrials.gov. The Effect of DA9301 on Tablet Computer-Induced Asthenopia. Available online: https://www.clinicaltrials.gov/study/NCT02641470 (accessed on 9 August 2023).
92. Ozlem, K.; Birkan, Y.; Mustafa, K.; Emin, K. Protective Effect of *Vaccinium myrtillus* on Ischemia- Reperfusion Injury in Rat Ovary. *Taiwan. J. Obstet. Gynecol.* **2018**, *57*, 836–841. [CrossRef]
93. Aqil, F.; Jeyabalan, J.; Agrawal, A.K.; Kyakulaga, A.H.; Munagala, R.; Parker, L.; Gupta, R.C. Exosomal Delivery of Berry Anthocyanidins for the Management of Ovarian Cancer. *Food Funct.* **2017**, *8*, 4100–4107. [CrossRef]
94. Anhê, F.F.; Varin, T.V.; Le Barz, M.; Pilon, G.; Dudonné, S.; Trottier, J.; St-Pierre, P.; Harris, C.S.; Lucas, M.; Lemire, M.; et al. Arctic Berry Extracts Target the Gut-Liver Axis to Alleviate Metabolic Endotoxaemia, Insulin Resistance and Hepatic Steatosis in Diet-Induced Obese Mice. *Diabetologia* **2018**, *61*, 919–931. [CrossRef] [PubMed]
95. Anhê, F.F.; Desjardins, Y.; Pilon, G.; Dudonné, S.; Genovese, M.I.; Lajolo, F.M.; Marette, A. Polyphenols and Type 2 Diabetes: A Prospective Review. *PharmaNutrition* **2013**, *1*, 105–114. [CrossRef]
96. Nguyen, B.; Bauman, A.; Gale, J.; Banks, E.; Kritharides, L.; Ding, D. Fruit and Vegetable Consumption and All-Cause Mortality: Evidence from a Large Australian Cohort Study. *Int. J. Behav. Nutr. Phys. Act.* **2016**, *13*, 9. [CrossRef] [PubMed]
97. Hoggard, N.; Cruickshank, M.; Moar, K.M.; Bestwick, C.; Holst, J.J.; Russell, W.; Horgan, G. A Single Supplement of a Standardised Bilberry (*Vaccinium myrtillus* L.) Extract (36% Wet Weight Anthocyanins) Modifies Glycaemic Response in Individuals with Type 2 Diabetes Controlled by Diet and Lifestyle. *J. Nutr. Sci.* **2013**, *2*, e22. [CrossRef]
98. Xiao, T.; Guo, Z.; Bi, X.; Zhao, Y. Polyphenolic Profile as Well as Anti-Oxidant and Anti-Diabetes Effects of Extracts from Freeze-Dried Black Raspberries. *J. Funct. Foods* **2017**, *31*, 179–187. [CrossRef]
99. Chan, S.W.; Chu, T.T.W.; Choi, S.W.; Benzie, I.F.F.; Tomlinson, B. Impact of Short-Term Bilberry Supplementation on Glycemic Control, Cardiovascular Disease Risk Factors, and Antioxidant Status in Chinese Patients with Type 2 Diabetes. *Phytother. Res.* **2021**, *35*, 3236–3245. [CrossRef]
100. Karcheva-Bahchevanska, D.P.; Lukova, P.K.; Nikolova, M.M.; Mladenov, R.D.; Iliev, I.N. Effect of Extracts of Bilberries (*Vaccinium myrtillus* L.) on Amyloglucosidase and α-Glucosidase Activity. *Folia Med.* **2017**, *59*, 197–202. [CrossRef]
101. Sun, X.H.; Zhou, T.T.; Wei, C.H.; Lan, W.Q.; Zhao, Y.; Pan, Y.J.; Wu, V.C.H. Antibacterial Effect and Mechanism of Anthocyanin Rich Chinese Wild Blueberry Extract on Various Foodborne Pathogens. *Food Control* **2018**, *94*, 155–161. [CrossRef]
102. Kim, J.; Kim, C.S.; Lee, Y.M.; Sohn, E.; Jo, K.; Kim, J.S. *Vaccinium myrtillus* Extract Prevents or Delays the Onset of Diabetes--Induced Blood-Retinal Barrier Breakdown. *Int. J. Food Sci. Nutr.* **2015**, *66*, 236–242. [CrossRef] [PubMed]
103. Pemmari, T.; Hämäläinen, M.; Ryyti, R.; Peltola, R.; Moilanen, E. Dried Bilberry (*Vaccinium myrtillus* L.) Alleviates the Inflammation and Adverse Metabolic Effects Caused by a High-Fat Diet in a Mouse Model of Obesity. *Int. J. Mol. Sci.* **2022**, *23*, 11021. [CrossRef]
104. Galicia-Garcia, U.; Benito-Vicente, A.; Jebari, S.; Larrea-Sebal, A.; Siddiqi, H.; Uribe, K.B.; Ostolaza, H.; Martín, C. Pathophysiology of Type 2 Diabetes Mellitus. *Int. J. Mol. Sci.* **2020**, *21*, 6275. [CrossRef] [PubMed]
105. ClinicalTrials.gov. Effects of Berries and Berry Fractions on Metabolic Diseases. Available online: https://www.clinicaltrials.gov/study/NCT01860547 (accessed on 9 August 2023).
106. ClinicalTrials.gov. The Health Effect of Diet Rich in Nordic Berries (Berry). Available online: https://www.clinicaltrials.gov/study/NCT01414647 (accessed on 10 August 2023).
107. ClinicalTrials.gov. Dietary Anthocyanins Improve Lipid Metabolism in a Dose—Dependent Manner. Available online: https://www.clinicaltrials.gov/study/NCT03415503 (accessed on 9 August 2023).
108. ClinicalTrials.gov. Safety and Efficacy of Herbal Tea in Type 2 Diabetics (DIABHerbMix). Available online: https://www.clinicaltrials.gov/study/NCT04054284 (accessed on 10 August 2023).
109. Bryl-Górecka, P.; Sathanoori, R.; Arevström, L.; Landberg, R.; Bergh, C.; Evander, M.; Olde, B.; Laurell, T.; Fröbert, O.; Erlinge, D. Bilberry Supplementation after Myocardial Infarction Decreases Microvesicles in Blood and Affects Endothelial Vesiculation. *Mol. Nutr. Food Res.* **2020**, *64*, 2000108. [CrossRef]
110. Ashour, O.M.; Elberry, A.A.; Alahdal, A.M.; Al Mohamadi, A.M.; Nagy, A.A.; Abdel-Naim, A.B.; Abdel-Sattar, E.A.; Mohamadin, A.M. Protective Effect of Bilberry (*Vaccinium myrtillus*) against Doxorubicin-Induced Oxidative Cardiotoxicity in Rats. *Med. Sci. Monit.* **2011**, *17*, 110–115. [CrossRef]
111. Habanova, M.; Saraiva, J.A.; Haban, M.; Schwarzova, M.; Chlebo, P.; Predna, L.; Gažo, J.; Wyka, J. Intake of Bilberries (*Vaccinium myrtillus* L.) Reduced Risk Factors for Cardiovascular Disease by Inducing Favorable Changes in Lipoprotein Profiles. *Nutr. Res.* **2016**, *36*, 1415–1422. [CrossRef] [PubMed]
112. Asgary, S.; Rafieiankopaei, M.; Sahebkar, A.; Shamsi, F.; Goli-malekabadi, N. Anti-Hyperglycemic and Anti-Hyperlipidemic Effects of *Vaccinium myrtillus* Fruit in Experimentally Induced Diabetes (Antidiabetic Effect of *Vaccinium myrtillus* Fruit). *J. Sci. Food Agric.* **2016**, *96*, 764–768. [CrossRef] [PubMed]
113. Li, J.; Zhao, R.; Zhao, H.; Chen, G.; Jiang, Y.; Lyu, X.; Wu, T. Reduction of Aging-Induced Oxidative Stress and Activation of Autophagy by Bilberry Anthocyanin Supplementation via the AMPK-MTOR Signaling Pathway in Aged Female Rats. *J. Agric. Food Chem.* **2019**, *67*, 7832–7843. [CrossRef]
114. Benassai, E.; Del Bubba, M.; Ancillotti, C.; Colzi, I.; Gonnelli, C.; Calisi, N.; Salvatici, M.C.; Casalone, E.; Ristori, S. Green and Cost-Effective Synthesis of Copper Nanoparticles by Extracts of Non-Edible and Waste Plant Materials from *Vaccinium* Species: Characterization and Antimicrobial Activity. *Mater. Sci. Eng. C Mater. Biol. Appl.* **2021**, *119*, 111453. [CrossRef]

115. Zhou, T.T.; Wei, C.H.; Lan, W.Q.; Zhao, Y.; Pan, Y.J.; Sun, X.H.; Wu, V.C.H. The Effect of Chinese Wild Blueberry Fractions on the Growth and Membrane Integrity of Various Foodborne Pathogens. *J. Food Sci.* **2020**, *85*, 1513–1522. [CrossRef]
116. Satoh, Y.; Ishihara, K. Investigation of the Antimicrobial Activity of Bilberry (*Vaccinium myrtillus* L.) Extract against Periodontopathic Bacteria. *J. Oral Biosci.* **2020**, *62*, 169–174. [CrossRef] [PubMed]
117. Bayar, Y.; Onaran, A.; Yilar, M.; Gul, F. Determination of the Essential Oil Composition and the Antifungal Activities of Bilberry (*Vaccinium myrtillus* L.) and Bay Laurel (*Laurus nobilis* L.). *J. Essent. Oil Bear. Plants* **2018**, *21*, 548–555. [CrossRef]
118. Lippert, E.; Ruemmele, P.; Obermeier, F.; Goelder, S.; Kunst, C.; Rogler, G.; Dunger, N.; Messmann, H.; Hartmann, A.; Endlicher, E. Anthocyanins Prevent Colorectal Cancer Development in a Mouse Model. *Digestion* **2017**, *95*, 275–280. [CrossRef] [PubMed]
119. Hong, J.; Kim, M.; Kim, B. The Effects of Anthocyanin-Rich Bilberry Extract on Transintestinal Cholesterol Excretion. *Foods* **2021**, *10*, 2852. [CrossRef] [PubMed]
120. Mauramo, M.; Onali, T.; Wahbi, W.; Vasara, J.; Lampinen, A.; Mauramo, E.; Kivimäki, A.; Martens, S.; Häggman, H.; Sutinen, M.; et al. Bilberry (*Vaccinium myrtillus* L.) Powder Has Anticarcinogenic Effects on Oral Carcinoma In Vitro and In Vivo. *Antioxidants* **2021**, *10*, 1319. [CrossRef]
121. Munagala, R.; Aqil, F.; Jeyabalan, J.; Agrawal, A.K.; Mudd, A.M.; Kyakulaga, A.H.; Singh, I.P.; Vadhanam, M.V.; Gupta, R.C. Exosomal Formulation of Anthocyanidins against Multiple Cancer Types. *Cancer Lett.* **2017**, *393*, 94–102. [CrossRef] [PubMed]
122. Kausar, H.; Jeyabalan, J.; Aqil, F.; Chabba, D.; Sidana, J.; Singh, I.P.; Gupta, R.C. Berry Anthocyanidins Synergistically Suppress Growth and Invasive Potential of Human Non-Small-Cell Lung Cancer Cells. *Cancer Lett.* **2012**, *325*, 54–62. [CrossRef] [PubMed]
123. ClinicalTrials.gov. Botanical Therapy in Treating Mucositis in Patients With Head and Neck Cancer Who Have Undergone Chemoradiation Therapy. Available online: https://www.clinicaltrials.gov/study/NCT01674374 (accessed on 9 August 2023).
124. American Herbal Pharmacopoeia. *Bilberry Fruit: Vaccinium myrtillus L.: Standards of Analysis, Quality Control, and Therapeutics*; American Herbal Pharmacopoeia: Scotts Valley, CA, USA, 2001; p. 25.
125. Biedermann, L.; Mwinyi, J.; Scharl, M.; Frei, P.; Zeitz, J.; Kullak-Ublick, G.A.; Vavricka, S.R.; Fried, M.; Weber, A.; Humpf, H.U.; et al. Bilberry Ingestion Improves Disease Activity in Mild to Moderate Ulcerative Colitis—An Open Pilot Study. *J. Crohns. Colitis* **2013**, *7*, 271–279. [CrossRef] [PubMed]
126. Karlsen, A.; Paur, I.; Bøhn, S.K.; Sakhi, A.K.; Borge, G.I.; Serafini, M.; Erlund, I.; Laake, P.; Tonstad, S.; Blomhoff, R. Bilberry Juice Modulates Plasma Concentration of NF-KappaB Related Inflammatory Markers in Subjects at Increased Risk of CVD. *Eur. J. Nutr.* **2010**, *49*, 345–355. [CrossRef]
127. Arevström, L.; Bergh, C.; Landberg, R.; Wu, H.; Rodriguez-Mateos, A.; Waldenborg, M.; Magnuson, A.; Blanc, S.; Fröbert, O. Freeze-Dried Bilberry (*Vaccinium myrtillus*) Dietary Supplement Improves Walking Distance and Lipids after Myocardial Infarction: An Open-Label Randomized Clinical Trial. *Nutr. Res.* **2019**, *62*, 13–22. [CrossRef]

Disclaimer/Publisher's Note: The statements, opinions and data contained in all publications are solely those of the individual author(s) and contributor(s) and not of MDPI and/or the editor(s). MDPI and/or the editor(s) disclaim responsibility for any injury to people or property resulting from any ideas, methods, instructions or products referred to in the content.

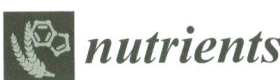

Review

Are We Ready to Recommend Capsaicin for Disorders Other Than Neuropathic Pain?

Janayne L. Silva, Elandia A. Santos and Jacqueline I. Alvarez-Leite *

Departamento de Bioquímica e Imunologia, Universidade Federal de Minas Gerais, Belo Horizonte 30161-970, MG, Brazil; janayneluihan@gmail.com (J.L.S.); elandianutri@gmail.com (E.A.S.)
* Correspondence: alvarez@ufmg.br

Abstract: Capsaicin, a lipophilic, volatile compound, is responsible for the pungent properties of chili peppers. In recent years, a significant increase in investigations into its properties has allowed the production of new formulations and the development of tools with biotechnological, diagnostic, and potential therapeutic applications. Most of these studies show beneficial effects, improving antioxidant and anti-inflammatory status, inducing thermogenesis, and reducing white adipose tissue. Other mechanisms, including reducing food intake and improving intestinal dysbiosis, are also described. In this way, the possible clinical application of such compound is expanding every year. This opinion article aims to provide a synthesis of recent findings regarding the mechanisms by which capsaicin participates in the control of non-communicable diseases such as obesity, diabetes, and dyslipidemia.

Keywords: capsaicin; pepper; diabetes; obesity; inflammation; gut microbiota

1. Introduction

Capsaicinoids are a group of lipophilic and volatile compounds with different pungency intensities characterized by a vanilloid ring. They have diverse biological activities and applications, from food flavoring to therapeutic adjuncts [1]. Among these, capsaicin (trans-8-methyl-*N*-vanilyl-6-nonenamide, $C_{18}H_{27}NO_3$) is the most pungent and abundant, accounting for about 70% of all capsaicinoids, followed by dihydrocapsaicin (~22%), nordihydrocapsaicin (~7%) [2]. The vanilloid ring has a high affinity for the Transient receptor potential vanilloid subtype 1 (TRPV1), a non-selective cationic channel widely distributed in different tissues. It is highly expressed in neural (peripheral and central) tissues, especially in C fibers, and, to a lesser extent, in the Aδ fibers of the nociceptive sensory pathway [3]. TRPV1 can also be found in other tissues, including adipose tissue [4], hepatocytes [5], immune system [6], and endothelial cells [7]. As a polymodal receptor, TRPV1 responds to a broad spectrum of physical and chemical stimuli such as heat, protons, and toxins. However, it exhibits affinity (in sub-μM order), sensitivity, and selectivity for capsaicin, its primary exogenous ligand [8]. A better understanding of the TRPV1–capsaicin interaction at molecular levels has guided pharmaceutical efforts towards the use of capsaicin in the treatment of pain, as well as helping to explore new clinical uses [9]. The biological activities of capsaicin include analgesic, anesthetic [10], anti-inflammatory [11], antioxidant [12], and thermogenic effects [13]. These activities are related to capsaicin's effects in reducing adiposity, blood pressure, blood glucose, and cholesterol levels [13,14]. Due to its pleiotropic action and high skin absorption, there is a growing interest in using capsaicin as a therapeutic alternative. Creams and patches with concentrations between 0.025–8% of capsaicin are commercially available for muscle or neuralgic pain management.

2. Metabolism and Bioactivity

Since capsaicin is a food compound, the natural route of capsaicin absorption is the oral via. However, its pungency limits the quantity of capsaicin administration, either in

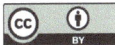

natura (in food) or as powder and capsules. Moreover, lipophilicity directly influences the activation kinetics of its receptor TRPV1 and, consequently, its ability to generate action potentials in excitable cells [15]. Thus, overcoming the capsaicin pungency maintaining its properties becomes a challenge. In this sense, capsinoids or non-pungent synthetic analogs of capsaicin, such as olvanil and arvanil (that bind efficiently to TRPV1), could replace capsaicin in some effects [16,17].

After oral ingestion, 50–90% of capsaicin is passively absorbed in the stomach, and its maximum concentration in blood is seen 1 h later [18] (Figure 1). First-pass metabolism occurs in the liver, mediated by the cytochrome P450 system, which generates metabolites such as 16-hydroxycapsaicin, 17-hydroxycapsaicin, nordihydrocapsaicin, 16,17-dehydrocapsaicin, vanillin, and vanilamine. In systemic circulation, capsaicin and its derived compounds are transported, linked to albumin, and distributed to organs and tissues [2].

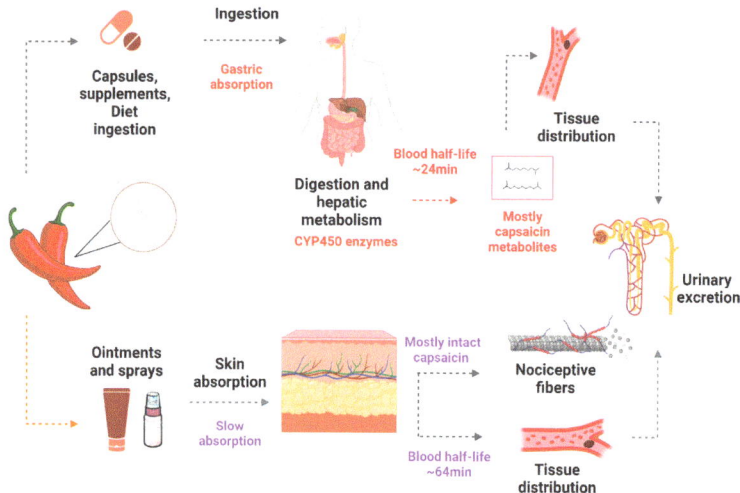

Figure 1. General metabolism of capsaicin orally or topically administered. Dietary capsaicin absorbed in the stomach reaches the hepatocytes via the portal system, where it is metabolized by the cytochrome P450 (CYP450) enzyme system. When given through topical administration, capsaicin is rapidly absorbed and undergoes slow biotransformation, mainly remaining intact, without hepatic biotransformation. After reaching systemic circulation, capsaicin and its metabolites are distributed to peripherical organs and trigger systemic effects. Finally, they are eliminated mainly through the kidneys. Created with BioRender.com.

When applied topically to the skin, capsaicin is rapidly absorbed and undergoes slow biotransformation, remaining primarily intact, with only a small part biotransformed into vanillin and vanillic acid. Unlike oral intake, topical applications prevent the hepatic metabolization of capsaicin, ensuring a greater bioavailability in target tissues [19]. The half-life of capsaicin by topical is 1 to 24 h, longer than oral intake, and its excretion is mainly by the renal according to [2,19].

After topical application, the absorbed capsaicin activates its receptor TRPV1, which causes the rapid influx of sodium ions (Na^+) and calcium (Ca^{2+}) from the extracellular environment to the cell interior. Then, a depolarization cascade is initiated and transmitted along sensory fibers from the spinal cord to the brain, causing pain sensation. A long-term refractory state follows the initial pain sensation, and the sensory neurons stop responding to an additional application of capsaicin in a process called "desensitization" [20,21] (Figure 1).

3. TRPV1-Dependent Mechanisms of Action

Capsaicin binds to the transmembrane segments of TRPV1 channels in a "tail up, head down" configuration and initiates calcium influx and desensitization of nerve fibers [8]. In the case of chronic use of capsaicin, during the first few applications, it promotes the release of the preformed substance P, a potent local pain signal, which causes an initial state of neurogenic inflammation. The depletion of substance P and inoperability of nociceptive cells due to the constant influx of calcium occur after repeated applications, which prevents the formation of more mediators and reduces the inflammatory state [22]. In summary, to minimize pain, capsaicin first causes hyperalgesia, which, by exhaustion, leads to desensitization and a state of analgesia [23].

The rapid ionic influx of Ca^{2+} caused by the TRPV1 activation generates activation of second messengers and modulation of several metabolic pathways. TRPV1 is also expressed in non-excitable cells, such as adipose tissue [4]. In this tissue, capsaicin can exert anti-obesogenic and thermoregulatory effects via TRPV1 activation [24] by increasing thermogenic gene expression such as uncoupling protein 1 (UCP-1), Sirtuin 1 (SIRT-1) [25] and peroxisome proliferator-activated receptor -γ (PPARγ) coactivator 1α (PGC-1α) [26,27]. These factors can interfere with lipid metabolism by suppressing inflammatory responses, increasing lipid oxidation, inhibiting adipogenesis, activating brown adipose tissue, and increasing satiety by interfering in the hypothalamic neuronal circuits [27,28].

The higher intracellular calcium concentration promoted by the Capsaicin-TRPV1 binding may increase the expression and activity of the endothelium-specific transcription factor (KLF2), which could increase the expression of the enzyme endothelial nitric oxide synthase (eNOS) and, consequently, the availability of nitric oxide (NO) (Figure 2). Moreover, capsaicin also induces expression [29] while decreasing the expression of inflammatory biomarkers such as IL-6, TNF, and CCL-2, associated with NF-κB inactivation [30]. Phosphorylation of Akt is also described after capsaicin treatment, which results in disruption of the NRF2/Keap complex and release of activated transcription factor NRF2 (Figure 2). This signaling triggers the transcription of heme-oxygenase1 genes, which are essential for heme degradation and prevention of oxidative damage [31]. Other antioxidant enzymes, such as superoxide dismutase (SOD), catalase, and glutathione peroxidase, as well as glutathione levels, may have their activities modified after oral treatment with capsaicin [32]. Figure 2 summarizes the main TRPV1-dependent effects of capsaicin.

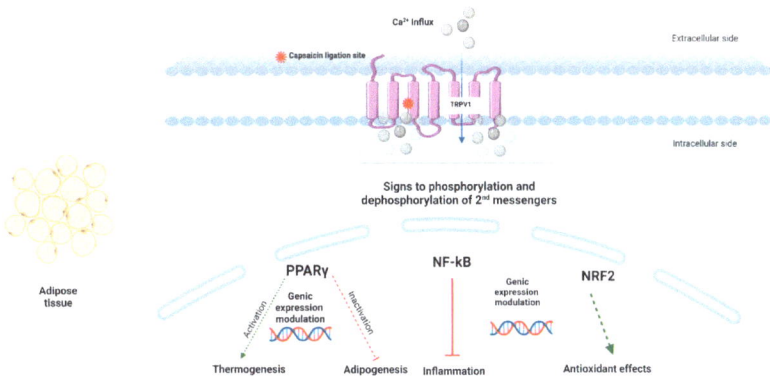

Figure 2. General scheme of the main effects described for the TRPV1-dependent action of capsaicin. The rapid influx of calcium caused by the binding of the capsaicin molecule to its receptor triggers a cascade of signals that include phosphorylation and dephosphorylation of second messengers and enzymes, regulating mainly the pathways of nociception (in neural tissue), thermogenesis, oxidative stress, inflammation, and adipogenesis in adipose tissue. Created with BioRender.com.

4. TRPV1-Independent Mechanisms of Action

Although TRPV1 is the central mediator of capsaicin's effects, studies suggest this receptor is not its only target (Figure 3). The activations of TRPV1-dependent or independent pathways by capsaicin are related to the dose of capsaicin and the site where capsaicin is acting [21]. For example, in the gastrointestinal tract, low concentrations of capsaicin (~1 µM) are reported to induce cell death by mechanisms involving a rapid and transient increase in TRPV1-dependent intracellular Ca^{2+}. However, higher concentrations of capsaicin ($\geq$10 µM) induce cell death through TRPV1-independent mechanisms involving mitochondrial dysfunction and plasma membrane depolarization [27].

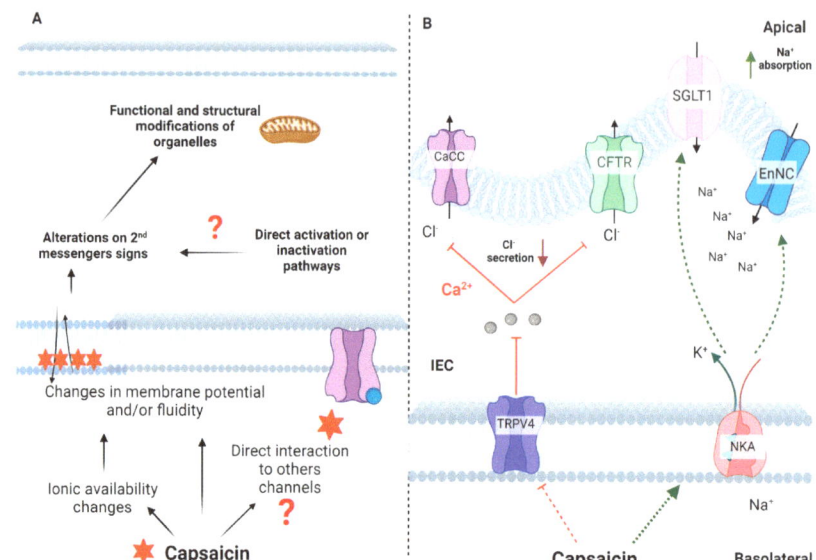

Figure 3. Main actions carried out by capsaicin independently of TRPV1. (**A**) Regardless of the presence of receptors, capsaicin could interact with biological membranes and modify membrane fluidity or potential, triggering signals conducted by the involved second messengers, which causes structural changes in cells and organelles, including mitochondria. These structural changes culminate in physiological responses in non-neuronal tissues that may be related to capsaicin's beneficial or adverse actions. Furthermore, it is suggested that capsaicin could also directly bind to receptors or channels other than TRPV1 and generate changes in the metabolic pathways related to these receptors. (**B**) In intestinal epithelial cells (IECs), capsaicin could induce changes in other ion channels, such as TRPV4, blocking their actions. This blockade attenuates Cl^- secretion and stimulates Na^+ absorption. NKA (Na/K ATPase); (ENaC) epithelial Na^+ channels; (CFTR) cystic fibrosis transmembrane conductance regulator; (SGLT1) Na^+-glucose cotransporter 1. Created with BioRender.com.

Despite extensive research, the exact mechanisms of non-neuronal and TRPV1-independent effects of capsaicin are poorly understood. A non-specific and receptor-independent effect, such as the induction of changes in membrane fluidity, is also dependent on membrane lipid composition [33]. Capsaicin can cause structural and physiological changes in organelles, such as mitochondria, by chemically affecting the structural properties of biological membranes. These changes occur because the physicochemical modifications in this nanoenvironment can alter the membrane potential and the ionic concentration and cause oxidative imbalance. These effects could culminate in apoptosis, as reported in pancreatic cancer cell lines [32].

The direct effects of capsaicin seem to be affected by the cell type, in addition to the dose and route of administration. Capsaicin acts not only through increases in Ca^{2+}

mediated by its binding to TRPV1 but also by modifying the availability and flux of other ions such as Na^+, K^+, and Ca^{2+} itself for other voltage-gated ion channels, ionic transporters, and possibly interacting directly with other channels and receptors [34].

It is suggested that capsaicin induces impaired hippocampal *Gamma oscillations* through a TRPV1-independent pathway involving Na^+/K^+ ATPase (NKA). Thus, using capsaicin to reduce these oscillations to levels of healthy controls could become a promising strategy in the face of psychiatric and neurological disorders that present this dysfunction as a characteristic [21].

Another possible TRPV1-independent effect of capsaicin is its oncoprotective action. In glioblastoma and colon cancer cells, capsaicin was able to induce apoptosis by increasing PPARγ expression independently of its vanilloid receptor [35]. Some of the TRPV1-independent effects of capsaicin may be related to its ability to activate or deactivate PPARs, particularly PPARγ [36]. PPARγ is predominantly expressed in adipose tissue and, to a lesser extent, in other tissues such as skeletal muscle and liver. Capsaicin is described as a PPARγ activator or inhibitor. This effect in modulating PPARγ seems to be dependent on several factors, such as the balance between the PPARs (which also include PPARα and PPARβ/δ) in the different metabolic states, the presence of TRPV1, the dose of capsaicin, and even the intestinal enterotype [37,38]. Therefore, the possibility of directing the actions of capsaicin in PPARγ for therapeutic purposes and, at the same time, minimizing side effects represent major challenges [39].

Dietary capsaicin can attenuate Cl^- secretion and stimulate Na^+ absorption by blocking TRPV4 channels while stimulating NKA activity in intestinal epithelial cells (IEC). The intracellular Ca^{2+} stimulates Cl^- secretion through the Ca^{2+}-dependent Cl^- secretion (CaCC) channel and apical cystic fibrosis transmembrane conductance regulator (CFTR). The blockade of TRPV4 caused by capsaicin decreases Ca^{2+} entry through this channel and reduces the stimulus for Cl^- secretion. In contrast, stimulation of basolateral NKA activity would establish an ionic gradient and driving force to promote apical Na^+ absorption via Na^+-glucose transporter 1 (SGLT1) and the epithelial apical Na^+ channel (ENaC) [40].

It is suggested that the protective effects of capsaicin against chemical carcinogens are mainly related to halogens metabolized by the cytochrome P450 (CYP450) enzyme system. Several mechanisms make capsaicin a promising agent against several types of cancer, as highlighted in a recent review [41]. Capsaicin acts by inhibiting the activity of these enzymes, which prevents the metabolization of halogens into highly reactive species. Thus, the chemoprotective role of capsaicin has been mainly associated with the ability to modulate CYP enzymes [42].

Recent approaches are centered on capsaicin's ability to modulate the intestinal microbiota. Capsaicin can influence intestinal microbiota by a mechanism not totally understood. It is suggested that regular treatment with capsaicin increases diversity in the gut microbiota and abundance of short-chain fatty acid (SCFA)-producing bacteria [43].

Moreover, capsaicin treatment prevents dysbiosis, gut barrier dysfunction, and low-grade chronic systemic inflammation [44] caused by dysbiosis. The ability of capsaicin to modulate the intestinal microbiota has been discussed not only as one of its TRPV1-independent effects but also as the basis for other beneficial systemic effects [45] on metabolic diseases [46] and cancer [47]. Nonetheless, although this is a promising field of research, the role of capsaicin on intestinal microbiota is still controversial [48]. Such studies were carried out primarily in experimental models; despite their promising effects, caution is needed when translating such effects into humans.

5. Anti-Inflammatory and Gastrointestinal Effects of Capsaicin

Capsaicin has been tested for preventing and treating intestinal pain and inflammation due to its functions in the gastrointestinal tract [49–51]. Its actions on gastrointestinal sensory neurons may be dependent or independent of TRPV1 in mammals. Capsaicin triggers a painful and burning sensation in a TRPV1-dependent manner. On the other hand, as cited before, capsaicin appears to induce changes in anion secretions and induction of apoptosis of cancer cells by mechanisms independent of TRPV1 [28,52]. However, little is known about the actions of capsaicin in the gastrointestinal tract independently of TRPV1 [40]. Recent evidence has shown an important role for TRPV4 channels in the pathogenesis of experimental ulcerative colitis because these channels regulate ion transport in the intestinal epithelium [40]. Capsaicin was able to inhibit Cl$^-$ secretion and promote Na$^+$ absorption by blocking TRPV4 channels. Moreover, the inactivation of TRPV4 channels by capsaicin in experimental colitis suppressed the overactivation of these channels that occurs in colitis [40].

Regarding anti-inflammatory effects, one of the main actions of capsaicin is the inhibition of the NFκ-B pathway that reduces proinflammatory cytokines (IL-6, TNF, and IL-1β) production and mRNA expression of the NLRP3 inflammasome, associated with a lower NFκB phosphorylation [53]. In addition, the reduction in the junctional protein E-cadherin, typical in *H. pylori* infection, was attenuated after capsaicin treatment. It occurred due to reduced expression of the gastric cancer biomarkers miR21 and miR223, which downregulate the E-cadherin expression [53].

However, the effects of capsaicin on inflammation can be modulated by the dose administered. Xiang et al. [54] investigated the effects of oral administration of 40, 60, and 80 mg/kg weight of capsaicin for 7 days on gastrointestinal health and intestinal microbiota, using specific pathogen-free (SPF) mice. They showed that intakes above 60 mg/kg seem harmful to the intestine. The administration of 80 mg/kg caused inflammatory cell infiltration and loss of mucus-producing goblet cells in the colon. Such inflammation was characterized by elevated levels of inflammatory cytokines, especially TNF and IL-β1, and lower levels of the anti-inflammatory cytokine IL-10, suggesting damage to the jejunum and colon at such a dose. In addition, there was an increase in serum levels of neuropeptides (SP and CGRP) related to visceral pain, causing additional damage to the gastrointestinal system in a TRPV1-dependent manner [54]. On the other hand, changes in the intestinal microbiota profile were observed when 40 mg/kg was assessed. The abundance of *Lactobacillus* in the jejunum and ileum associated with capsaicin treatment was related to higher levels of IL-10, suggesting that the microbiota modulation by capsaicin may induce changes in the intestinal inflammatory environment.

In an experimental model of colorectal cancer, Cheng et al. [48] administered 300 mg/kg of capsaicin for 12 weeks to mice before the intraperitoneal injection of EGFP-labelled CT26 cells. Mice presented a proinflammatory microenvironment with increased cytokines IL-12, TNF, and IFN in the liver and IL-6 in the blood. In addition, there was an increase in neutrophils, macrophages, and monocyte infiltration associated with a reduction in the thickness of the intestinal mucus barrier, bacterial translocation, and destruction of the vascular epithelial barrier. The authors suggested that intake of high-dose CAP over the long term could increase the risk of metastasis in colorectal cancer [48]. However, the results contradict other studies indicating capsaicin could suppress tumor cell growth [54–56]. As discussed above, some effects of capsaicin are dose-dependent and may differ according to its concentration and time of use. For instance, there is no reason to recommend or avoid using capsaicin-rich foods in those with intestinal diseases [27,48,55–57].

6. Capsaicin and Non-Communicable Chronic Diseases

Capsaicin has been suggested as a potential alternative treatment for diabetes due to its influence on glucose metabolism [32]. The in vitro study of Bort et al. [36] using C1C12-derived myotubes cultured with 100 and 200 μM of capsaicin found an increase in intracellular calcium induced by CAP-TRPV1 binding. It could stimulate intracellular signaling pathways through calcium/calmodulin-dependent protein kinase kinase 2 (CAMKK2), which, in turn, phosphorylates AMP-activated protein kinase (AMPK), a regulatory kinase involved in glucose and lipid metabolisms. This action would improve insulin sensitivity due to increased fatty acid oxidation, insulin secretion, glucose uptake, and reduction in inflammatory factors [36].

Capsaicin was also related to increased glucose uptake in a TRPV1-independent, TRPV4-dependent manner, stimulating the co-transport of Na-glucose. In TRPV4 knockout mice, Na^+ uptake was increased compared to the wild type, in which CAP was also shown to be able to potentiate the action of blocking TRPV4 and Na absorption via the Na-glucose cotransporter (SGLT1) [40,58].

In diabetic rats, oral administration of 0.5 g/kg of capsaicin for 8 weeks reduced cholesterolemia, triglyceridemia, and cardiac fibrosis [59]. An analysis of the heart showed increased expression of TRPV1 and eNOS associated with increased levels of nitric oxide and reduced reactive oxygen species (ROS). Similar results were obtained when vascular endothelial cells from these animals were treated with different concentrations of glucose and capsaicin [59].

Individuals with chronic diseases such as diabetes are more prone to vascular senescence, manifested by accelerated vascular stiffness and atherosclerosis. Senescent endothelial cells show loss of proliferation potential, decreased vasodilation, and proinflammatory and pro-arteriosclerotic phenotype [60]. In this sense, the beneficial effects of capsaicin at different concentrations (0.3 μM, 1.0 μM, and 3.0 μM) on the senescence of HUVEC cells exposed to 5 and 33 mM of glucose were studied. The findings showed a capsaicin-induced increase in sirtuin 1 (SIRT1), a protein that prevents endothelial senescence induced by intermittent hyperglycemia. In addition to increasing SIRT1 levels, capsaicin was able to suppress p21, a protein associated with ROS production and senescence. Thus, it was suggested that capsaicin could be a potential adjuvant in treating vascular aging in diabetes [60].

Reports of the action of capsaicin in atherosclerosis development are numerous, mainly due to the improvement in lipid profile, inflammation, and endothelial dysfunction [46,60–63]. Dai et al. [46] studied the role of the microbiota in the anti-atherosclerotic effect of oral capsaicin (0.01% w/w) in ApoE knockout mice fed a high-fat diet (HFD) and demonstrated that the reduction in LDL-c and increase in HDL-c was associated with reductions in atherogenesis shown by the reduction in the lesion area on aortic sinus and greater stability of atherosclerotic plaques. In the context of inflammation, capsaicin improved the HFD-induced inflammatory response in the intestinal mucosa, as seen by the reduction in inflammatory biomarkers IL-6 and LPS. In addition, capsaicin administration also altered the composition of the intestinal microbiota and metabolomic profiles, which could contribute to improving atherosclerosis. The microbiota's relevant role in capsaicin's action was confirmed when these effects disappeared in antibiotic-treated animals [46].

Regarding experimental studies on body weight control, Song et al. [64] showed that diets with low (0.01%) or high (0.02%) capsaicin supplementation could not prevent weight gain in ob/ob mice but inhibited increased fasting blood glucose and improved insulin sensitivity. Despite the absence of effects on body weight, capsaicin, in both concentrations, increased fecal levels of butyrate (short-chain fatty acid produced by microbiota fermentation) and blood GLP-1 while decreasing blood levels of ghrelin and inflammatory cytokines [64]. Although both levels of supplementation failed to alter the α and β diversity of the intestinal microbiota, there was an increase in the *Firmicutes/Bacteroidetes* fila ratio. At the genus level, an increase in the abundance of Roseburia was found, related to lower blood glucose levels, and a decrease in the abundance of *Bacteroides* and *Parabacteroides* associated with higher blood glucose [64].

Together, these data corroborate previous studies showing the influence of the microbiota-modulating action in the hypoglycemic and anti-inflammatory effects of Capsaicin [27,48,49,65]. Nonetheless, although these preclinical studies show encouraging results, they must be confirmed through long-lasting controlled trials.

7. Effect of Capsaicin on Metabolic Syndrome and Obesity

Many studies with capsaicin have been performed in rodents, and the resulting transposition to humans is not always possible, including dose matching for humans. In this way, Szallasi et al. [66] estimated the correspondence of dietary capsaicin intake from rats to humans. They concluded that a dose of 50 mg/kg of supplemented capsaicin for rats (about 250 g of body weight) would be equivalent to 12.5 mg/day for humans, an intake higher than the average consumption in Korea, estimated in 2.17 mg of Capsaicin [67]. Furthermore, the 0.01% capsaicin supplementation in diet, used in several experimental models, is also above the average intake in most countries that consume spicy meals. Thus, studies on realistic amounts of capsaicin supplementation or foods rich in capsaicinoids should be conducted. Moreover, these studies should consider individual differences, such as the presence or absence of obesity and its metabolic consequences.

The described beneficial properties of capsaicin occur due to a wide variety of properties, which goes beyond the metabolism and expands its field of use from packaging conservation to effects on human health [68,69].

The metabolic actions of capsaicin, mainly related to antioxidant, anti-inflammatory, and thermogenic properties, make capsaicin a promising adjuvant in treating and preventing metabolic syndrome, obesity, and associated comorbidities such as dyslipidemia and diabetes mellitus [69–72].

A previous scope review analyzed publications about capsaicin receptors signaling for its antiobesity properties [73]. The analysis showed that, besides TRPV1, capsaicin could also act as an agonist for PPARs, especially PPARγ, on fat metabolism [36,74]. Given the role of PPARγ in the transcriptional regulation of adipogenesis, this would be one of the potential pathways for the antiobesity action of Caps. Activation of PPARγ by capsaicin has also been associated with its beneficial action on obesity, reducing inflammatory markers and inducing the expression and synthesis of adiponectin in mouse adipocytes [73].

Thus, capsaicin signaling in obesity and fat metabolism is mainly described as TRPV1-dependent [25,75–78], although some studies presented TRPV1-independent actions, including activation of PPARγ [4,76,79,80]. In fact, independently of capsaicin signaling, several mechanisms mediate the action of capsaicin in weight loss, mostly linked to its ability to increase thermogenesis, induce satiety, and modify the obesogenic microbiota.

Although several reviews have been published in recent years about the effect of capsaicin, capsinoids, and spicy foods on obesity [24,41,66,81,82], we are far from the confirmatory answer to if this action occurs in the general as well as in the affected population, what the magnitude of this action is, if it is safe, and what the optimal therapeutic dose and treatment duration are.

7.1. Effects of Capsaicin on Food Intake and Satiety

Capsaicin, through its binding to albumin, reaches the adrenal gland, which induces the release of catecholamines. It has been shown that capsaicin can increase lipolysis in adipocytes and stimulate fat oxidation by activating the sympathetic nervous system [83]. This situation may affect tissues such as brown and white adipose tissue involved in body weight control. In white adipose tissue, capsaicin can exert several actions, increasing lipolysis and reducing lipogenesis [84,85] and, thus, reducing adipocyte volume and, consequently, adiposity [86]. In brown adipose tissue, capsaicin activates browning by increasing UCP1 expression, mitochondrial biogenesis, energy expenditure, and glycerol recycling [85,87,88].

Studies in animal models have suggested that capsaicin may increase satietogenic hormones such as glucagon-like protein 1 (GLP-1) and the gastric inhibitory peptide (GIP) [89]. The intense concentration of TRPV1 in the nervous system, mainly in the hypothalamus, supports the possible relationship between capsaicin and changes in hunger/satiety control. However, the role of capsaicin in increasing these incretins in clinical studies is still inconsistent. In this way, some reviews assessed the effect of capsaicin and spicy food on cognition, food preferences, and satiety induction [24,81,90–92]. Although an increase in GLP-1 was seen after a capsaicin-supplemented meal [93], a more recent study using intraduodenal infusion of capsaicin in volunteers without obesity did not observe an increase in plasma concentrations of GLP-1 and PYY [94].

Rigamonti et al. [95] assessed the acute effect of capsaicin on appetite-regulating gastrointestinal peptides on the energy balance of young subjects with obesity. They showed that capsaicin (2 mg), provided during an "ad libitum" dinner, did not change circulating levels of ghrelin, GLP-1, peptide YY, or satiety after food. Nonetheless, the pre-post meal difference in rest metabolism was higher in those receiving capsaicin. The authors suggest capsaicin could act as a metabolic activator rather than a hypophagic inducer [95]. In another study, supplementation for 8 weeks with 12 mg/day of capsiate, a non-pungent analog of capsaicin, increased body weight by 1 kg. However, this increase was due to increased upper body strength compared to placebo [96].

It is interesting to note that the effect of capsaicin may change between individuals, depending on body weight. It was the result of a meta-analysis that found that after ingestion of capsaicin or capsinoids, there is a modest increase in energy expenditure of around 58 kcal/day and a reduction in the respiratory quotient, suggesting increased lipid oxidation in individuals with BMI > 25 kg/m^2 [97]. In those with BMI < 25 kg/m^2, capsaicin or capsinoids did not affect energy expenditure or respiratory quotient. In this way, research addressing the long-term effect of capsaicin in individuals with and without obesity should be conducted, analyzing the effects on food intake, satiety, and intestinal hormone production. The diet composition should also be considered since it affects hormone release and central food control.

7.2. Effect of Capsaicin on Obesogenic Dysbiosis

The effects of capsaicin in favoring healthy gut microbiota have been demonstrated in experimental animals [98–101] and in vitro studies [43,102], with a lag in the literature regarding clinical studies. One factor in chronic low-grade inflammation linked to obesity is metabolic endotoxemia, resulting in intestinal dysbiosis. Kang et al. [103] demonstrated that mice fed a high-fat diet supplemented with capsaicin exhibited lower levels of metabolic endotoxemia and chronic inflammation associated with lower body weight gain. Other findings in the gastrointestinal tract were increased abundance of butyrate-producing *Ruminococcaceae* and *Lachnospiraceae*, and low levels of S24-7 lipopolysaccharide (LPS)-producing bacteria and inhibition of type 1 cannabinoid receptors (CB1). Interestingly, when the microbiota from the capsaicin-treated animals was transferred to germ-free mice fed a high-fat diet, the recipient mice maintained the protective effects.

Furthermore, when microbiota depletion was induced by an antibiotic cocktail, there was a loss of capsaicin protection against obesity [103]. However, Manca et al. [104], in an exploratory clinical study with women presenting overweight and obesity, showed that the oral administration of capsicum extract capsules for 12 weeks produced a modest increase in the relative abundance of the genus *Flavonifractor*. The rise in the *Flavonifractor* genus may be related to its ability to metabolize flavonoids such as curcumin, with which capsaicin has structural homology. Species belonging to this genus, such as *F. plautii*, have been involved in reducing inflammation [105].

Xia et al. [59] cultivated human fecal microbiota from healthy volunteers with red pepper (2%) for 24 h and found an increase in acetate and propionate concentrations compared with control cultures. *Subdoligranulum* spp.-, *Blautia* spp.-, *Faecalibacterium prausnitzii*-, *P. vulgatus*-, and *Prevotella copri*-like bacteria were defined as red pepper-responsive indigenous gut bacteria. The authors concluded that red pepper increases the short-chain fatty acid-producing bacteria and other beneficial bacteria in human fecal cultures. A similar result was seen in the study of Mahalak et al. [43], showing that capsaicin increases the diversity of human microbiota and SCFA abundance. These studies could explain the beneficial health effects of capsaicin in obesity and other non-communicable chronic diseases. The influence of capsaicin on glucose homeostasis and obesity by modulation of the gut microbiota is summarized in Figure 4.

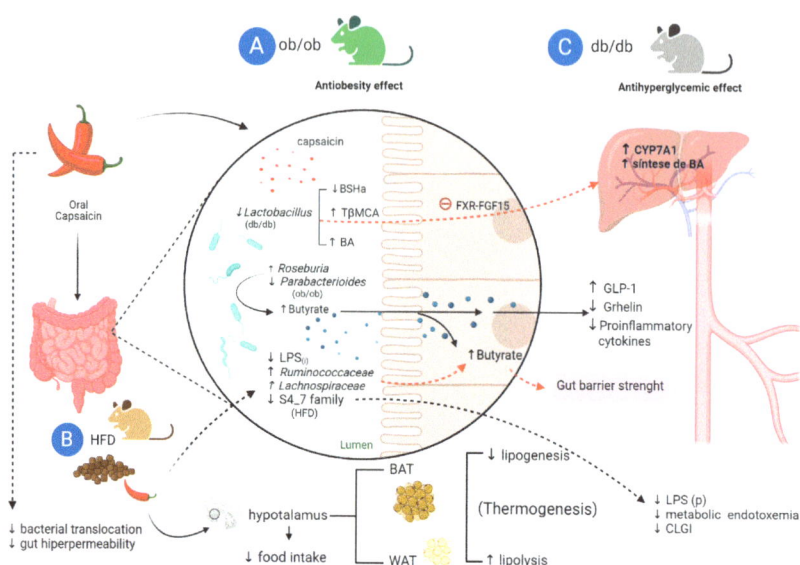

Figure 4. Influence of dietary capsaicin on glucose homeostasis and obesity via modulation of the gut microbiota. (**A**). capsaicin increases the abundance of Roseburia. It decreases the abundance of Bacteroides and Parabacterioides in obese diabetic mice (ob/ob), leading to an increase in butyrate and GLP-1 and a decrease in total plasma ghrelin and also and proinflammatory cytokines. (**B**). The antiobesity effects of capsaicin in mice fed a high-fat diet (HFD) modulate the gut–brain (hypothalamus) axis by decreasing food intake. In addition, capsaicin induces browning, favoring the formation of brown adipose tissue (BAT) and stimulating lipolysis of white adipose tissue (WAT). Capsaicin reduces the abundance of Gram-negative bacteria that secrete intestinal lipopolysaccharide (LPS(i)) and increases the abundance of butyrogenic bacteria (Ruminococcacea and Lachnospiraceae) and, consequently, butyrate. This effect attenuates the increased intestinal permeability and bacterial translocation caused by HFD and suppresses cannabinoid intestinal receptor type 1 (CB1(i)) expression. Thus, dietary capsaicin strengthens the intestinal barrier due to the increase in butyrate production, decrease in LPS(i) and plasma LPS (LPS(p)) with reduction in metabolic endotoxemia and chronic low-grade inflammation (CLGI) (**C**). The antihyperglycemic effect of capsaicin is due to a decrease in the abundance of Lactobacillus in diabetic mice (db/db), causing a reduction in the activity of bile salt hydrolase (BSHa) and an increase in the levels of conjugated bile acids (BA) in the intestine and of β-muricholic tauro acid (TβMCA), a farsenoid receptor antagonist (FXR), leading to the suppression of the FXR-FGF15 axis and a positive regulation of the expression of cholesterol 7 hydroxylase (CYP7A 1) stimulating the hepatic synthesis of BA. Created with BioRender.com.

In conclusion, clinical studies exploring the role of intestinal microbiota on the capsaicin effect, as well as the effect of capsaicin on the microbiome and intestinal microbiota balance, are necessary to assess the impact of this interaction on several metabolic conditions.

7.3. Effect of Non-Pungent Capsinoids and Spice Foods

Capsiate, dihydrocapsiate, and nordihydrocapsiate belong to the family capsinoids with a molecular structure similar to capsaicin. Like capsaicin, capsinoids bind TRPV1 in the intestinal epithelium. However, they do not activate TRPV1 in the oral cavity. Hereafter, they can induce their biological effects without producing pungency. In this way, capsinoids such as capsiate could be, as occurs with capsaicin, a promising agent for treating obesity.

Gupta et al. [71], in a review of the benefits of capsiate, concluded that it shares several properties with capsaicin, including increased satiety and reduced body weight. Likewise, Zsiborás et al. [97], in their meta-analysis, concluded that the metabolic effects not only of capsaicin but also of capsiate are significant in individuals with high BMI. However, in the same year, Szallasi et al. [66], analyzing clinical studies carried out with capsiate, did not observe a significant influence of non-pungent capsinoids on body weight and obesity.

Some reviews and clinical studies carried out with red [71,84,106] or black pepper [107,108] have observed beneficial effects on human health. Since capsaicin and chili peppers are the main components that give spicy characteristics to foods, it could be expected to associate the increase in spicy food consumption with the increase in capsaicin's beneficial effects. In this way, Yang et al. [109] examined the association between the frequency of spicy food intake and abdominal obesity in a Chinese population of 40,877 individuals. Interestingly, the results showed that the higher consumption of spicy foods was associated with increased abdominal adiposity. However, other factors besides capsaicin content, such as total caloric and nutrient intakes, physical activity, and comorbidities, among others, could have contributed to this result.

Similar results were found in a meta-analysis to evaluate the association between consumption of spicy foods and overweight/obesity, high blood pressure, and blood lipid profile [67]. The results showed that greater consumption of spicy foods was associated with an increased risk of overweight/obesity, an increased LDL-c, and a modest reduction in HDL-c. However, the consumption of spicy foods was negatively correlated with hypertension. Another study [110] analyzed the profile of spicy food consumption in a Chinese population. The results showed that the more frequent consumption and intense pungency of spicy foods were positively correlated with a preference for deep-fried food, salty snakes, alcohol and tea drinking, and tobacco smoking. These results highlight the importance of distinguishing between isolated capsaicin and pepper-containing foods' effects.

In addition to capsaicinoids and capsinoids, peppers are sources of nutrients and other bioactive components such as flavonoids, phenolic compounds, carotenoids, and ascorbic acid. These compounds aggregate and enhance several properties in peppers beyond capsaicin effects [92,111]. Other issues, such as the cultural consumption of pepper and the genetic characteristics of the studied populations, can influence the results. In this sense, clinical studies in populations from countries with the highest levels of per capita pepper consumption, such as Bulgaria (21 mg/day), Singapore (14 mg/day), and Vietnam (0.4 mg/day), as well as studies that consider different genetic characteristics, such as the presence of polymorphisms or different proteoforms of vanilloid receptors, can provide important findings and a better understanding of the role of capsaicin in health and diseases.

We can conclude that using capsinoids and pepper to improve chronic diseases is still controversial, mainly considering spicy foods in epidemiological studies. In this way, it is not possible to recommend or avoid spicy foods for such diseases.

8. Adverse Effects

Capsaicin is not free from adverse effects, especially when given topically. The most common effects, considering all routes of administration, are burning sensation, pruritus, edema at the administration site, and pain [112]. Muscle aches, chills, nasopharyngitis, sinusitis, bronchitis, cough and dyspnea, fever, tachycardia, dizziness and headache, hypertension, nausea, and vomiting are also described, although less common. Rarer complications include dysgeusia, hypoesthesia, peripheral edema, peripheral sensory neuropathy, and throat irritation [112]. Nonetheless, most effects may disappear during treatment.

9. Conclusions

Studies using capsaicinoids and capsinoids as adjuvants in obesity, diabetes, dyslipidemia, or cancer therapy are increasing in the literature. Although capsaicin is already approved as a topical treatment for neuropathic pain, its use in non-communicable diseases has not been properly and extensively studied to permit us an incontestable conclusion. Most of these studies show beneficial properties, improving antioxidant and anti-inflammatory status, inducing thermogenesis, and reducing white adipose tissue. Other mechanisms are also described, including reducing food intake and improving intestinal dysbiosis. Although some clinical studies lead us to the benefits of capsaicin supplementation, few studies were performed over 12 weeks in a population affected by these diseases. We should also further explore the route of administration for each disease since the metabolism of capsaicin depends on its route of administration.

Regarding obesity, several reviews have been published in recent years on the effect of capsaicin, capsinoids, and spicy foods on weight loss, making the indication as an adjuvant in this disease likely in the medium term. Type 2 diabetes and dyslipidemia are closely linked to obesity and, consequently, could be beneficiated by capsaicin supplementation. However, at the moment, there is still a lack of information about the following: 1—whether capsaicin action is similar in the general population and those affected by the disease; 2—the optimal therapeutic dose; 3—the duration of treatment; and 4—the safety of long-term administration. Even less is known about the effects of capsaicin on the gut microbiota and how this could reflect on metabolic diseases. In this way, many studies are still needed to characterize its action on dysbiosis. Regarding the role of capsaicin in cancer prevention, we are only in the first steps. Much remains to be researched, including understanding whether capsaicin is a cancer-protective or -promoting agent.

Furthermore, non-pungent capsinoids or synthetic analogs can conveniently substitute capsaicin. However, meta-analyses, although mostly showing beneficial effects in obesity, diabetes, dyslipidemia, and cancer, still need confirmation from new clinical trials.

Therefore, the answer to the question "Are we ready to recommend capsaicin for disorders other than neuropathic pain?" is no, we are not. We are close, but not ready yet, to including capsaicin supplements or creams as an adjunct in treating obesity and type 2 diabetes. Furthermore, we are far from fully understanding the role of capsaicin in other non-communicable diseases.

Author Contributions: Conceptualization, J.I.A.-L.; writing—original draft preparation, J.L.S., E.A.S. and J.I.A.-L.; writing—review and editing, J.L.S., E.A.S. and J.I.A.-L.; supervision, J.I.A.-L. All authors have read and agreed to the published version of the manuscript.

Funding: The authors thank the Conselho Nacional de Desenvolvimento Científico e Tecnológico (CNPq) for the research fellowship of J.I.A.L. (#310571/2020-0) and for the Ph.D. scholarship of J.L.S.

Conflicts of Interest: The authors declare no conflict of interest.

References

1. Rogers, J.; Urbina, S.L.; Taylor, L.W.; Wilborn, C.D.; Purpura, M.; Jäger, R.; Juturu, V. Capsaicinoids supplementation decreases percent body fat and fat mass: Adjustment using covariates in a post hoc analysis. *BMC Obes.* **2018**, *5*, 22. [CrossRef]
2. Chanda, S.; Bashir, M.; Babbar, S.; Koganti, A.; Bley, K. In vitro hepatic and skin metabolism of capsaicin. *Drug Metab. Dispos.* **2008**, *36*, 670–675. [CrossRef] [PubMed]
3. Stienstra, R.; Saudale, F.; Duval, C.; Keshtkar, S.; Groener, J.E.M.; Van Rooijen, N.; Staels, B.; Kersten, S.; Müller, M. Kupffer cells promote hepatic steatosis via interleukin-1β-dependent suppression of peroxisome proliferator-activated receptor α activity. *Hepatology* **2010**, *51*, 511–522. [CrossRef] [PubMed]
4. Kida, R.; Yoshida, H.; Murakami, M.; Shirai, M.; Hashimoto, O.; Kawada, T.; Matsui, T.; Funaba, M. Direct action of capsaicin in brown adipogenesis and activation of brown adipocytes. *Cell Biochem. Funct.* **2016**, *34*, 34–41. [CrossRef] [PubMed]
5. Tao, L.; Yang, G.; Sun, T.; Jie, T.; Zhu, C.; Yu, H.; Cheng, Y.; Yang, Z.; Xu, M.; Jiang, Y.; et al. Capsaicin receptor TRPV1 maintains quiescence of hepatic stellate cells in the liver via recruitment of SARM1. *J. Hepatol.* **2023**, *78*, 805–819. [CrossRef] [PubMed]
6. Bertin, S.; Aoki-Nonaka, Y.; De Jong, P.R.; Nohara, L.L.; Xu, H.; Stanwood, S.R.; Srikanth, S.; Lee, J.; To, K.; Abramson, L.; et al. The ion channel TRPV1 regulates the activation and proinflammatory properties of CD4[+] T cells. *Nat. Immunol.* **2014**, *15*, 1055–1063. [CrossRef]
7. Negri, S.; Faris, P.; Rosti, V.; Antognazza, M.R.; Lodola, F.; Moccia, F. Endothelial TRPV1 as an Emerging Molecular Target to Promote Therapeutic Angiogenesis. *Cells* **2020**, *9*, 1341. [CrossRef]
8. Yang, F.; Xiao, X.; Cheng, W.; Yang, W.; Yu, P.; Song, Z.; Yarov-Yarovoy, V.; Zheng, J. Structural mechanism underlying capsaicin binding and activation of the TRPV1 ion channel. *Nat. Chem. Biol.* **2015**, *11*, 518–524. [CrossRef]
9. Forstenpointner, J.; Naleschinski, D.; Wasner, G.; Hüllemann, P.; Binder, A.; Baron, R. Sensitized vasoactive C-nociceptors: Key fibers in peripheral neuropathic pain. *Pain Rep.* **2019**, *4*, e709. [CrossRef]

10. Irving, G.A.; Backonja, M.; Rauck, R.; Webster, L.R.; Tobias, J.K.; Vanhove, G.F. NGX-4010, a capsaicin 8% dermal patch, administered alone or in combination with systemic neuropathic pain medications, reduces pain in patients with postherpetic neuralgia. *Clin. J. Pain* **2012**, *28*, 101–107. [CrossRef]
11. Huang, C.-J.; Pu, C.-M.; Su, S.-Y.; Lo, S.-L.; Lee, C.H.; Yen, Y.-H. Improvement of wound healing by capsaicin through suppression of the inflammatory response and amelioration of the repair process. *Mol. Med. Rep.* **2023**, *28*, 1–13. [CrossRef]
12. Batiha, G.E.S.; Alqahtani, A.; Ojo, O.A.; Shaheen, H.M.; Wasef, L.; Elzeiny, M.; Ismail, M.; Shalaby, M.; Murata, T.; Zaragoza-Bastida, A.; et al. Biological Properties, Bioactive Constituents, and Pharmacokinetics of Some *Capsicum* spp. and Capsaicinoids. *Int. J. Mol. Sci.* **2020**, *21*, 5179. [CrossRef]
13. Thongin, S.; Den-udom, T.; Uppakara, K.; Sriwantana, T.; Sibmooh, N.; Laolob, T.; Boonthip, C.; Wichai, U.; Muta, K.; Ketsawatsomkron, P. Beneficial effects of capsaicin and dihydrocapsaicin on endothelial inflammation, nitric oxide production and antioxidant activity. *Biomed. Pharmacother.* **2022**, *154*, 113521. [CrossRef]
14. Nawaka, N.; Wanmasae, S.; Makarasen, A.; Dechtrirat, D.; Techasakul, S.; Jeenduang, N. Allicin and Capsaicin Ameliorated Hypercholesterolemia by Upregulating LDLR and Downregulating PCSK9 Expression in HepG2 Cells. *Int. J. Mol. Sci.* **2022**, *23*, 14299. [CrossRef]
15. Ursu, D.; Knopp, K.; Beattie, R.E.; Liu, B.; Sher, E. Pungency of TRPV1 agonists is directly correlated with kinetics of receptor activation and lipophilicity. *Eur. J. Pharmacol.* **2010**, *641*, 114–122. [CrossRef]
16. Lim, S.G.; Seo, S.E.; Jo, S.; Kim, K.H.; Kim, L.; Kwon, O.S. Highly Efficient Real-Time TRPV1 Screening Methodology for Effective Drug Candidates. *ACS Omega* **2022**, *7*, 36441–36447. [CrossRef]
17. Marzęda, P.; Wróblewska-Łuczka, P.; Florek-Łuszczki, M.; Drozd, M.; Góralczyk, A.; Łuszczki, J.J. Comparison of the Anticancer Effects of Arvanil and Olvanil When Combined with Cisplatin and Mitoxantrone in Various Melanoma Cell Lines-An Isobolographic Analysis. *Int. J. Mol. Sci.* **2022**, *23*, 14192. [CrossRef] [PubMed]
18. Suresh, D.; Srinivasan, K. Tissue distribution & elimination of capsaicin, piperine & curcumin following oral intake in rats. *Indian J. Med. Res.* **2010**, *131*, 682–691. [PubMed]
19. Christensen, J.D.; Lo Vecchio, S.; Andersen, H.H.; Elberling, J.; Arendt-Nielsen, L. Effect of Topical Analgesia on Desensitization Following 8% Topical Capsaicin Application. *J. Pain* **2021**, *22*, 778–788. [CrossRef] [PubMed]
20. van Neerven, S.G.A.; Mouraux, A. Capsaicin-Induced Skin Desensitization Differentially Affects A-Delta and C-Fiber-Mediated Heat Sensitivity. *Front. Pharmacol.* **2020**, *11*, 615. [CrossRef]
21. Balleza-Tapia, H.; Dolz-Gaiton, P.; Andrade-Talavera, Y.; Fisahn, A. Capsaicin-Induced Impairment of Functional Network Dynamics in Mouse Hippocampus via a TrpV1 Receptor-Independent Pathway: Putative Involvement of Na$^+$/K$^+$-ATPase. *Mol. Neurobiol.* **2020**, *57*, 1170–1185. [CrossRef] [PubMed]
22. Lawrence, G.W.; Zurawski, T.H.; Dong, X.; Oliver Dolly, J. Population Coding of Capsaicin Concentration by Sensory Neurons Revealed Using Ca^{2+} Imaging of Dorsal Root Ganglia Explants from Adult pirt-GCaMP3 Mouse. *Cell. Physiol. Biochem.* **2021**, *55*, 428–448.
23. Arora, V.; Campbell, J.N.; Chung, M.K. Fight fire with fire: Neurobiology of capsaicin-induced analgesia for chronic pain. *Pharmacol. Ther.* **2021**, *220*, 107743. [CrossRef] [PubMed]
24. Irandoost, P.; Lotfi Yagin, N.; Namazi, N.; Keshtkar, A.; Farsi, F.; Mesri Alamdari, N.; Vafa, M. The effect of Capsaicinoids or Capsinoids in red pepper on thermogenesis in healthy adults: A systematic review and meta-analysis. *Phyther. Res.* **2021**, *35*, 1358–1377. [CrossRef]
25. Baskaran, P.; Krishnan, V.; Ren, J.; Thyagarajan, B. Capsaicin induces browning of white adipose tissue and counters obesity by activating TRPV1 channel-dependent mechanisms. *Br. J. Pharmacol.* **2016**, *173*, 2369–2389. [CrossRef]
26. Ghorbanpour, A.; Salari, S.; Baluchnejadmojarad, T.; Roghani, M. Capsaicin protects against septic acute liver injury by attenuation of apoptosis and mitochondrial dysfunction. *Heliyon* **2023**, *9*, e14205. [CrossRef] [PubMed]
27. Xiang, Y.; Xu, X.; Zhang, T.; Wu, X.; Fan, D.; Hu, Y.; Ding, J.; Yang, X.; Lou, J.; Du, Q.; et al. Beneficial effects of dietary capsaicin in gastrointestinal health and disease. *Exp. Cell Res.* **2022**, *417*, 113227. [CrossRef]
28. Bouyer, P.G.; Tang, X.; Weber, C.R.; Shen, L.; Turner, J.R.; Matthews, J.B. Capsaicin induces NKCC1 internalization and inhibits chloride secretion in colonic epithelial cells independently of TRPV1. *Am. J. Physiol. Gastrointest. Liver Physiol.* **2013**, *304*, G142–G156. [CrossRef]
29. Ching, L.C.; Kou, Y.R.; Shyue, S.K.; Su, K.H.; Wei, J.; Cheng, L.C.; Yu, Y.B.; Pan, C.C.; Lee, T.S. Molecular mechanisms of activation of endothelial nitric oxide synthase mediated by transient receptor potential vanilloid type 1. *Cardiovasc. Res.* **2011**, *91*, 492–501. [CrossRef]
30. Kang, J.H.; Kim, C.S.; Han, I.S.; Kawada, T.; Yu, R. Capsaicin, a spicy component of hot peppers, modulates adipokine gene expression and protein release from obese-mouse adipose tissues and isolated adipocytes, and suppresses the inflammatory responses of adipose tissue macrophages. *FEBS Lett.* **2007**, *581*, 4389–4396. [CrossRef]
31. Joung, E.J.; Li, M.H.; Lee, H.G.; Somparn, N.; Jung, Y.S.; Na, H.K.; Kim, S.H.; Cha, Y.N.; Surh, Y.J. Capsaicin induces heme oxygenase-1 expression in HepG2 cells via activation of PI3K-Nrf2 signaling: NAD(P)H:quinone oxidoreductase as a potential target. *Antioxid. Redox Signal.* **2007**, *9*, 2087–2098. [CrossRef] [PubMed]
32. Pramanik, K.C.; Boreddy, S.R.; Srivastava, S.K. Role of mitochondrial electron transport chain complexes in capsaicin mediated oxidative stress leading to apoptosis in pancreatic cancer cells. *PLoS ONE* **2011**, *6*, e20151. [CrossRef]

33. Sharma, N.; Phan, H.T.T.; Yoda, T.; Shimokawa, N.; Vestergaard, M.C.; Takagi, M. Effects of Capsaicin on Biomimetic Membranes. *Biomimetics* 2019, *4*, 17. [CrossRef] [PubMed]
34. Isaev, D.; Yang, K.H.S.; Shabbir, W.; Howarth, F.C.; Oz, M. Capsaicin Inhibits Multiple Voltage-Gated Ion Channels in Rabbit Ventricular Cardiomyocytes in TRPV1-Independent Manner. *Pharmaceuticals* 2022, *15*, 1187. [CrossRef] [PubMed]
35. Szoka, L.; Palka, J. Capsaicin up-regulates pro-apoptotic activity of thiazolidinediones in glioblastoma cell line. *Biomed. Pharmacother.* 2020, *132*, 110741. [CrossRef]
36. Bort, A.; Sánchez, B.G.; Mateos-Gómez, P.A.; Díaz-Laviada, I.; Rodríguez-Henche, N. Capsaicin targets lipogenesis in hepG2 cells through AMPK activation, AKT inhibition and ppars regulation. *Int. J. Mol. Sci.* 2019, *20*, 1660. [CrossRef]
37. Wagner, N.; Wagner, K.D. The Role of PPARs in Disease. *Cells* 2020, *9*, 2367. [CrossRef]
38. Kang, C.; Zhang, Y.; Zhu, X.; Liu, K.; Wang, X.; Chen, M.; Wang, J.; Chen, H.; Hui, S.; Huang, L.; et al. Healthy Subjects Differentially Respond to Dietary Capsaicin Correlating with Specific Gut Enterotypes. *J. Clin. Endocrinol. Metab.* 2016, *101*, 4681–4689. [CrossRef]
39. Zeng, H.; Shi, N.; Peng, W.; Yang, Q.; Ren, J.; Yang, H.; Chen, L.; Chen, Y.; Guo, J. Effects of Capsaicin on Glucose Uptake and Consumption in Hepatocytes. *Molecules* 2023, *28*, 5258. [CrossRef]
40. Wan, H.; Chen, X.Y.; Zhang, F.; Chen, J.; Chu, F.; Sellers, Z.M.; Xu, F.; Dong, H. Capsaicin inhibits intestinal Cl^- secretion and promotes Na^+ absorption by blocking TRPV4 channels in healthy and colitic mice. *J. Biol. Chem.* 2022, *298*, 101847. [CrossRef]
41. Adetunji, T.L.; Olawale, F.; Olisah, C.; Adetunji, A.E.; Aremu, A.O. Capsaicin: A Two-Decade Systematic Review of Global Research Output and Recent Advances Against Human Cancer. *Front. Oncol.* 2022, *12*, 908487. [CrossRef]
42. Babbar, S.; Chanda, S.; Bley, K. Inhibition and induction of human cytochrome P450 enzymes in vitro by capsaicin. *Xenobiotica* 2010, *40*, 807–816. [CrossRef] [PubMed]
43. Mahalak, K.K.; Bobokalonov, J.; Firrman, J.; Williams, R.; Evans, B.; Fanelli, B.; Soares, J.W.; Kobori, M.; Liu, L. Analysis of the Ability of Capsaicin to Modulate the Human Gut Microbiota In Vitro. *Nutrients* 2022, *14*, 1283. [CrossRef] [PubMed]
44. Kang, Y.; Cai, Y. Gut microbiota and obesity: Implications for fecal microbiota transplantation therapy. *Hormones* 2017, *16*, 223–234. [CrossRef] [PubMed]
45. Wang, F.; Huang, X.; Chen, Y.; Zhang, D.; Chen, D.; Chen, L.; Lin, J. Study on the Effect of Capsaicin on the Intestinal Flora through High-Throughput Sequencing. *ACS Omega* 2020, *5*, 1246–1253. [CrossRef]
46. Dai, Z.; Li, S.; Meng, Y.; Zhao, Q.; Zhang, Y.; Suonan, Z.; Sun, Y.; Shen, Q.; Liao, X.; Xue, Y. Capsaicin Ameliorates High-Fat Diet-Induced Atherosclerosis in ApoE−/− Mice via Remodeling Gut Microbiota. *Nutrients* 2022, *14*, 4334. [CrossRef]
47. Garufi, A.; Pistritto, G.; Cirone, M.; D'Orazi, G. Reactivation of mutant p53 by capsaicin, the major constituent of peppers. *J. Exp. Clin. Cancer Res.* 2016, *35*, 1–9. [CrossRef]
48. Cheng, P.; Wu, J.; Zong, G.; Wang, F.; Deng, R.; Tao, R.; Qian, C.; Shan, Y.; Wang, A.; Zhao, Y.; et al. Capsaicin shapes gut microbiota and pre-metastatic niche to facilitate cancer metastasis to liver. *Pharmacol. Res.* 2023, *188*, 106643. [CrossRef]
49. Rosca, A.E.; Iesanu, M.I.; Zahiu, C.D.M.; Voiculescu, S.E.; Paslaru, A.C.; Zagrean, A.M. Capsaicin and gut microbiota in health and disease. *Molecules* 2020, *25*, 5681. [CrossRef]
50. Braga Ferreira, L.G.; Faria, J.V.; dos Santos, J.P.S.; Faria, R.X. Capsaicin: TRPV1-independent mechanisms and novel therapeutic possibilities. *Eur. J. Pharmacol.* 2020, *887*, 173356. [CrossRef]
51. Zhang, L.; Lu, W.; Lu, C.; Guo, Y.; Chen, X.; Chen, J.; Xu, F.; Wan, H.; Dong, H. Beneficial effect of capsaicin via TRPV4/EDH signals on mesenteric arterioles of normal and colitis mice. *J. Adv. Res.* 2022, *39*, 291–303. [CrossRef] [PubMed]
52. Holzer, P. Vanilloid receptor TRPV1: Hot on the tongue and inflaming the colon. *Neurogastroenterol. Motil.* 2004, *16*, 697–699. [CrossRef] [PubMed]
53. Saha, K.; Sarkar, D.; Khan, U.; Karmakar, B.C.; Paul, S.; Mukhopadhyay, A.K.; Dutta, S.; Bhattacharya, S. Capsaicin Inhibits Inflammation and Gastric Damage during H. pylori Infection by Targeting NF-kB–miRNA Axis. *Pathogens* 2022, *11*, 641. [CrossRef] [PubMed]
54. Xiang, Q.; Tang, X.; Cui, S.; Zhang, Q.; Liu, X.; Zhao, J.; Zhang, H.; Mao, B.; Chen, W. Capsaicin, the Spicy Ingredient of Chili Peppers: Effects on Gastrointestinal Tract and Composition of Gut Microbiota at Various Dosages. *Foods* 2022, *11*, 686. [CrossRef]
55. Liu, Y.P.; Dong, F.X.; Chai, X.; Zhu, S.; Zhang, B.L.; Gao, D.S. Role of Autophagy in Capsaicin-Induced Apoptosis in U251 Glioma Cells. *Cell. Mol. Neurobiol.* 2016, *36*, 737–743. [CrossRef]
56. Zheng, L.; Chen, J.; Ma, Z.; Liu, W.; Yang, F.; Yang, Z.; Wang, K.; Wang, X.; He, D.; Li, L.; et al. Capsaicin enhances anti-proliferation efficacy of pirarubicin via activating TRPV1 and inhibiting PCNA nuclear translocation in 5637 cells. *Mol. Med. Rep.* 2016, *13*, 881–887. [CrossRef]
57. Liang, W.; Lan, Y.; Chen, C.; Song, M.; Xiao, J.; Huang, Q.; Cao, Y.; Ho, C.-T.; Lu, M. Modulating effects of capsaicin on glucose homeostasis and the underlying mechanism. *Crit. Rev. Food Sci. Nutr.* 2023, *63*, 3634–3652. [CrossRef]
58. Ferdowsi, P.V.; Ahuja, K.D.K.; Beckett, J.M.; Myers, S. TRPV1 Activation by Capsaicin Mediates Glucose Oxidation and ATP Production Independent of Insulin Signalling in Mouse Skeletal Muscle Cells. *Cells* 2021, *10*, 1560. [CrossRef]
59. Xia, Y.; Lee, G.; Yamamoto, M.; Takahashi, H.; Kuda, T. Detection of indigenous gut bacteria related to red chilli pepper (*Capsicum annuum*) in murine caecum and human faecal cultures. *Mol. Biol. Rep.* 2022, *49*, 10239–10250. [CrossRef]
60. Zhu, S.L.; Wang, M.L.; He, Y.T.; Guo, S.W.; Li, T.T.; Peng, W.J.; Luo, D. Capsaicin ameliorates intermittent high glucose-mediated endothelial senescence via the TRPV1/SIRT1 pathway. *Phytomedicine* 2022, *100*, 154081. [CrossRef]

61. Zhou, Y.; Wang, X.; Guo, L.; Chen, L.; Zhang, M.; Chen, X.; Li, J.; Zhang, L. TRPV1 activation inhibits phenotypic switching and oxidative stress in vascular smooth muscle cells by upregulating PPARα. *Biochem. Biophys. Res. Commun.* **2021**, *545*, 157–163. [CrossRef] [PubMed]
62. Zhang, S.; Wang, D.; Huang, J.; Hu, Y.; Xu, Y. Application of capsaicin as a potential new therapeutic drug in human cancers. *J. Clin. Pharm. Ther.* **2020**, *45*, 16–28. [CrossRef] [PubMed]
63. McCarty, M.F.; DiNicolantonio, J.J.; O'Keefe, J.H. Capsaicin may have important potential for promoting vascular and metabolic health: Table 1. *Open Hear.* **2015**, *2*, e000262. [CrossRef] [PubMed]
64. Song, J.-X.X.; Ren, H.; Gao, Y.-F.F.; Lee, C.-Y.Y.; Li, S.-F.F.; Zhang, F.; Li, L.; Chen, H. Dietary Capsaicin Improves Glucose Homeostasis and Alters the Gut Microbiota in Obese Diabetic ob/ob Mice. *Front. Physiol.* **2017**, *8*, 602. [CrossRef] [PubMed]
65. Xue, M.; Ji, X.; Xue, C.; Liang, H.; Ge, Y.; He, X.; Zhang, L.; Bian, K.; Zhang, L. Caspase-dependent and caspase-independent induction of apoptosis in breast cancer by fucoidan via the PI3K/AKT/GSK3β pathway in vivo and in vitro. *Biomed. Pharmacother.* **2017**, *94*, 898–908. [CrossRef]
66. Szallasi, A. Capsaicin for Weight Control: "Exercise in a Pill" (or Just Another Fad)? *Pharmaceuticals* **2022**, *15*, 851. [CrossRef]
67. Wang, M.; Huang, W.; Xu, Y. Effects of spicy food consumption on overweight/obesity, hypertension and blood lipids in China: A meta-analysis of cross-sectional studies. *Nutr. J.* **2023**, *22*, 29. [CrossRef]
68. Baenas, N.; Belović, M.; Ilic, N.; Moreno, D.A.; García-Viguera, C. Industrial use of pepper (*Capsicum annum* L.) derived products: Technological benefits and biological advantages. *Food Chem* **2019**, *274*, 872–885. [CrossRef]
69. Wang, F.; Xue, Y.; Fu, L.; Wang, Y.; He, M.; Zhao, L.; Liao, X. Extraction, purification, bioactivity and pharmacological effects of capsaicin: A review. *Crit. Rev. Food Sci. Nutr.* **2022**, *62*, 5322–5348. [CrossRef]
70. Uarrota, V.G.; Maraschin, M.; de Bairros, Â.d.F.M.; Pedreschi, R. Factors affecting the capsaicinoid profile of hot peppers and biological activity of their non-pungent analogs (Capsinoids) present in sweet peppers. *Crit. Rev. Food Sci. Nutr.* **2021**, *61*, 649–665. [CrossRef]
71. Gupta, R.; Kapoor, B.; Gulati, M.; Kumar, B.; Gupta, M.; Singh, S.K.; Awasthi, A. Sweet pepper and its principle constituent capsiate: Functional properties and health benefits. *Crit. Rev. Food Sci. Nutr.* **2022**, *62*, 7370–7394. [CrossRef] [PubMed]
72. Sanati, S.; Razavi, B.M.; Hosseinzadeh, H. A review of the effects of *Capsicum annuum* L. and its constituent, capsaicin, in metabolic syndrome. *Iran. J. Basic Med. Sci.* **2018**, *21*, 439–448. [PubMed]
73. Ávila, D.L.; Nunes, N.A.M.; Almeida, P.H.R.F.; Gomes, J.A.S.; Rosa, C.O.B.; Alvarez-Leite, J.I. Signaling Targets Related to Antiobesity Effects of Capsaicin: A Scoping Review. *Adv. Nutr.* **2021**, *12*, 2232–2243. [CrossRef]
74. Sanjay, M.; Sharma, A.; Lee, H.J. Role of Phytoconstituents as PPAR Agonists: Implications for Neurodegenerative Disorders. *Biomedicines* **2021**, *9*, 1914. [CrossRef] [PubMed]
75. Krishnan, V.; Baskaran, P.; Thyagarajan, B. Troglitazone activates TRPV1 and causes deacetylation of PPARγ in 3T3-L1 cells. *Biochim. Biophys. Acta Mol. Basis Dis.* **2019**, *1865*, 445–453. [CrossRef]
76. Baboota, R.K.; Singh, D.P.; Sarma, S.M.; Kaur, J.; Sandhir, R.; Boparai, R.K.; Kondepudi, K.K.; Bishnoi, M. Capsaicin induces "Brite" phenotype in differentiating 3T3-L1 preadipocytes. *PLoS ONE* **2014**, *9*, e103093. [CrossRef]
77. Zhang, L.L.; Liu, D.Y.; Ma, L.Q.; Luo, Z.D.; Cao, T.B.; Zhong, J.; Yan, Z.C.; Wang, L.J.; Zhao, Z.G.; Zhu, S.J.; et al. Activation of transient receptor potential vanilloid type-1 channel prevents adipogenesis and obesity. *Circ. Res.* **2007**, *100*, 1063–1070. [CrossRef]
78. Chen, J.; Li, L.; Li, Y.; Liang, X.; Sun, Q.; Yu, H.; Zhong, J.; Ni, Y.; Chen, J.; Zhao, Z.; et al. Activation of TRPV1 channel by dietary capsaicin improves visceral fat remodeling through connexin43-mediated Ca^{2+} Influx. *Cardiovasc. Diabetol.* **2015**, *14*, 1–14. [CrossRef]
79. Kida, R.; Noguchi, T.; Murakami, M.; Hashimoto, O.; Kawada, T.; Matsui, T.; Funaba, M. Supra-pharmacological concentration of capsaicin stimulates brown adipogenesis through induction of endoplasmic reticulum stress. *Sci. Rep.* **2018**, *8*, 845. [CrossRef]
80. Fan, L.; Xu, H.; Yang, R.; Zang, Y.; Chen, J.; Qin, H. Combination of Capsaicin and Capsiate Induces Browning in 3T3-L1 White Adipocytes via Activation of the Peroxisome Proliferator-Activated Receptor γ/β3-Adrenergic Receptor Signaling Pathways. *J. Agric. Food Chem.* **2019**, *67*, 6232–6240. [CrossRef]
81. Thornton, T.; Mills, D.; Bliss, E. Capsaicin: A Potential Treatment to Improve Cerebrovascular Function and Cognition in Obesity and Ageing. *Nutrients* **2023**, *15*, 1537. [CrossRef] [PubMed]
82. Oz, M.; Lorke, D.E.; Howarth, F.C. Transient receptor potential vanilloid 1 (TRPV1)-independent actions of capsaicin on cellular excitability and ion transport. *Med. Res. Rev.* **2023**, *43*, 1038–1067. [CrossRef] [PubMed]
83. Ludy, M.J.; Moore, G.E.; Mattes, R.D. The Effects of Capsaicin and Capsiate on Energy Balance: Critical Review and Meta-analyses of Studies in Humans. *Chem. Senses* **2012**, *37*, 103–121. [CrossRef] [PubMed]
84. Oh, M.-J.; Lee, H.-B.; Yoo, G.; Park, M.; Lee, C.-H.; Choi, I.; Park, H.-Y. Anti-obesity effects of red pepper (*Capsicum annuum* L.) leaf extract on 3T3-L1 preadipocytes and high fat diet-fed mice. *Food Funct.* **2023**, *14*, 292–304. [CrossRef]
85. Lu, M.; Cao, Y.; Xiao, J.; Song, M.; Ho, C.T. Molecular mechanisms of the anti-obesity effect of bioactive ingredients in common spices: A review. *Food Funct.* **2018**, *9*, 4569–4581. [CrossRef] [PubMed]
86. Mosqueda-Solís, A.; Sánchez, J.; Portillo, M.P.; Palou, A.; Picó, C. Combination of capsaicin and hesperidin reduces the effectiveness of each compound to decrease the adipocyte size and to induce browning features in adipose tissue of western diet fed rats. *J. Agric. Food Chem.* **2018**, *66*, 9679–9689. [CrossRef]
87. Silvester, A.J.; Aseer, K.R.; Yun, J.W. Dietary polyphenols and their roles in fat browning. *J. Nutr. Biochem.* **2019**, *64*, 1–12. [CrossRef]

88. Takeda, Y.; Dai, P. Capsaicin directly promotes adipocyte browning in the chemical compound-induced brown adipocytes converted from human dermal fibroblasts. *Sci. Rep.* **2022**, *12*, 6612. [CrossRef]
89. Wang, Y.; Tang, C.; Tang, Y.; Yin, H.; Liu, X. Capsaicin has an anti-obesity effect through alterations in gut microbiota populations and short-chain fatty acid concentrations. *Food Nutr. Res.* **2020**, *64*. [CrossRef]
90. Siebert, E.; Lee, S.Y.; Prescott, M.P. Chili pepper preference development and its impact on dietary intake: A narrative review. *Front. Nutr.* **2022**, *9*, 1039207. [CrossRef]
91. Sirotkin, A.V. Peppers and Their Constituents against Obesity. *Biol. Futur.* **2023**. Epub ahead of print. [CrossRef] [PubMed]
92. Azlan, A.; Sultana, S.; Huei, C.S.; Razman, M.R. Antioxidant, Anti-Obesity, Nutritional and Other Beneficial Effects of Different Chili Pepper: A Review. *Molecules* **2022**, *27*, 898. [CrossRef] [PubMed]
93. Smeets, A.J.; Westerterp-Plantenga, M.S. The acute effects of a lunch containing capsaicin on energy and substrate utilisation, hormones, and satiety. *Eur. J. Nutr.* **2009**, *48*, 229–234. [CrossRef] [PubMed]
94. Van Avesaat, M.; Troost, F.J.; Westerterp-Plantenga, M.S.; Helyes, Z.; Le Roux, C.W.; Dekker, J.; Masclee, A.A.M.; Keszthelyi, D. Capsaicin-induced satiety is associated with gastrointestinal distress but not with the release of satiety hormones. *Am. J. Clin. Nutr.* **2016**, *103*, 305–313. [CrossRef]
95. Rigamonti, A.E.; Casnici, C.; Marelli, O.; De Col, A.; Tamini, S.; Lucchetti, E.; Tringali, G.; De Micheli, R.; Abbruzzese, L.; Bortolotti, M.; et al. Acute administration of capsaicin increases resting energy expenditure in young obese subjects without affecting energy intake, appetite, and circulating levels of orexigenic/anorexigenic peptides. *Nutr. Res.* **2018**, *52*, 71–79. [CrossRef]
96. de Moura e Silva, V.E.L.; Cholewa, J.M.; Jäger, R.; Zanchi, N.E.; de Freitas, M.C.; de Moura, R.C.; Barros, E.M.L.; Antunes, B.M.; Caperuto, E.C.; Ribeiro, S.L.G.; et al. Chronic capsiate supplementation increases fat-free mass and upper body strength but not the inflammatory response to resistance exercise in young untrained men: A randomized, placebo-controlled and double-blind study. *J. Int. Soc. Sports Nutr.* **2021**, *18*, 50. [CrossRef]
97. Zsiborás, C.; Mátics, R.; Hegyi, P.; Balaskó, M.; Pétervári, E.; Szabó, I.; Sarlós, P.; Mikó, A.; Tenk, J.; Rostás, I.; et al. Capsaicin and capsiate could be appropriate agents for treatment of obesity: A meta-analysis of human studies. *Crit. Rev. Food Sci. Nutr.* **2018**, *58*, 1419–1427. [CrossRef]
98. Wang, D.; Guo, S.; He, H.; Gong, L.; Cui, H. Gut Microbiome and Serum Metabolome Analyses Identify Unsaturated Fatty Acids and Butanoate Metabolism Induced by Gut Microbiota in Patients with Chronic Spontaneous Urticaria. *Front. Cell. Infect. Microbiol.* **2020**, *10*, 24. [CrossRef]
99. Kumar, V.; Kumar, V.; Mahajan, N.; Kaur, J.; Devi, K.; Dharavath, R.N.; Singh, R.P.; Kondepudi, K.K.; Bishnoi, M. Mucin secretory action of capsaicin prevents high fat diet-induced gut barrier dysfunction in C57BL/6 mice colon. *Biomed. Pharmacother.* **2022**, *145*, 112452. [CrossRef]
100. Xia, J.; Gu, L.; Guo, Y.; Feng, H.; Chen, S.; Jurat, J.; Fu, W.; Zhang, D. Gut Microbiota Mediates the Preventive Effects of Dietary Capsaicin Against Depression-like Behavior Induced by Lipopolysaccharide in Mice. *Front. Cell. Infect. Microbiol.* **2021**, *11*, 627608. [CrossRef]
101. Xia, Y.; Kuda, T.; Yamamoto, M.; Yano, T.; Nakamura, A.; Takahashi, H. The effect of Sichuan pepper on gut microbiota in mice fed a high-sucrose and low-dietary fibre diet. *Appl. Microbiol. Biotechnol.* **2023**, *107*, 2627–2638. [CrossRef] [PubMed]
102. Chen, X.; Pan, S.; Li, F.; Xu, X.; Xing, H. Plant-Derived Bioactive Compounds and Potential Health Benefits: Involvement of the Gut Microbiota and Its Metabolic Activity. *Biomolecules* **2022**, *12*, 1871. [CrossRef]
103. Kang, C.; Wang, B.; Kaliannan, K.; Wang, X.; Lang, H.; Hui, S.; Huang, L.; Zhang, Y.; Zhou, M.; Chen, M.; et al. Gut microbiota mediates the protective effects of dietary capsaicin against chronic low-grade inflammation and associated obesity induced by high-fat diet. *MBio* **2017**, *8*, 10–1128. [CrossRef]
104. Manca, C.; Lacroix, S.; Pérusse, F.; Flamand, N.; Chagnon, Y.; Drapeau, V.; Tremblay, A.; Di Marzo, V.; Silvestri, C. Oral Capsaicinoid Administration Alters the Plasma Endocannabinoidome and Fecal Microbiota of Reproductive-Aged Women Living with Overweight and Obesity. *Biomedicines* **2021**, *9*, 1246. [CrossRef] [PubMed]
105. Mikami, A.; Ogita, T.; Namai, F.; Shigemori, S.; Sato, T.; Shimosato, T. Oral administration of Flavonifractor plautii attenuates inflammatory responses in obese adipose tissue. *Mol. Biol. Rep.* **2020**, *47*, 6717–6725. [CrossRef] [PubMed]
106. Ao, Z.; Huang, Z.; Liu, H. Spicy Food and Chili Peppers and Multiple Health Outcomes: Umbrella Review. *Mol. Nutr. Food Res.* **2022**, *66*, 2200167. [CrossRef]
107. Zanzer, Y.C.; Plaza, M.; Dougkas, A.; Turner, C.; Östman, E. Black pepper-based beverage induced appetite-suppressing effects without altering postprandial glycaemia, gut and thyroid hormones or gastrointestinal well-being: A randomized crossover study in healthy subjects. *Food Funct.* **2018**, *9*, 2774–2786. [CrossRef] [PubMed]
108. Ashokkumar, K.; Murugan, M.; Dhanya, M.K.; Pandian, A.; Warkentin, T.D. Phytochemistry and therapeutic potential of black pepper [*Piper nigrum* (L.)] essential oil and piperine: A review. *Clin. Phytoscience* **2021**, *7*, 1–11. [CrossRef]
109. Yang, X.; Tang, W.; Mao, D.; Liu, X.; Qian, W.; Dai, Y.; Chen, L.; Ding, X. Spicy food consumption is associated with abdominal obesity among Chinese Han population aged 30–79 years in the Sichuan Basin: A population-based cross-sectional study. *BMC Public Health* **2022**, *22*, 1881. [CrossRef]
110. Wen, Q.; Wei, Y.; Du, H.; Lv, J.; Guo, Y.; Bian, Z.; Yang, L.; Chen, Y.Y.; Chen, Y.Y.; Shi, L.; et al. Characteristics of spicy food consumption and its relation to lifestyle behaviours: Results from 0.5 million adults. *Int. J. Food Sci. Nutr.* **2021**, *72*, 569–576. [CrossRef]

111. Duranova, H.; Valkova, V.; Gabriny, L. Chili peppers (*Capsicum* spp.): The spice not only for cuisine purposes: An update on current knowledge. *Phytochem. Rev.* **2022**, *21*, 1379–1413. [CrossRef]
112. Bode, A.M.; Dong, Z. The Two Faces of Capsaicin. *Cancer Res.* **2011**, *71*, 2809–2814. [CrossRef] [PubMed]

Disclaimer/Publisher's Note: The statements, opinions and data contained in all publications are solely those of the individual author(s) and contributor(s) and not of MDPI and/or the editor(s). MDPI and/or the editor(s) disclaim responsibility for any injury to people or property resulting from any ideas, methods, instructions or products referred to in the content.

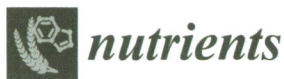

Review

The Pharmacological Properties of Red Grape Polyphenol Resveratrol: Clinical Trials and Obstacles in Drug Development

Mohd Farhan [1,*] and Asim Rizvi [2]

[1] Department of Basic Sciences, Preparatory Year Deanship, King Faisal University, Al Ahsa 31982, Saudi Arabia
[2] Department of Biochemistry, Faculty of Life Sciences, Aligarh Muslim University, Aligarh 202002, India; rizvirizviasim@gmail.com
* Correspondence: mfarhan@kfu.edu.sa

Abstract: Resveratrol is a stilbenoid from red grapes that possesses a strong antioxidant activity. Resveratrol has been shown to have anticancer activity, making it a promising drug for the treatment and prevention of numerous cancers. Several in vitro and in vivo investigations have validated resveratrol's anticancer capabilities, demonstrating its ability to block all steps of carcinogenesis (such as initiation, promotion, and progression). Additionally, resveratrol has been found to have auxiliary pharmacological effects such as anti-inflammatory, cardioprotective, and neuroprotective activity. Despite its pharmacological properties, several obstacles, such as resveratrol's poor solubility and bioavailability, as well as its adverse effects, continue to be key obstacles to drug development. This review critically evaluates the clinical trials to date and aims to develop a framework to develop resveratrol into a clinically viable drug.

Keywords: polyphenol; red grape; resveratrol; physiological effects; pharmacological activity

1. Introduction

The natural polyphenol resveratrol (*trans*-3,5,4′-trihydroxystilbene) is a stilbenoid. In 1939, Takaoka was the first to successfully extract resveratrol from Veratrum grandiflorum. [1,2]. The skin of red grapes contains the highest concentration of resveratrol. It has also been shown that certain foods, including tea, blueberries, pomegranates, almonds, pistachios, and dark chocolate, contain resveratrol (Figure 1) [3,4].

Resveratrol comprises a phenol ring connected to a catechol by an ethylene bridge. Two isomeric variants of resveratrol, *cis*- and *trans*-resveratrol, can be distinguished based on their chemical structure (Figure 2). The *trans* form predominates in terms of frequency, and it has been attributed to a variety of biological actions, including the induction of cell cycle arrest, differentiation, apoptosis, and the inhibition of the proliferation of cancer cells [3–5].

Resveratrol has been shown to have a broad range of therapeutic effects, such as its anti-inflammatory, antioxidant, platelet-inhibiting, hyperlipidemic, immunomodulatory, anti-carcinogenic, cardioprotective, vasodilatory, and neuroprotective activity [5–9]. It has been reported that resveratrol can sustain or improve human cerebrovascular functions [10], *modulate* in vitro angiogenesis by altering vascular endothelial growth factor (VEGF) expression and the formation of new vascular networks [11], stimulate human immune cell functions [12], boost rat cell viability and proliferation [13], reduce mitochondrial respiratory dysfunction, and boost cellular reprogramming in human fibroblasts derived from patients with a mammalian target of rapamycin (mTOR) pathway deficiency [14]. Resveratrol has been shown to also have neuroprotective [15], hepatoprotective [16], and cardioprotective [17,18] effects. In particular, the polyphenol appears to ameliorate the main risk factors of cardiovascular diseases (CVDs) because it can enhance endothelial function, scavenge reactive oxygen species (ROS), reduce inflammation, inhibit platelet aggregation, and improve the lipid profile, among other things [19,20]. In addition, redox-associated

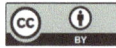

mechanisms were suggested as potential mechanisms through which resveratrol exerts its cardioprotective effects. These redox-associated mechanisms include the maintenance of mitochondrial function during hypoxia/reoxygenation-induced oxidative stress [21], the overexpression of antioxidant enzymes, like peroxidase and superoxide dismutase (SOD) [22], and the regulation of nitric oxide (NO) generation [23].

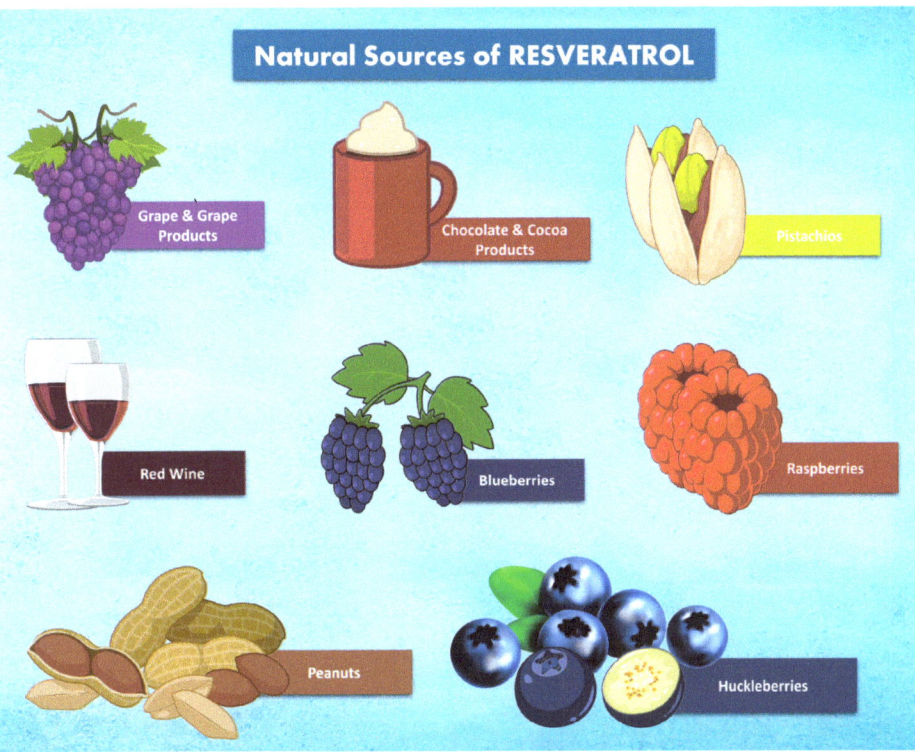

Figure 1. Several resveratrol-containing foodstuffs.

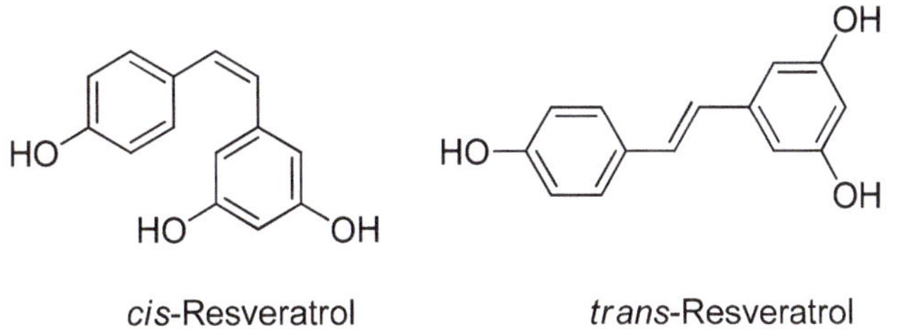

Figure 2. The chemical structure of resveratrol (*cis* and *trans* forms).

Resveratrol has been demonstrated to be safe for human consumption in several studies [24,25], although there have also been reports of harmful effects of *resveratrol* in vitro and in vivo [26]. For instance, when resveratrol was given in large quantities, it showed systemic suppression of P450 cytochromes [2]. Several pharmacological interactions involving resveratrol were also discovered and because of the potential for these interactions to reduce the efficacy of the medication, they are considered hazardous [27]. High-dose resveratrol has hormetic effects in vitro (micromolar range in cell culture media) and in vivo (nanomolar range in the blood) [28–30], including pro-oxidant effects [29–34], but it also has toxic side effects, such as disrupting the thyroid and causing goiter if used for an extended period of time. Thus, it is important to identify the actual biologically effective concentration range at which this compound should be supplemented in human subjects [35,36]. Further studies on pharmacological interactions would allow researchers to address these interactions and understand their cost-to-benefit ratio.

Resveratrol Bioavailability and Metabolism

There are a number of obstacles in the way of resveratrol being used commercially as a pharmaceutical agent, the most significant of which include resveratrol's limited bioavailability and quick metabolism. These two factors may reduce resveratrol's [2,37] effects in vivo. With only a few traces of un-metabolized resveratrol detectable in the plasma after an oral dose of 25 mg [37], it is clear that resveratrol has a very limited bioavailability in the body. Although more than 70% of resveratrol is absorbed in the digestive tract, it is rapidly consumed through three separate metabolic routes after ingestion. According to recent research [38], the bioavailability of resveratrol is determined by its extremely quick sulfate conjugation in the intestine/liver (Figure 3).

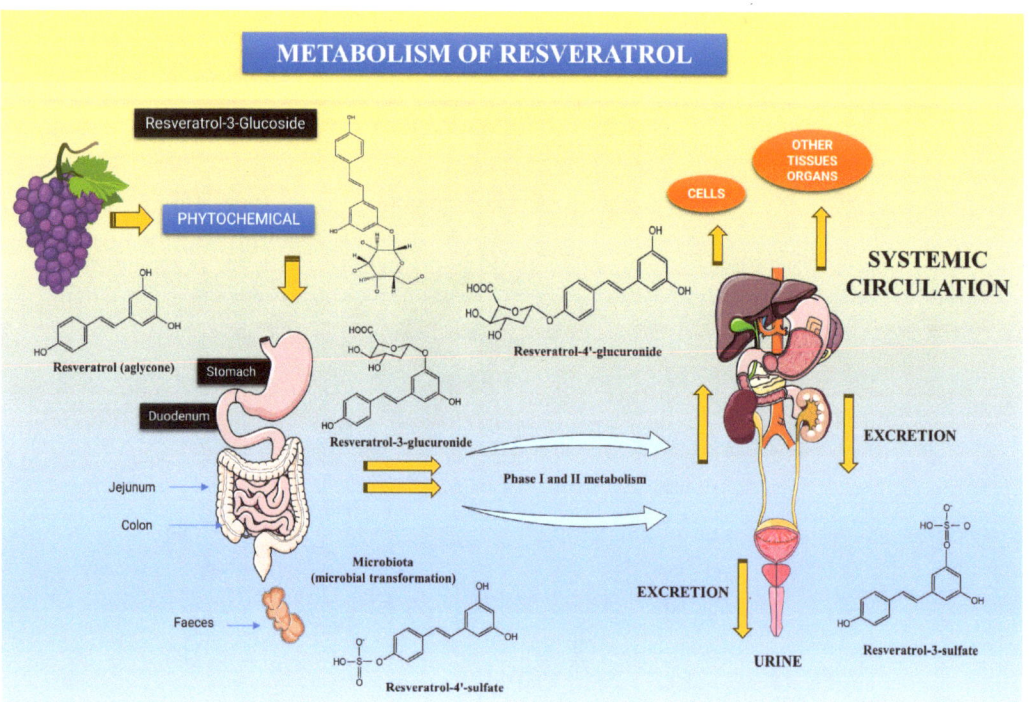

Figure 3. The absorption of resveratrol in the gastrointestinal tract of humans.

The fact that resveratrol is only marginally soluble in water (0.05 mg/mL) hinders its absorption. pH and temperature have significant effects on the stability and solubility of resveratrol [39]. In this context, studies found that the solubility of resveratrol is 64 µg/mL at a pH of 1.2, 61 µg/mL at a pH of 6.8, and 50 µg/mL above a pH of 7.4. Once dissolved in water, resveratrol is only stable at ambient temperature or body temperature under acidic conditions; at higher pH levels, the stilbene is destroyed at an exponential rate. We can infer that resveratrol is most stable in its liquid state when kept at a low pH, cool temperature, and away from oxygen and light [39].

After being ingested, resveratrol moves through the body either through passive diffusion or by forming complexes with transporters such as integrins, albumin, and low-density lipoprotein (LDL) [2,40,41]. Although resveratrol seems to be stable in the stomach's acidic environment, it may be hydrolyzed to oligomeric phenolics or undergo isomeric conversion. In addition, resveratrol's glycosylation by resident bacteria in the stomach can result in the absorption-competent stilbenoid glucoside piceid (resveratrol-3-O-beta-glucoside) [2,42]. Intestinal and hepatic conjugation processes also contribute to resveratrol modification. Benzoic, phenylacetic, and propionic acids can be metabolized from resveratrol by intestinal bacteria, whereas phase II metabolism in the liver results in glucuronidated, sulfated, and methylated metabolites that are known to retain some of the biological activity of the parent chemical [2,41,43,44].

The affinity of resveratrol for transport proteins is also connected to its biological effects in vivo. There is a lot of evidence that resveratrol can form complexes with plasma transport proteins, such as human serum albumin (HSA) and lipoproteins, which promote resveratrol stability and activity [45–48]. To enter various tissues, resveratrol forms complexes with HSA [49,50]. HSA is required in circulation to bind resveratrol, transport it, enhance its uptake by cells, and redistribute it to different cell types [2,48]. In this regard, it has previously been established that epigallocatechin gallate (EGCG), another naturally occurring polyphenolic antioxidant from green tea, can also be bound and stabilized by HSA under aqueous physiological conditions. Consequently, HSA and other plasma proteins may play a pivotal role in mediating the in vivo physiologic effects of resveratrol. Dihydro-resveratrol glucuronides, resveratrol glucuronides, and glucosides are all metabolites of resveratrol, and it is known that resveratrol induces its own metabolism, which raises the activity of phase II hepatic detoxifying enzymes. High levels of these metabolites are detected in human plasma and urine [51,52]. This suggests that free resveratrol may be released locally from these metabolites, as its half-life and plasma concentrations were shown to be 10 times higher than the natural resveratrol component [2,44,53].

2. Resveratrol: Pharmacology and Therapeutic Potential

Some of the most prominent biological actions of resveratrol and its therapeutic potential are summarized in Figure 4 and Table 1. The subsequent sub-sections will elucidate the pharmacological effects associated with moderate consumption of resveratrol with special reference to anti-diabetic effects, cardiovascular effects, neuroprotective functions, and anticancer properties.

Table 1. A summary of resveratrol's various pharmacological properties.

Pharmacology	Reference
Anticancer	[54–56]
Analgesic and Anti-inflammatory	[57–59]
Anti-diabetic	[60–62]
Neuroprotection	[63–65]
Antiviral	[66–68]
Anti-obesity	[69–71]
Cardioprotection	[72–74]
Antioxidant	[75–77]
Anti-aging	[78–80]
Nephroprotection	[81–83]

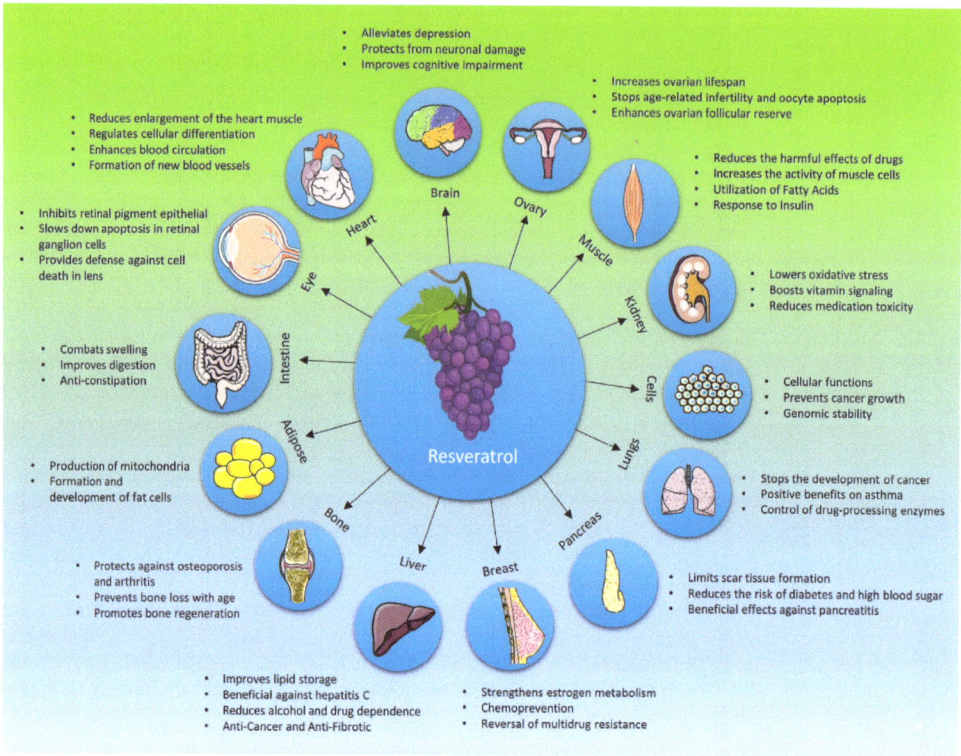

Figure 4. The health benefits of resveratrol consumption in humans.

2.1. Resveratrol in Cardiovascular Health

Heart disease and stroke are the leading causes of death and disability in developed nations [84]. Atherosclerosis is the leading cause of cardiovascular disorders affecting the coronary arteries. Light to moderate alcohol use has been linked to a lower risk of developing type 2 diabetes, increased HDL cholesterol, and decreased lipid oxidative stress. Red wine is superior to other alcoholic beverages in lowering the risk of developing coronary heart disease. It is possible that the synergistic effects of both resveratrol and alcohol come into play in such an action [85].

Resveratrol has been shown in preclinical trials to inhibit LDL oxidation [86]. The effect of red wine on cholesterol is multifaceted, with resveratrol playing a role in hepatic cholesterol and lipoprotein metabolism. The process lowers plasma cholesterol by decreasing cholesterol absorption and its transportation to the liver. Additional effects of resveratrol on cardiovascular disease risk variables include upregulating lipoprotein lipase activity and downregulating low-density lipoprotein circulation [87]. Resveratrol also affects apolipoproteins A and B. In a study, researchers looked at how moderate consumption of red wine, dealcoholized red wine, and gin affected glucose metabolism and lipid profile [88]. Sixty-seven males with a high cardiovascular risk were enrolled in the trial. For four weeks, everyone received 30 g of alcohol each day, which is the same as a standard glass of dealcoholized red wine. A decrease in the Homeostatic Model Assessment for Insulin Resistance (HOMA-IR) and mean-adjusted plasma insulin were observed following wine and dealcoholized wine consumption, while increases in high-density lipoprotein cholesterol, apolipoprotein A-I, and A-II were observed following gin and red wine consumption, and a decrease in lipoprotein was observed following red wine consumption [88]. Paraoxonase 1 is a hydrolytic enzyme that contributes to the protective functions of high-density lipoprotein. A moderate intake of red wine was found to positively alter paraoxonase 1 activity in a healthy Mexican population [89]. A group of researchers [90] looked at the phenomenon of subclinical coronary atherosclerosis. Carotid and femoral artery plaque were measured in this predominantly male sample following polyphenol consumption. Both femoral and carotid subclinical atherosclerosis risk decreased in correlation with increased consumption of flavonoids, while femoral subclinical atherosclerosis risk decreased in correlation with increased consumption of stilbenes. Red wine polyphenols were studied for their potential to counteract age-related declines in vascular function and physical exercise capacity in rats of varying ages (12, 20, and 40 weeks). From week 16 through week 40, rats were treated with either red wine polyphenols or apocynin (an antioxidant and NDPH oxidase inhibitor). Both supplements were found to be effective in reducing endothelial dysfunction, oxidative stress, and abnormal protein expression. Finally, polyphenols in red wine protect against endothelium dysfunction that comes with aging [86]. Seventeen dyslipidaemic postmenopausal women were studied to determine the effects of acute ingestion of red wine and dealcoholized red wine on postprandial lipid and lipoprotein metabolism [86]. Over a six-hour period, acute consumption worsened postprandial lipaemia and increased insulin secretion, but it had no effect on postprandial triglyceride, chylomicrons, or insulin homeostasis. Therefore, it is reasonable to anticipate that long-term use of resveratrol may be good for cardiovascular health [86]. In a particular study, it was shown that moderate consumption of red wine among an elderly population with high cardiovascular risk was associated with a decreased likelihood of metabolic syndrome, abnormal waist circumference, low concentrations of high-density lipoprotein cholesterol, high blood pressure, and hyperglycemia, in comparison to individuals who did not consume red wine [91].

2.2. Resveratrol for the Treatment and Prevention of Cancer

Cancer is a leading cause of death all over the world. Each year, it impacts over 6 million people [86]. Chemoprevention is promising for preventing cancer by utilizing either natural or synthetic drugs, or a combination of the two [92]. Resveratrol present in food and drink is thought to be responsible for lowering cancer risk. Stilbenes have been shown to prevent cancer in cell cultures and animals exposed to cancer cells or carcinogenic substances [86]. Colorectal cancer is the third most common kind of cancer, affecting an estimated 1.8 million individuals annually. In most cases, oncogenic mutations accumulate over time in non-cancerous polyps in the intestinal epithelium lining the colon or rectum. If these benign polyps are not caught early enough, they can develop into malignant adenomatous polyps. This development is significantly influenced by environmental factors like nutrition, smoking, alcohol usage, and inactivity. Several studies [93,94] point to the importance of a healthy diet (such as the Mediterranean diet) as a preventative measure against numerous diseases. Cancer prevention is aided by eating foods high in polyphenols and monounsaturated fats, such as those found in the Mediterranean diet [95].

Resveratrol has been investigated for its apoptotic effects on human colon cancer cells (SNU-C4) [96]. Through chromatin condensation and apoptotic body formation, the results demonstrated that resveratrol (100 g/mL) promoted apoptosis in SNU-C4 cells. Resveratrol was found to decrease Bcl-2 expression while increasing Bax and Caspase-3 expression compared to a control group [86]. In order to prevent colon cancer in animals, scientists looked into resveratrol-rich plant extracts like those found in red wine, pomegranate, white grape, and rosemary [97]. Workshop-made cured pork, which is known to promote colon carcinogenesis, had the extracts added to it. Both normal rats and rats provoked by azoxymethane received supplements for a total of 100 days. The number of mucin-depleted foci per colon was found to decrease in response to dry red wine, pomegranate extract, and tocopherol. Incorporating these extracts into cured meat has been proposed as a means of lowering the risk of colorectal cancer associated with eating processed meat [86,97]. It was also determined whether or not red wine extracts were effective in inhibiting the growth of colon cancer cells in vitro and colonic aberrant crypt foci in vivo [98]. Red wine extracts with greater anti-proliferative activity were examined in cells, and the ability to inhibit the development of aberrant crypt foci in mice was found to be the product of a lengthy vinification procedure. Synergistic anti-proliferative effects were also observed between quercetin and *trans*-resveratrol [98].

2.3. Resveratrol in Diabetes

The scientific community is becoming increasingly interested in substances that may have anti-diabetic effects. There is hope that such molecules can serve as the foundation for future therapeutic and preventative pharmaceuticals [99]. According to the World Health Organization, almost 500 million individuals will have diabetes mellitus by the year 2025. This condition is part of a more complex metabolic syndrome. Retinal, renal, limb, cardiac, nervous system, and vascular malfunctions, as well as compromised quality of life, and ultimately death, are all associated with this condition [86]. The risk of developing type 2 diabetes is reduced with moderate wine drinking, according to a number of studies [86,100].

In animal studies, simulating type 1 diabetes, a wine concentrate supplemented with natural polyphenols reduced hyperglycemia, brought hemoglobin and erythrocyte counts back to normal, and increased cell survival. Treatment with wine concentrate decreased the activity of catalase and glutathione peroxidase and raised the activity of superoxide dismutase in the plasma of rats with experimental diabetes mellitus [99]. In vitro research [101] looked into the potential anti-diabetic effects of Portuguese red wine. The results demonstrated that both the dealcoholized red wine and the four fractions of red wine produced through solid-phase extraction exhibited potent inhibitory effects against amylase and glucosidase. Monomeric and oligomeric flavan-3-ol molecules are primarily responsible for these actions [86,101]. Researchers examined the effects of co-digesting red wine with models of glucose and whey protein on the digestion, bioavailability, and colonic metabolism of the wine's polyphenols and constituents. The most significant finding was a decrease in glucose bioaccessibility, which provides more evidence that moderate wine drinking has hypoglycemic effects. Additionally, protein breakdown was slowed, and short-chain fatty acid synthesis (particularly butyric acid) was elevated [102].

2.4. Resveratrol in Neuroprotection

The neuroprotective effects of resveratrol have been the subject of multiple investigations. Pretreatment with resveratrol protected neural stem cells from oxygen–glucose deprivation and activated nuclear factor erythroid 2-related factor 2 (Nrf2) [103]. Piceatoannol, a resveratrol metabolite, prevented glutamate-induced cell death in HT22 neuronal cells [104]. When resveratrol was given to rats, the pre-induction of cerebral ischemia led to the rats' oxidation indicators dropping, and their superoxide dismutase activity was restored [105]. Glutathione peroxidase and glutathione reductase are necessary for maintaining glutathione in a reduced state. Drinking red wine boosted the enzymes of glutathione metabolism [106]. Red wine powder (freeze-dried with maltodextrin and gum arabic) [107] protects human neuroblastoma SH-SY5Y cell viability when treated with 6-hydroxydopamine. Indeed, red wine powder at a concentration of 150 ng GAE/mL ensured that 88.3% of cells would survive after being exposed to 6-hydroxydopamine cytotoxicity. Polyphenols with numerous hydroxyl groups are effective at preventing the production of mono- and di-adducts that contribute to the formation of advanced glycation end products. This is an effective means of protecting against neurodegenerative disorders [108]. Some of the possible pathways for resveratrol action in different disorders are summarized in Figure 5.

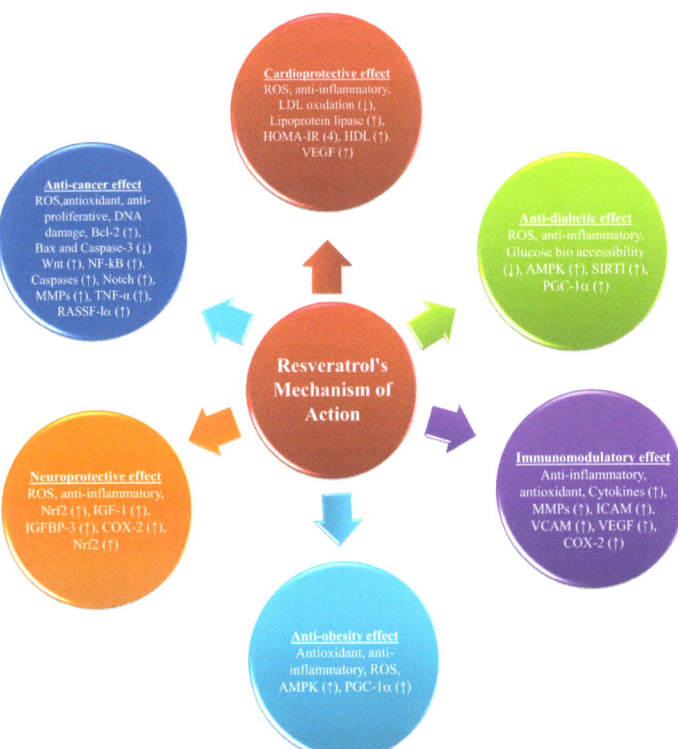

Figure 5. The current knowledge of the action of resveratrol and its prospective therapeutic mechanisms (↑) up and (↓) down; nuclear factor-kB (NF-kB), matrix metalloproteinases (MMPs), 5′-AMP-activated protein kinase (AMPK), intercellular adhesion molecule (ICAM), vascular cell adhesion molecule (VCAM), sirtuin type 1 (SIRT1), tumor necrosis factor α (TNF-α), peroxisome proliferator-activated receptor-γ coactivator 1α (PGC-1α), insulin-like growth factor 1 (IGF-1), insulin-like growth factor-binding protein (IGFBP-3), ras association domain family 1 isoform A (RASSF-1α), pAkt, vascular endothelial growth factor (VEGF), cyclooxygenase 2 (COX-2), nuclear factor erythroid 2-related factor 2 (Nrf2), and Kelch-like ECH-associated protein 1 (Keap1), Homeostatic Model Assessment for Insulin Resistance (HOMA-IR), low-density lipoprotein (LDL), high-density lipoprotein (HDL), wingless-related integration site (Wnt), B-cell lymphoma 2 (Bcl-2), Bcl-2-associated X protein (Bax).

3. Human Clinical Trials of Resveratrol

Resveratrol shows promise as a compound that can help cells keep its metabolic balance. Researchers conducted numerous clinical investigations to verify the therapeutic effects of resveratrol on vascular metabolic illnesses in order to better understand its clinical transformative value. This resulted in 244 finished clinical trials and 27 ongoing trials by the end of 2019 [109]. Numerous diseases and disorders, such as diabetes, obesity, cancer, neurological, and cardiovascular diseases, have been the focus of clinical trials investigating the preventive and therapeutic effects of resveratrol. Preclinical and clinical studies have shown that resveratrol can modulate a wide variety of signaling molecules, including wingless-related integration site (Wnt), nuclear factor-kB (NF-kB), cytokines, caspases, Notch, matrix metalloproteinases (MMPs), 5′-AMP-activated protein kinase (AMPK), intercellular adhesion molecule (ICAM), vascular cell adhesion molecule (VCAM), sirtuin type 1 (SIRT1), tumor necrosis factor α (TNF-α), peroxisome proliferator-activated receptor-γ coactivator 1α (PGC-1α), insulin-like growth factor 1 (IGF-1), insulin-like growth factor-binding protein (IGFBP-3), ras association domain family 1 isoform A (RASSF-1α), pAkt, vascular endothelial growth factor (VEGF), cyclooxygenase 2 (COX-2), nuclear factor erythroid 2-related factor 2 (Nrf2), and Kelch-like ECH-associated protein 1 (Keap1) [109,110]. The ability of resveratrol to interact with numerous targets, such as kinases, receptors, and signaling molecules, is the likely explanation for its pleiotropic behavior [109,110]. The major resveratrol clinical trials are listed below in Table 2.

Table 2. A review of the clinical trials on resveratrol's potential as a therapeutic molecule.

Clinical Condition	Cohort Size (Numbers)	Resveratrol Dose and Duration	Principal Outcomes of Resveratrol Treatment	Reference
Atherosclerosis	Individuals diagnosed with nonalcoholic fatty liver disease were randomly assigned to either a placebo (n = 25) or resveratrol (n = 25) group	600 mg/day, 84 days	Plasma ox-LDL, LDL-C/HDL-C, and LDL-C/ox-LDL levels showed no changes	[111]
	Individuals in good health were randomly assigned to either a resveratrol (n = 24) or a calorie restriction (n = 24) group	500 mg/day, 30 days	A rise in plasma TC and non-HDL cholesterol but no change in plasma TG, HDL-C, LDL-C, or apolipoprotein A1	[112]
	Randomized groups of patients with carotid stenosis >70% and a request for surgical intervention were given either Cardioaspirin® and Aterofisiol® (n = 107) or Cardioaspirin® and placebo (n = 107)	20 mg/day, 25 days	Decreased dry weight of lipid and cholesterol in removed plaques (0.232 ± 0.018 vs. 0.356 ± 0.022; 0.036 ± 0.006 vs. 0.053 ± 0.007 mg/mg dry weight, respectively)	[113]
	Randomized placebo (n = 28) and resveratrol (n = 28) groups of patients with type 2 diabetes mellitus and coronary heart disease	500 mg/day, 30 days	No change in plasma TG, TC, or LDL-C; HDL-C plasma levels increased; TC/HDL-C plasma levels dropped	[114]
	Stable coronary artery disease patients (n = 10) were given placebo or resveratrol treatments	330 mg/day, 3 days	Coronary artery bypass graft patients had higher FMD than those who had undergone percutaneous coronary intervention, whereas percutaneous coronary intervention patients showed no difference in FMD	[115]
Hypertension	Patients with hypertension (n = 24) given a placebo or resveratrol	300 mg, acute supplementation	Increased FMD in women and individuals with higher LDL-C	[116]
	Patients with hypertension (n = 18) given a placebo or isolated phytochemicals	60 mg/day, 28 days	Decreased diastolic blood pressure	[117]
	Peripheral artery disease patients were split into two groups and given either a standard balloon angioplasty (n = 75) or a resveratrol drug-coated balloon (n = 78)	0.9 µg/mm^2, 728 days	Target lesion revascularization was reduced, and patients were able to walk further after treatment than those who received standard balloon angioplasty	[118]

Table 2. Cont.

Clinical Condition	Cohort Size (Numbers)	Resveratrol Dose and Duration	Principal Outcomes of Resveratrol Treatment	Reference
Diabetes	A prospective, open-label, randomized controlled experiment involving 62 patients with type 2 diabetes	250 mg/day, 90 days	Decreases in hemoglobin A1c, systolic blood pressure, total cholesterol, and total protein indicate better glycemic control	[119]
	Placebo-treated (n = 38) and resveratrol-treated (n = 38) patients with type 2 diabetes	1000 mg/day, 56 days	Changes in plasma HDL-C, TG, TC, and LDL-C were not significant, whereas plasma glucose was reduced	[120]
	A randomized, placebo-controlled, double-blind investigation of 19 patients with type 2 diabetes	5 mg twice daily, 30 days	Glucose and insulin levels dropped, glucose spikes after meals were postponed, and ortho-tyrosine was excreted in the urine	[121]
	Nonalcoholic fatty liver disease patients who were overweight and randomly assigned to either a placebo (n = 8) or resveratrol (n = 8) group	1500 mg/day, 180 days	Very low-density lipoprotein TG secretion. Oxidation, and clearance rates were not affected, neither at baseline nor in response to insulin	[122]
	Type 2 diabetes patients in whom the disease is under control (n = 17) were given either placebo or resveratrol	150 mg/day, 30 days	Insulin sensitivity in the liver and the rest of the body did not change, nor did the amount of fat stored in the liver	[123]
	Placebo- and resveratrol-treated patients with type 2 diabetes (n = 14)	1000 mg/day, 35 days	Glycemic control and glucagon-like peptide 1 secretion did not vary	[124]
	Treatment with resveratrol or a placebo in elderly people with glucose intolerance (n = 30)	2–3 g/day, 42 days	Reactive hyperemia index rises, but blood pressure and plasma lipid levels remain unchanged	[125]
	Diabetic patients at high risk (n = 8) treated with placebo and resveratrol	150 mg/day, 34 days	There was no difference in the absorption of 18F-fluorodeoxyglucose or the inflammation of arteries	[126]
Obesity	Children and adolescents with obesity were split into two groups: those who took a resveratrol supplement (n = 16) and those who took a placebo (n = 11)	20 mg/day, 180 days	Enhanced hyperemic delta flow 6 months after post-occlusive release	[127]
	Obese older people (n = 22) were divided into two groups: those given placebo or resveratrol with curcumin	200 mg, 30 min before consuming the high-fat meal	Post-meal soluble vascular cell adhesion molecule-1 response was reduced, but other inflammatory indicators and adhesion molecules in the blood were unaffected	[128]

Table 2. Cont.

Clinical Condition	Cohort Size (Numbers)	Resveratrol Dose and Duration	Principal Outcomes of Resveratrol Treatment	Reference
Obesity	Placebo ($n = 10$), 300 mg ($n = 10$), and 1000 mg ($n = 9$) resveratrol groups were used to test the effects of resveratrol on the weight and health of older, overweight persons	300 and 1000 mg/day, 90 days	The 1000 mg resveratrol group had higher levels of soluble vascular cell adhesion molecule-1 and total plasminogen activator inhibitor than the 300 mg resveratrol and placebo groups	[129]
Neurodegenerative diseases	102 people with early-onset Huntington's disease (HD)	40 mg twice a day, 365 days	Not known yet	[130]
	120 patients with mild to moderate dementia most likely due to Alzheimer's disease (AD)	500 mg/day with dose escalation of up to 1000 mg twice/day, 365 days	Nausea, weight loss, and diarrhea are the only reported side effects of resveratrol, which is safe and well-tolerated. CSF Aβ40 and Aβ42 biomarkers show no improvement. Enhanced decline in brain volume	[131]
	27 people with mild to moderate AD	Resveratrol, glucose, and malate supp. delivered in grape juice, 365 days	At modest doses, resveratrol is safe and well-tolerated. The Mini-Mental State Exam and the AD Assessment Scale for Cognition scores did not significantly change	[130]
Cancer	14 patients with prostate cancer	500, 1000, 2000, 3000, or 4000 mg of MPX. Every 500 mg MPX has 4.4 µg resveratrol, 60–930 days (depending on the patient)	Increased PSADT	[132]
	A single-center, randomized, placebo-controlled trial of 66 people with prostate cancer	150 mg or 1000 mg daily, 120 days	A drop in androstenedione, and dehydroepiandrosterone (DHEAS). The PSA and prostate size remained unchanged	[133]
	Phase 1 trial of nine patients with colorectal cancer; randomized, placebo-controlled, double-blind	5.0 g SRT501, 14 days before surgery	Elevated levels of activated caspase-3 (apoptosis)	[134]
	Cases of colorectal cancer in 20 patients	500 or 1000 mg, 8 days prior to surgery	Ki-67 staining decreases, indicating a decrease in tumor cell growth	[135]
	Randomized, double-blind, placebo-controlled clinical study for breast cancer in 39 people	5 or 50 mg twice daily, 90 days	Decreased $RASSF$-1α methylation	[136]

TG: triglyceride; TC: total cholesterol; HDL-C: high-density lipoprotein cholesterol; ox-LDL: oxidized low-density lipoprotein; LDL-C: low-density lipoprotein cholesterol; FMD: flow-mediated dilatation; PSA: prostate-specific antigen; MPX: pulverized muscadine grape skin, which contains resveratrol; PSA: doubling time.

4. Resveratrol as an Adjuvant

Contradictory findings in in vivo investigations on resveratrol have been reported, and this discrepancy has been linked to the drug's low bioavailability, On the other hand, supplementary treatment can help with resveratrol's subpar bioavailability. Therapeutic benefits can be increased by the synergistic interaction of resveratrol and other bioactive components and micronutrients [137]. This is likely due to an increase in resveratrol bioavailability and a broadening of the metabolic effects of the combined agents. Polyphenols are able to link and interact with other compounds using their hydroxyl groups, which allows them to control the efficacy of other chemicals, including proteins and nutrients [2,138]. Compared to free polyphenols, polyphenol complexes might be more bioavailable, soluble, and absorbable in the small intestine due to their stabilized chemical structure [139]. A potential benefit of combining resveratrol with other treatment modalities is that polyphenol complexes can target numerous metabolic pathways. It is true that resveratrol combined with various therapeutic modalities has been shown to have favorable benefits in a variety of diseases and conditions, including cancer [138].

It has been suggested that the combination of vitamins with polyphenols not only results in synergistic biological effects but also stabilizes, maintains, and supports the action of polyphenols. Combining resveratrol with vitamin D3 has been shown to increase resveratrol's estrogenic activity and modify ER-mediated transcription [137]. In diabetic nephropathy, resveratrol, and vitamin D3 were found to have synergistic benefits. Combining resveratrol with vitamin D3 has been proven to suppress TNF-α and IL-6 expression more than either medicine alone [140]. The combination of glucan, vitamin C, and resveratrol exhibited a higher suppression of breast and lung tumor growth in in vivo models compared to the individual drugs [138,141].

To combat human papillomavirus (HPV)-positive head and neck squamous cell carcinoma, researchers examined the efficacy of a tri-combination (TriCurin) of three polyphenols (curcumin derived from spice turmeric, resveratrol, and epicatechin gallate from green tea). TriCurin inhibited tumor growth by 85% when administered intratumorally in vivo, and it lowered cell viability, clonogenic survival, and tumor sphere formation in vitro while greatly increasing apoptosis [142]. TriCurin also increased p53 protein levels and decreased HPV16 E6 and E7 [142,143]. In a separate investigation, resveratrol and epicatechin gallate were found to trigger apoptosis in prostate cancer cells at dosages as low as 100 microM [144]. CruciferexTM, a substance derived from cruciferous vegetables, was used in a study of human head and neck squamous carcinoma. CruciferexTM contains a mixture of various polyphenols, including resveratrol. Matrix metalloproteinase (MMP) secretion and cell proliferation were both greatly slowed by the polyphenol mixture [145].

Given the prevalence of cancer and other disorders that require the targeting of several molecular pathways simultaneously, the findings of this study indicate that the combination of polyphenols such as resveratrol, nutrients, and other treatments with additive and/or complementary effects may offer a promising approach to achieve synergistic actions.

5. Resveratrol Based Nanoformulations

Various drug carriers have been tried and are being used to improve the poor bioavailability and stability of resveratrol, resulting in a reduced requirement to consume large resveratrol doses and fewer unwanted effects. These can take the form of emulsions, nanoparticles, or liposomes [146,147]. Lipophilic pharmaceuticals can be better stabilized and bioavailable, water-soluble, safe, biodistributed, and biocompatible when encapsulated in solid lipid nanoparticles [148]. The oral bioavailability of resveratrol was improved by up to 335.7 percent when it was loaded into poly-lactic-co-glycolic acid (PLGA) nanoparticles before being administered to rats [149]. The therapeutic potential and efficacy of resveratrol were further increased by nanoparticle formulations, in particular its in vivo anticancer activity in a variety of cancer types. Tumor size was reduced in studies of gliomas, ovarian cancer, and colorectal cancer when resveratrol was administered [150,151]. High-loading resveratrol-loaded gelatin nanoparticles were found to induce cell death via changes in p53, p21, caspase-3, Bax, Bcl-2, and NF-kB expression when utilized in a coculture setting [152]. Using a rat embryonic cardiomyocyte (H9C2) model, researchers discovered that Curcumin-Resveratrol-mP127 (co-loaded curcumin and resveratrol at a molar ratio of 5:1 in Pluronic® F127 micelles) proved cardioprotective by inhibiting apoptosis and reactive oxygen species (ROS) [153]. In addition to cancer treatment, resveratrol has shown therapeutic effects in treating various diseases, therefore further improvements in resveratrol carrier delivery should help mitigate the negative effects of large dosages of resveratrol.

Children with chronic liver illness have stunted growth and development because of poor nutrient absorption [154]. An increase in morbidity and mortality is related to malnutrition, which is an unfavorable prognostic factor in liver transplantation [155]. Current vitamin E supplementation guidelines recommend giving children D-α-tocopheryl-polyethylene-glycol-succinate (TPGS) orally to increase their chances of survival and overall health, although TPGS alone does not prevent spinocerebellar degeneration or lipid peroxidation [156,157]. Micelles loaded with resveratrol have shown a protective action in the liver, boosting the efficacy of TPGS [158]. Through a phase-solubility analysis, the researchers determined that TPGS was suitable for encapsulating resveratrol in micelles; next, resveratrol TPGS formulations were made through solvent casting and solvent diffusion evaporation. Low polydispersity, a somewhat neutral Zeta potential, and small mean diameters (12 nm) were all characteristics of resveratrol TPGS colloidal dispersions [159]. Infrared spectroscopy and differential scanning calorimetry both validated the formulations' strong drug loading capacity and stable drug release. Resveratrol TPGSs showed reduced toxicity on HaCaT cells compared to empty TPGSs while maintaining the same level of antioxidant activity as pure resveratrol as measured by the DPPH assay. The antioxidant activity of resveratrol and the reduced surfactant toxicity on normal cells suggest that resveratrol TPGS micelles may be able to overcome the obstacles of conventional liver disease therapy [159,160]. Table 3 details the encouraging results obtained from a variety of nanoformulation methods for increasing resveratrol's biological activity.

Table 3. Recent nanoformulation-based advances in boosting resveratrol's biological activity.

Nanoformulation Method	Study Model	Outcome	Reference
Resveratrol medication delivery systems based on self-emulsification	In vitro, in vivo (rats)	Enhanced pharmacokinetics, decreased metabolism, and enhanced solubility	[161]
Micellar solubilization of resveratrol	Twelve healthy volunteers (oral administration)	Increased oral bioavailability	[162]
Suspension of free resveratrol, resveratrol-filled nanoparticles, and layer-by-layer nanoparticles	In vivo (Wistar rats, oral administration, 20 mg/kg)	Systemic exposure was increased when resveratrol was encapsulated in layer-by-layer nanoparticles with resveratrol nanocores	[163]
Nanoparticle delivery method based on oat-shellac proteins	In vitro, in vivo (rat model)	Resveratrol was buffered in the stomach acid and released gradually into the small intestine. Transport and absorption by cells are enhanced relative to free resveratrol. Enhancement in bioavailability	[164]
Resveratrol nanoencapsulation in casein	In vitro, in vivo (rats)	Oral administration in rats: remained in the gut and reached intestinal epithelium. Produced high plasma levels of resveratrol (sustained for at least 8 h) and similar results for its metabolites. Oral bioavailability was 10 times higher compared to an oral solution of resveratrol	[165]

Table 3. *Cont.*

Nanoformulation Method	Study Model	Outcome	Reference
Trans-resveratrol nanocrystals	In vitro, in vivo (rats)	Increased oral bioavailability	[166]
Nanoparticles of human serum albumin coupled with glycyrrhizic acid and loaded with resveratrol	In vivo (rats; single-dose tail vein injection)	The absorption rate of resveratrol was increased. High levels of resveratrol were found in most of the rats' vital organs. The highest levels were found in the liver, suggesting that a delivery method that focuses on the liver could be effective	[167]
Trans-resveratrol-loaded mixed micelles	In vivo (rats; intravenous administration)	Enhanced pharmacokinetic parameters. Improved brain targeting	[168]
Resveratrol bovine serum albumin nanoparticles (RES-BSANP)	In vivo (nude mice; intraperitoneal injection)	Enhanced dilution and soluble in water. Cancer development was suppressed in hairless mice bearing human ovarian primary tumors	[169]
Folate-conjugated HSA nanoparticles	HePG2 liver cancer cells	Showed decreased resveratrol release and increased cytotoxicity	[170]
Piperine-loaded mixed micelles	MCF-7 breast cancer cells	Improved cytotoxicity	[171]
Sericin nanoparticles	Caco-2 cells colorectal cancer cells	Strong cytotoxic against Caco-2 cells	[172]
Folic acid-targeted micelles	MCF-7 breast cancer cells	Increased cytotoxicity was achieved due to the sustained release of encapsulated resveratrol provided by the nano-formulation.	[173]

6. Toxicity and Adverse Effects of Resveratrol

Resveratrol is known for its antioxidant and chemopreventive properties. However, some investigations have shown that it may act as a pro-oxidizing agent [4,29,30], which may paradoxically affect disease pathogenesis. Resveratrol's antioxidant activity is a consequence of ROS scavenging [174,175] and antioxidant defense upregulation [176]. Resveratrol may modulate gene and protein expression through redox-sensitive intracellular pathways in tissues and cells. Thus, gene expression modifications and increased antioxidant defense system action lead to cell survival and adaptability in oxidative environments [4,177,178]. Resveratrol can also be auto-oxidized to semiquinones and the comparatively stable 4'-phenoxyl radical, producing ROS under certain enzymatic conditions [179]. pH and hydroxyl anions or organic bases affect polyphenol oxidative processes [180].

A study examined the dose–time dependency of acute resveratrol injection on lipoperoxidation levels in male rats' hearts, livers, and kidneys synchronized with a 12 h dark–light cycle. Resveratrol was an antioxidant in the dark and a pro-oxidant in the light, possibly reflecting the changing ratio of pro- and antioxidant activities in various organs during a 24 h cycle or postprandial oxidative burst [181]. Dietary polyphenols, including resveratrol, have impressive antioxidant and cytotoxic properties. Since every antioxidant is a redox agent, it can become a pro-oxidant, causing lipid peroxidation and DNA damage under certain conditions. Thus, pro-oxidant action may contribute to resveratrol's anticancer and apoptotic activities [182]. Resveratrol's pro-oxidant action can damage DNA and stop the cell cycle [178].

Resveratrol can influence many pathways simultaneously, resulting in diverse or even opposite biological effects depending on concentration or treatment period. Although a dose-dependent resveratrol pro-oxidative action causes oxidative stress in cells over short periods of time, less cytotoxicity was identified at the same dose but with longer exposure times. This suggests that surviving cells were more resistant to resveratrol-induced damage, which decreased over time [4,183]. Low resveratrol doses (0.1–1.0 μg/mL) increase cell proliferation, but higher doses (10.0–100.0 μg/mL) cause apoptosis and reduce mitotic activity in human tumors and endothelial cells [184]. Studies have shown that resveratrol has a dual effect on HT-29 colon cancer cells, with low concentrations (1 and 10 μmol/L) increasing cell number and higher doses (50 or 100 μmol/L) decreasing cell number and increasing apoptotic or necrotic cell percentage [185].

Resveratrol is interesting for drug research because it does not have any harmful or debilitating side effects. Resveratrol dosages have been varied in in vivo and in vitro experiments. However, the best dose and route must be determined according to the patient's needs. In addition, resveratrol causes cell death in tumor tissues but not in normal tissues [182]. The tumor-specific absorption of resveratrol is due to variations in cellular targets and gene expression in cancer cells. It has been shown [186] that lower resveratrol levels may be beneficial, but higher amounts kill tumor cells by pro-apoptotic signaling.

It has also been shown that resveratrol causes cell death in tumor tissues while having little to no effect on healthy neighboring tissues [187]. Because of variations in accessible cellular targets and gene expression, resveratrol is tumor-specific in that its absorption by normal cells is significantly lower than cancer cells. It has been hypothesized that modest dosages of resveratrol may have health benefits, whereas high amounts destroy tumor cells through pro-apoptotic actions [186].

The short-term use (1.0 g) of resveratrol appears to be safe. However, patients with nonalcoholic fatty liver disease may have nausea, vomiting, diarrhea, and liver impairment at dosages of 2.5 g or more per day [188]. Curiously, in long-term clinical trials [189], no serious adverse effects were reported. In fact, a single 5 g dose of resveratrol or a part of that dose spread out over numerous days has been shown to be safe and well-tolerated [190]. It is important to note, though, that these findings may be replicable among sick individuals because the research was conducted on healthy populations. Orally administered resveratrol is metabolized by gut microbiota [191], making it difficult to determine which effects are solely due to resveratrol or both resveratrol and its metabolites, further complicating our understanding of resveratrol dose-dependency and administration route [191].

High doses of resveratrol have been shown to inhibit cell growth and trigger apoptosis in normal cells, confirming the compound's biphasic actions throughout a wide range of concentrations [192]. Rapid activation of mitogen-activated protein kinase (MAPK) by resveratrol is dependent on MEK-1, Src, matrix metalloproteinase, and the epidermal growth factor receptor. Nanomolar doses (i.e., magnitude less than that required for ER genomic activity) and concentrations possibly/transiently obtained in serum after oral red wine ingestion [193] activate MAPK and endothelial nitric-oxide synthase (eNOS). Mice as young as one years old benefit from resveratrol's anti-aging properties when consumed in low dosages. Mice fed a dosage of 1800 mg/kg of resveratrol died after three to four months [194]. Despite the common occurrence of diarrhea, studies on the steady-state pharmacokinetics and tolerability of 2000 mg *trans*-resveratrol indicated that it was well-tolerated by healthy subjects [195]. This dosage was given twice a day with meals, quercetin, and alcohol.

Studies highlighting the health advantages of resveratrol all point to the importance of dose and age in eliciting such benefits. Another study that looked at the effects of resveratrol on insulin resistance caused by both aging and re-nutrition found that it increased insulin sensitivity in elderly mice fed a standard diet but had no effect on the insulin resistance status of elderly mice fed a high-protein diet [4]. On the other hand, resveratrol was harmful, lowering aortic distensibility and boosting inflammation and superoxide generation. These results suggest that resveratrol is helpful in a malnourished state of physiological aging, but that it may increase atherogenesis-associated risk factors when combined with high-protein diets in elderly mice, possibly by triggering vascular alterations that are themselves a risk factor for the cardiovascular system [196], which remains to be proven without reasonable doubt.

The biological effects of resveratrol are strongly linked to a hormetic effect (as discussed in the introduction), with low doses generally having beneficial effects and high doses having toxic effects. This biphasic effect on the cellular redox state, which is an antioxidant at low doses and a pro-oxidant at high doses, is believed to be responsible for resveratrol's hormetic property [2,4]. However, studies on resveratrol have mainly focused on short-term outcomes, leading to controversy [4]. The primary focus should be on resveratrol dosage and interaction with the environment's redox state, especially when precise redox modulation is needed for physiological function or to prevent harmful effects. More extensive studies in complex models are needed to validate current findings. Despite numerous human and animal studies supporting resveratrol's beneficial properties, there are not enough clinical studies reporting resveratrol's harmful effects, and the molecular mechanism of resveratrol's action needs to be better identified.

7. Conclusions and Future Perspectives

This article provides a summary of the research on the health benefits and mechanism of action behind red grape polyphenol resveratrol, including its effects on cardiovascular disease, cancer prevention and therapy, neuroprotection, and diabetes. Studies on both animals and humans show that resveratrol, when consumed in moderation, can have positive health effects. But in order to make resveratrol more promising pharmaceutically, adjustments must be made to its structure and bioavailability. The potential of resveratrol in the treatment and prevention of various diseases warrants further investigation. Additionally, resveratrol's biochemical mechanism of action has to be thoroughly elucidated. Most importantly, more standardized clinical trial designs are needed to adequately examine the benefits of resveratrol and establish its mechanisms of therapy and prevention of disease.

Author Contributions: All authors have read and agreed to the published version of the manuscript.

Funding: This work was supported by the Deanship of Scientific Research, Vice Presidency for Graduate Studies and Scientific Research, King Faisal University, Saudi Arabia (Grant No. 4585).

Institutional Review Board Statement: Not applicable.

Informed Consent Statement: Not applicable.

Data Availability Statement: Not applicable.

Conflicts of Interest: The author declares no conflict of interest.

References

1. Takaoka, M. Resveratrol, a new phenolic compound, from Veratrum grandiflorum. *J. Chem. Soc. Jpn.* **1939**, *60*, 1090–1100.
2. Shaito, A.; Posadino, A.M.; Younes, N.; Hasan, H.; Halabi, S.; Alhababi, D.; Al-Mohannadi, A.; Abdel-Rahman, W.M.; Eid, A.H.; Nasrallah, G.K.; et al. Potential Adverse Effects of Resveratrol: A Literature Review. *Int. J. Mol. Sci.* **2020**, *21*, 2084. [CrossRef]
3. Akinwumi, B.C.; Bordun, K.M.; Anderson, H.D. Biological activities of stilbenoids. *Int. J. Mol. Sci.* **2018**, *19*, 792. [CrossRef] [PubMed]
4. Salehi, B.; Mishra, A.P.; Nigam, M.; Sener, B.; Kilic, M.; Sharifi-Rad, M.; Fokou, P.V.T.; Martins, N.; Sharifi-Rad, J. Resveratrol: A Double-Edged Sword in Health Benefits. *Biomedicines* **2018**, *6*, 91. [CrossRef] [PubMed]
5. Colica, C.; Milanović, M.; Milić, N.; Aiello, V.; De Lorenzo, A.; Abenavoli, L. A Systematic Review on Natural Antioxidant Properties of Resveratrol. *Nat. Prod. Commun.* **2018**, *13*, 1934578X1801300923. [CrossRef]
6. Duta-Bratu, C.-G.; Nitulescu, G.M.; Mihai, D.P.; Olaru, O.T. Resveratrol and Other Natural Oligomeric Stilbenoid Compounds and Their Therapeutic Applications. *Plants* **2023**, *12*, 2935. [CrossRef]
7. Pannu, N.; Bhatnagar, A. Resveratrol: From enhanced biosynthesis and bioavailability to multitargeting chronic diseases. *Biomed. Pharm.* **2019**, *109*, 2237–2251. [CrossRef]
8. Andrade, S.; Ramalho, M.J.; Pereira, M.D.C.; Loureiro, J.A. Resveratrol Brain Delivery for Neurological Disorders Prevention and Treatment. *Front. Pharm.* **2018**, *9*, 1261. [CrossRef] [PubMed]
9. Xiao, Q.; Zhu, W.; Feng, W.; Lee, S.S.; Leung, A.W.; Shen, J.; Gao, L.; Xu, C. A Review of Resveratrol as a Potent Chemoprotective and Synergistic Agent in Cancer Chemotherapy. *Front. Pharmacol.* **2019**, *9*, 1534. [CrossRef]
10. Rodrigo-Gonzalo, M.J.; González-Manzano, S.; Mendez-Sánchez, R.; Santos-Buelga, C.; Recio-Rodríguez, J.I. Effect of Polyphenolic Complements on Cognitive Function in the Elderly: A Systematic Review. *Antioxidants* **2022**, *11*, 1549. [CrossRef] [PubMed]

11. García-Caballero, M.; Torres-Vargas, J.A.; Marrero, A.D.; Martínez-Poveda, B.; Medina, M.Á.; Quesada, A.R. Angioprevention of Urologic Cancers by Plant-Derived Foods. *Pharmaceutics* **2022**, *14*, 256. [CrossRef]
12. Zhang, L.Z.; Gong, J.G.; Li, J.H.; Hao, Y.S.; Xu, H.J.; Liu, Y.C.; Feng, Z.H. Dietary resveratrol supplementation on growth performance, immune function and intestinal barrier function in broilers challenged with lipopolysaccharide. *Poult. Sci.* **2023**, *102*, 102968. [CrossRef] [PubMed]
13. Moreira-Pinto, B.; Costa, L.; Felgueira, E.; Fonseca, B.M.; Rebelo, I. Low Doses of Resveratrol Protect Human Granulosa Cells from Induced-Oxidative Stress. *Antioxidants* **2021**, *10*, 561. [CrossRef]
14. Almannai, M.; El-Hattab, A.W.; Ali, M.; Soler-Alfonso, C.; Scaglia, F. Clinical trials in mitochondrial disorders, an update. *Mol. Genet. Metab.* **2020**, *131*, 1–13. [CrossRef] [PubMed]
15. Babylon, L.; Schmitt, F.; Franke, Y.; Hubert, T.; Eckert, G.P. Effects of Combining Biofactors on Bioenergetic Parameters, Aβ Levels and Survival in Alzheimer Model Organisms. *Int. J. Mol. Sci.* **2022**, *23*, 8670. [CrossRef] [PubMed]
16. Reda, D.; Elshopakey, G.E.; Mahgoub, H.A.; Risha, E.F.; Khan, A.A.; Rajab, B.S.; El-Boshy, M.E.; Abdelhamid, F.M. Effects of resveratrol against induced metabolic syndrome in rats: Role of oxidative stress, inflammation, and insulin resistance. *Evid. Based Complement. Altern. Med. eCAM* **2022**, *2022*, 3362005. [CrossRef] [PubMed]
17. Efimova, S.S.; Ostroumova, O.S. Modulation of the Dipole Potential of Model Lipid Membranes with Phytochemicals: Molecular Mechanisms, Structure–Activity Relationships, and Implications in Reconstituted Ion Channels. *Membranes* **2023**, *13*, 453. [CrossRef]
18. Hrelia, S.; Di Renzo, L.; Bavaresco, L.; Bernardi, E.; Malaguti, M.; Giacosa, A. Moderate Wine Consumption and Health: A Narrative Review. *Nutrients* **2023**, *15*, 175. [CrossRef]
19. Yang, C.; Tian, X.; Han, Y.; Shi, X.; Wang, H.; Li, H. Extracts of Dunkelfelder Grape Seeds and Peel Increase the Metabolic Rate and Reduce Fat Deposition in Mice Maintained on a High-Fat Diet. *Foods* **2023**, *12*, 3251. [CrossRef]
20. Martins, D.; Garcia, L.R.; Queiroz, D.A.R.; Lazzarin, T.; Tonon, C.R.; Balin, P.d.S.; Polegato, B.F.; de Paiva, S.A.R.; Azevedo, P.S.; Minicucci, M.F.; et al. Oxidative Stress as a Therapeutic Target of Cardiac Remodeling. *Antioxidants* **2022**, *11*, 2371. [CrossRef]
21. Arinno, A.; Apaijai, N.; Chattipakorn, S.C.; Chattipakorn, N. The roles of resveratrol on cardiac mitochondrial function in cardiac diseases. *Eur. J. Nutr.* **2021**, *60*, 29–44. [CrossRef]
22. Chedea, V.S.; Tomoiaga, L.L.; Macovei, S.O.; Magureanu, D.C.; Iliescu, M.L.; Bocsan, I.C.; Buzoianu, A.D.; Vosloban, C.M.; Pop, R.M. Antioxidant/pro-oxidant actions of polyphenols from grapevine and wine by-products-base for complementary therapy in ischemic heart diseases. *Front. Cardiovasc. Med.* **2021**, *8*, 750508. [CrossRef]
23. Raj, P.; Thandapilly, S.J.; Wigle, J.; Zieroth, S.; Netticadan, T. A Comprehensive Analysis of the Efficacy of Resveratrol in Atherosclerotic Cardiovascular Disease, Myocardial Infarction and Heart Failure. *Molecules* **2021**, *26*, 6600. [CrossRef]
24. Arias-Sánchez, R.A.; Torner, L.; Fenton Navarro, B. Polyphenols and Neurodegenerative Diseases: Potential Effects and Mechanisms of Neuroprotection. *Molecules* **2023**, *28*, 5415. [CrossRef]
25. Jomova, K.; Raptova, R.; Alomar, S.Y.; Alwasel, S.H.; Nepovimova, E.; Kuca, K.; Valko, M. Reactive oxygen species, toxicity, oxidative stress, and antioxidants: Chronic diseases and aging. *Arch. Toxicol.* **2023**, *97*, 2499–2574. [CrossRef]
26. Li, C.; Wang, Z.; Lei, H.; Zhang, D. Recent progress in nanotechnology-based drug carriers for resveratrol delivery. *Drug Deliv.* **2023**, *30*, 2174206. [CrossRef] [PubMed]
27. Iweala, E.J.; Oluwapelumi, A.E.; Dania, O.E.; Ugbogu, E.A. Bioactive Phytoconstituents and Their Therapeutic Potentials in the Treatment of Haematological Cancers: A Review. *Life* **2023**, *13*, 1422. [CrossRef] [PubMed]
28. Posadino, A.M.; Giordo, R.; Cossu, A.; Nasrallah, G.K.; Shaito, A.; Abou-Saleh, H.; Eid, A.H.; Pintus, G. Flavin Oxidase-Induced ROS Generation Modulates PKC Biphasic Effect of Resveratrol on Endothelial Cell Survival. *Biomolecules* **2019**, *9*, 209. [CrossRef]
29. Wani, S.A.; Khan, L.A.; Basir, S.F. Quercetin and resveratrol ameliorate nickel-mediated hypercontraction in isolated wistar rat aorta. *J. Smooth Muscle Res. = Nihon Heikatsukin Gakkai Kikanshi* **2022**, *58*, 89–105. [CrossRef] [PubMed]
30. Roumes, H.; Goudeneche, P.; Pellerin, L.; Bouzier-Sore, A.-K. Resveratrol and Some of Its Derivatives as Promising Prophylactic Treatments for Neonatal Hypoxia-Ischemia. *Nutrients* **2022**, *14*, 3793. [CrossRef]
31. Rojas-Aguilar, F.A.; Briones-Aranda, A.; Jaramillo-Morales, O.A.; Romero-Nava, R.; Esquinca-Avilés, H.A.; Espinosa-Juárez, J.V. The Additive Antinociceptive Effect of Resveratrol and Ketorolac in the Formalin Test in Mice. *Pharmaceuticals* **2023**, *16*, 1078. [CrossRef]
32. Ramli, I.; Posadino, A.M.; Giordo, R.; Fenu, G.; Fardoun, M.; Iratni, R.; Eid, A.H.; Zayed, H.; Pintus, G. Effect of Resveratrol on Pregnancy, Prenatal Complications and Pregnancy-Associated Structure Alterations. *Antioxidants* **2023**, *12*, 341. [CrossRef]
33. Cortés-Espinar, A.J.; Ibarz-Blanch, N.; Soliz-Rueda, J.R.; Bonafos, B.; Feillet-Coudray, C.; Casas, F.; Bravo, F.I.; Calvo, E.; Ávila-Román, J.; Mulero, M. Rhythm and ROS: Hepatic Chronotherapeutic Features of Grape Seed Proanthocyanidin Extract Treatment in Cafeteria Diet-Fed Rats. *Antioxidants* **2023**, *12*, 1606. [CrossRef] [PubMed]
34. Jiang, H.; Ni, J.; Hu, L.; Xiang, Z.; Zeng, J.; Shi, J.; Chen, Q.; Li, W. Resveratrol May Reduce the Degree of Periodontitis by Regulating ERK Pathway in Gingival-Derived MSCs. *Int. J. Mol. Sci.* **2023**, *24*, 11294. [CrossRef] [PubMed]
35. Danailova, Y.; Velikova, T.; Nikolaev, G.; Mitova, Z.; Shinkov, A.; Gagov, H.; Konakchieva, R. Nutritional Management of Thyroiditis of Hashimoto. *Int. J. Mol. Sci.* **2022**, *23*, 5144. [CrossRef]
36. Giuliani, C.; Iezzi, M.; Ciolli, L.; Hysi, A.; Bucci, I.; Di Santo, S.; Rossi, C.; Zucchelli, M.; Napolitano, G. Resveratrol has anti-thyroid effects both in vitro and in vivo. *Food Chem. Toxicol.* **2017**, *107*, 237–247. [CrossRef]
37. Fragopoulou, E.; Gkotsi, K.; Petsini, F.; Gioti, K.; Kalampaliki, A.D.; Lambrinidis, G.; Kostakis, I.K.; Tenta, R. Synthesis and Biological Evaluation of Resveratrol Methoxy Derivatives. *Molecules* **2023**, *28*, 5547. [CrossRef]

38. Iqbal, I.; Wilairatana, P.; Saqib, F.; Nasir, B.; Wahid, M.; Latif, M.F.; Iqbal, A.; Naz, R.; Mubarak, M.S. Plant Polyphenols and Their Potential Benefits on Cardiovascular Health: A Review. *Molecules* **2023**, *28*, 6403. [CrossRef]
39. Sun, W.; Shahrajabian, M.H. Therapeutic Potential of Phenolic Compounds in Medicinal Plants—Natural Health Products for Human Health. *Molecules* **2023**, *28*, 1845. [CrossRef]
40. Delmas, D.; Aires, V.; Limagne, E.; Dutartre, P.; Mazue, F.; Ghiringhelli, F.; Latruffe, N. Transport, stability, and biological activity of resveratrol. *Ann. N. Y. Acad. Sci.* **2011**, *1215*, 48–59. [CrossRef] [PubMed]
41. Burkon, A.; Somoza, V. Quantification of free and protein-bound trans-resveratrol metabolites and identification of trans-resveratrol-C/O-conjugated diglucuronides—Two novel resveratrol metabolites in human plasma. *Mol. Nutr. Food Res.* **2008**, *52*, 549–557. [CrossRef] [PubMed]
42. Rotches-Ribalta, M.; Andres-Lacueva, C.; Estruch, R.; Escribano, E.; Urpi-Sarda, M. Pharmacokinetics of resveratrol metabolic profile in healthy humans after moderate consumption of red wine and grape extract tablets. *Pharmacol. Res.* **2012**, *66*, 375–382. [CrossRef]
43. Wang, P.; Sang, S. Metabolism and pharmacokinetics of resveratrol and pterostilbene. *Biofactors* **2018**, *44*, 16–25. [CrossRef] [PubMed]
44. Baur, J.A.; Sinclair, D.A. Therapeutic potential of resveratrol: The in vivo evidence. *Nat. Rev. Drug Discov.* **2006**, *5*, 493–506. [CrossRef]
45. Rezende, J.P.; Hudson, E.A.; De Paula, H.M.C.; Meinel, R.S.; Da Silva, A.D.; Da Silva, L.H.M.; Pires, A. Human serum albumin-resveratrol complex formation: Effect of the phenolic chemical structure on the kinetic and thermodynamic parameters of the interactions. *Food Chem.* **2020**, *307*, 125514. [CrossRef] [PubMed]
46. Fan, Y.; Liu, Y.; Gao, L.; Zhang, Y.; Yi, J. Improved chemical stability and cellular antioxidant activity of resveratrol in zein nanoparticle with bovine serum albumin-caffeic acid conjugate. *Food Chem.* **2018**, *261*, 283–291. [CrossRef] [PubMed]
47. Geng, T.; Zhao, X.; Ma, M.; Zhu, G.; Yin, L. Resveratrol-Loaded Albumin Nanoparticles with Prolonged Blood Circulation and Improved Biocompatibility for Highly Effective Targeted Pancreatic Tumor Therapy. *Nanoscale Res. Lett.* **2017**, *12*, 437. [CrossRef] [PubMed]
48. Pantusa, M.; Bartucci, R.; Rizzuti, B. Stability of trans-resveratrol associated with transport proteins. *J. Agric. Food Chem.* **2014**, *62*, 4384–4391. [CrossRef]
49. Walle, T.; Hsieh, F.; DeLegge, M.H.; Oatis, J.E., Jr.; Walle, U.K. High absorption but very low bioavailability of oral resveratrol in humans. *Drug Metab. Dispos.* **2004**, *32*, 1377–1382. [CrossRef] [PubMed]
50. Szymkowiak, I.; Kucinska, M.; Murias, M. Between the Devil and the Deep Blue Sea—Resveratrol, Sulfotransferases and Sulfatases—A Long and Turbulent Journey from Intestinal Absorption to Target Cells. *Molecules* **2023**, *28*, 3297. [CrossRef]
51. Wang, Q.; Yu, Q.; Wu, M. Antioxidant and neuroprotective actions of resveratrol in cerebrovascular diseases. *Front. Pharmacol.* **2022**, *13*, 948889. [CrossRef] [PubMed]
52. Szczepańska, P.; Rychlicka, M.; Groborz, S.; Kruszyńska, A.; Ledesma-Amaro, R.; Rapak, A.; Gliszczyńska, A.; Lazar, Z. Studies on the Anticancer and Antioxidant Activities of Resveratrol and Long-Chain Fatty Acid Esters. *Int. J. Mol. Sci.* **2023**, *24*, 7167. [CrossRef] [PubMed]
53. Trius-Soler, M.; Pratico, G.; Gurdeniz, G.; Garcia-Aloy, M.; Canali, R.; Fausta, N.; Brouwer-Brolsma, E.M.; Andres-Lacueva, C.; Dragsted, L.O. Biomarkers of moderate alcohol intake and alcoholic beverages: A systematic literature review. *Genes Nutr.* **2023**, *18*, 7. [CrossRef]
54. Karabekir, S.C.; Ozgorgulu, A. Possible protective effects of resveratrol in hepatocellular carcinoma. *Iran. J. Basic Med. Sci.* **2020**, *23*, 71–78. [PubMed]
55. Florio, R.; De Filippis, B.; Veschi, S.; di Giacomo, V.; Lanuti, P.; Catitti, G.; Brocco, D.; di Rienzo, A.; Cataldi, A.; Cacciatore, I.; et al. Resveratrol Derivative Exhibits Marked Antiproliferative Actions, Affecting Stemness in Pancreatic Cancer Cells. *Int. J. Mol. Sci.* **2023**, *24*, 1977. [CrossRef]
56. Peterle, L.; Sanfilippo, S.; Borgia, F.; Li Pomi, F.; Vadalà, R.; Costa, R.; Cicero, N.; Gangemi, S. The Role of Nutraceuticals and Functional Foods in Skin Cancer: Mechanisms and Therapeutic Potential. *Foods* **2023**, *12*, 2629. [CrossRef]
57. Wang, G.; Hu, Z.; Song, X.; Cui, Q.; Fu, Q.; Jia, R.; Zou, Y.; Li, L.; Yin, Z. Analgesic and Anti-Inflammatory Activities of Resveratrol through Classic Models in Mice and Rats. *Evid. Based Complement. Alternat. Med.* **2017**, *2017*, 5197567. [CrossRef] [PubMed]
58. Almatroodi, S.A.; Alsahli, M.A.; Aljohani, A.S.M.; Alhumaydhi, F.A.; Babiker, A.Y.; Khan, A.A.; Rahmani, A.H. Potential Therapeutic Targets of Resveratrol, a Plant Polyphenol, and Its Role in the Therapy of Various Types of Cancer. *Molecules* **2022**, *27*, 2665. [CrossRef] [PubMed]
59. De Sá Coutinho, D.; Pacheco, M.T.; Frozza, R.L.; Bernardi, A. Anti-Inflammatory Effects of Resveratrol: Mechanistic Insights. *Int. J. Mol. Sci.* **2018**, *19*, 1812. [CrossRef]
60. Silva, A.F.R.; Silva-Reis, R.; Ferreira, R.; Oliveira, P.A.; Faustino-Rocha, A.I.; Pinto, M.d.L.; Coimbra, M.A.; Silva, A.M.S.; Cardoso, S.M. The Impact of Resveratrol-Enriched Bread on Cardiac Remodeling in a Preclinical Model of Diabetes. *Antioxidants* **2023**, *12*, 1066. [CrossRef] [PubMed]
61. García-Martínez, B.I.; Ruiz-Ramos, M.; Pedraza-Chaverri, J.; Santiago-Osorio, E.; Mendoza-Núñez, V.M. Hypoglycemic Effect of Resveratrol: A Systematic Review and Meta-Analysis. *Antioxidants* **2021**, *10*, 69. [CrossRef] [PubMed]
62. Moon, D.O. A comprehensive review of the effects of resveratrol on glucose metabolism: Unveiling the molecular pathways and therapeutic potential in diabetes management. *Mol. Biol. Rep.* **2023**, *50*, 8743–8755. [CrossRef] [PubMed]

63. Rahman, M.H.; Akter, R.; Bhattacharya, T.; Abdel-Daim, M.M.; Alkahtani, S.; Arafah, M.W.; Al-Johani, N.S.; Alhoshani, N.M.; Alkeraishan, N.; Alhenaky, A.; et al. Resveratrol and neuroprotection: Impact and its therapeutic potential in Alzheimer's disease. *Front. Pharmacol.* **2020**, *11*, 619024. [CrossRef]
64. Xiang, L.; Wang, Y.; Liu, S.; Liu, B.; Jin, X.; Cao, X. Targeting Protein Aggregates with Natural Products: An Optional Strategy for Neurodegenerative Diseases. *Int. J. Mol. Sci.* **2023**, *24*, 11275. [CrossRef] [PubMed]
65. Dos Santos, M.G.; Schimith, L.E.; Andre-Miral, C.; Muccillo-Baisch, A.L.; Arbo, B.D.; Hort, M.A. Neuroprotective effects of resveratrol in in vivo and in vitro experimental models of parkinson's disease: A systematic review. *Neurotox. Res.* **2022**, *40*, 319–345. [CrossRef]
66. Filardo, S.; Di Pietro, M.; Mastromarino, P.; Sessa, R. Therapeutic potential of resveratrol against emerging respiratory viral infections. *Pharmacol. Ther.* **2020**, *214*, 107613. [CrossRef] [PubMed]
67. Abba, Y.; Hassim, H.; Hamzah, H.; Noordin, M.M. Antiviral Activity of Resveratrol against Human and Animal Viruses. *Adv. Virol.* **2015**, *2015*, 184241. [CrossRef]
68. Yoon, J.; Ku, D.; Lee, M.; Lee, N.; Im, S.G.; Kim, Y. Resveratrol Attenuates the Mitochondrial RNA-Mediated Cellular Response to Immunogenic Stress. *Int. J. Mol. Sci.* **2023**, *24*, 7403. [CrossRef] [PubMed]
69. Carpéné, C.; Les, F.; Cásedas, G.; Peiro, C.; Fontaine, J.; Chaplin, A.; Mercader, J.; López, V. Resveratrol Anti-Obesity Effects: Rapid Inhibition of Adipocyte Glucose Utilization. *Antioxidants* **2019**, *8*, 74. [CrossRef]
70. Zhou, L.; Xiao, X.; Zhang, Q.; Zheng, J.; Deng, M. Deciphering the anti-obesity benefits of resveratrol: The "gut microbiota-adipose tissue" axis. *Front. Endocrinol.* **2019**, *10*, 413. [CrossRef]
71. Vrânceanu, M.; Hegheș, S.-C.; Cozma-Petruț, A.; Banc, R.; Stroia, C.M.; Raischi, V.; Miere, D.; Popa, D.-S.; Filip, L. Plant-Derived Nutraceuticals Involved in Body Weight Control by Modulating Gene Expression. *Plants* **2023**, *12*, 2273. [CrossRef] [PubMed]
72. Gal, R.; Deres, L.; Toth, K.; Halmosi, R.; Habon, T. The Effect of Resveratrol on the Cardiovascular System from Molecular Mechanisms to Clinical Results. *Int. J. Mol. Sci.* **2021**, *22*, 10152. [CrossRef]
73. Kazemirad, H.; Kazerani, H.R. Cardioprotective effects of resveratrol following myocardial ischemia and reperfusion. *Mol. Biol. Rep.* **2020**, *47*, 5843–5850. [CrossRef]
74. Menezes-Rodrigues, F.S.; Errante, P.R.; Araujo, E.A.; Fernandes, M.P.P.; Silva, M.M.D.; Pires-Oliveira, M.; Scorza, C.A.; Scorza, F.A.; Taha, M.O.; Caricati-Neto, A. Cardioprotection stimulated by resveratrol and grape products prevents lethal cardiac arrhythmias in an animal model of ischemia and reperfusion. *Acta Cir. Bras.* **2021**, *36*, e360306. [CrossRef]
75. Bohara, R.A.; Tabassum, N.; Singh, M.P.; Gigli, G.; Ragusa, A.; Leporatti, S. Recent Overview of Resveratrol's Beneficial Effects and Its Nano-Delivery Systems. *Molecules* **2022**, *27*, 5154. [CrossRef] [PubMed]
76. Wijekoon, C.; Netticadan, T.; Siow, Y.L.; Sabra, A.; Yu, L.; Raj, P.; Prashar, S. Potential Associations among Bioactive Molecules, Antioxidant Activity and Resveratrol Production in *Vitis vinifera* Fruits of North America. *Molecules* **2022**, *27*, 336. [CrossRef]
77. Gu, T.; Wang, N.; Wu, T.; Ge, Q.; Chen, L. Antioxidative stress mechanisms behind resveratrol: A multidimensional analysis. *J. Food Qual.* **2021**, *2021*, 5571733. [CrossRef]
78. Zhou, D.D.; Luo, M.; Huang, S.Y.; Saimaiti, A.; Shang, A.; Gan, R.Y.; Li, H.B. Effects and mechanisms of resveratrol on aging and age-related diseases. *Oxidative Med. Cell. Longev.* **2021**, *2021*, 9932218. [CrossRef] [PubMed]
79. Pyo, I.S.; Yun, S.; Yoon, Y.E.; Choi, J.W.; Lee, S.J. Mechanisms of aging and the preventive effects of resveratrol on age-related diseases. *Molecules* **2020**, *25*, 4649. [CrossRef]
80. Leis, K.; Pisanko, K.; Jundziłł, A.; Mazur, E.; Mêcińska-Jundziłł, K.; Witmanowski, H. Resveratrol as a factor preventing skin aging and affecting its regeneration. *Postep. Dermatol. Alergol.* **2022**, *39*, 439–445. [CrossRef]
81. Gowd, V.; Kang, Q.; Wang, Q.; Wang, Q.; Chen, F.; Cheng, K.W. Resveratrol: Evidence for its nephroprotective effect in diabetic nephropathy. *Adv. Nutr.* **2020**, *11*, 1555–1568. [CrossRef] [PubMed]
82. Jin, Q.; Liu, T.; Qiao, Y.; Liu, D.; Yang, L.; Mao, H.; Ma, F.; Wang, Y.; Peng, L.; Zhan, Y. Oxidative stress and inflammation in diabetic nephropathy: Role of polyphenols. *Front. Immunol.* **2023**, *14*, 1185317. [CrossRef] [PubMed]
83. Cheng, K.; Song, Z.; Chen, Y.; Li, S.; Zhang, Y.; Zhang, H.; Zhang, L.; Wang, C.; Wang, T. Resveratrol Protects Against Renal Damage via Attenuation of Inflammation and Oxidative Stress in High-Fat-Diet-Induced Obese Mice. *Inflammation* **2018**, *42*, 937–945. [CrossRef] [PubMed]
84. Ahmadi, A.; Jamialahmadi, T.; Sahebkar, A. Polyphenols and atherosclerosis: A critical review of clinical effects on LDL oxidation. *Pharmacol. Res.* **2022**, *184*, 106414. [CrossRef] [PubMed]
85. Castaldo, L.; Narváez, A.; Izzo, L.; Graziani, G.; Gaspari, A.; Di Minno, G.; Ritieni, A. Red Wine Consumption and Cardiovascular Health. *Molecules* **2019**, *24*, 3626. [CrossRef] [PubMed]
86. Buljeta, I.; Pichler, A.; Šimunović, J.; Kopjar, M. Beneficial Effects of Red Wine Polyphenols on Human Health: Comprehensive Review. *Curr. Issues Mol. Biol.* **2023**, *45*, 782–798. [CrossRef]
87. Rasines-Perea, Z.; Teissedre, P.-L. Grape Polyphenols' Effects in Human Cardiovascular Diseases and Diabetes. *Molecules* **2017**, *22*, 68. [CrossRef] [PubMed]
88. Chiva-Blanch, G.; Urpi-Sarda, M.; Ros, E.; Valderas-Martinez, P.; Casas, R.; Arranz, S.; Guillén, M.; Lamuela-Raventós, R.M.; Llorach, R.; Andres-Lacueva, C.; et al. Effects of red wine polyphenols and alcohol on glucose metabolism and the lipid profile: A randomized clinical trial. *Clin. Nutr.* **2013**, *32*, 200–206. [CrossRef]

89. Navarro-García, F.; Ponce-Ruíz, N.; Rojas-García, A.E.; Ávila-Villarreal, G.; Herrera-Moreno, J.F.; Barrón-Vivanco, B.S.; Bernal-Hernández, Y.Y.; González-Arias, C.A.; Medina-Díaz, I.M. The Role of Nutritional Habits and Moderate Red Wine Consumption in PON1 Status in Healthy Population. *Appl. Sci.* **2021**, *11*, 9503. [CrossRef]
90. Salazar, H.M.; de Deus Mendonça, R.; Laclaustra, M.; Moreno-Franco, B.; Åkesson, A.; Guallar-Castillón, P.; Donat-Vargas, C. The intake of flavonoids, stilbenes, and tyrosols, mainly consumed through red wine and virgin olive oil, is associated with lower carotid and femoral subclinical atherosclerosis and coronary calcium. *Eur. J. Nutr.* **2022**, *61*, 2697–2709. [CrossRef]
91. Tresserra-Rimbau, A.; Medina-Remón, A.; Lamuela-Raventós, R.M.; Bulló, M.; Salas-Salvadó, J.; Corella, D.; Fitó, M.; Gea, A.; Gómez-Gracia, E.; Lapetra, J.; et al. Moderate red wine consumption is associated with a lower prevalence of the metabolic syndrome in the PREDIMED population. *Br. J. Nutr.* **2015**, *113*, 121–130. [CrossRef] [PubMed]
92. Surh, Y.J. Cancer chemoprevention with dietary phytochemicals. *Nat. Rev. Cancer* **2003**, *3*, 768–780. [CrossRef] [PubMed]
93. Amor, S.; Châlons, P.; Aires, V.; Delmas, D. Polyphenol Extracts from Red Wine and Grapevine: Potential Effects on Cancers. *Diseases* **2018**, *6*, 106. [CrossRef] [PubMed]
94. Bray, F.; Ferlay, J.; Soerjomataram, I.; Siegel, R.L.; Torre, L.A.; Jemal, A. Global cancer statistics 2018: GLOBOCAN estimates of incidence and mortality worldwide for 36 cancers in 185 countries. *CA: Cancer J. Clin.* **2018**, *68*, 394–424. [CrossRef]
95. Liu, L.; Jin, R.; Hao, J.; Zeng, J.; Yin, D.; Yi, Y.; Zhu, M.; Mandal, A.; Hua, Y.; Ng, C.K.; et al. Consumption of the Fish Oil High-Fat Diet Uncouples Obesity and Mammary Tumor Growth through Induction of Reactive Oxygen Species in Protumor Macrophages. *AACR* **2020**, *80*, 2564–2574. [CrossRef] [PubMed]
96. Kim, M.-J.; Kim, Y.-J.; Park, H.-J.; Chung, J.-H.; Leem, K.-H.; Kim, H.-K. Apoptotic effect of red wine polyphenols on human colon cancer SNU-C4 cells. *Food Chem. Toxicol.* **2006**, *44*, 898–902. [CrossRef]
97. Bastide, N.M.; Naud, N.; Nassy, G.; Vendeuvre, J.-L.; Taché, S.; Guéraud, F.; Hobbs, D.A.; Kuhnle, G.G.; Corpet, D.; Pierre, F.H.F. Red Wine and Pomegranate Extracts Suppress Cured Meat Promotion of Colonic Mucin-Depleted Foci in Carcinogen-Induced Rats. *Nutr. Cancer* **2017**, *69*, 289–298. [CrossRef]
98. Mazué, F.; Delmas, D.; Murillo, G.; Saleiro, D.; Limagne, E.; Latruffe, N. Differential protective effects of red wine polyphenol extracts (RWEs) on colon carcinogenesis. *Food Funct.* **2014**, *5*, 663–670. [CrossRef]
99. Sabadashka, M.; Hertsyk, D.; Strugała-Danak, P.; Dudek, A.; Kanyuka, O.; Kucharska, A.Z.; Kaprelyants, L.; Sybirna, N. Anti-Diabetic and Antioxidant Activities of Red Wine Concentrate Enriched with Polyphenol Compounds under Experimental Diabetes in Rats. *Antioxidants* **2021**, *10*, 1399. [CrossRef]
100. Martin, M.A.; Goy, L.; Ramos, S. Protective effects of tea, red wine and cocoa in diabetes. Evidences from human studies. *Food Chem. Toxicol.* **2017**, *109*, 302–314. [CrossRef]
101. Xia, X.; Sun, B.; Li, W.; Zhang, X.; Zhao, Y. Anti-diabetic activity phenolic constituents from red wine against α-glucosidase and α-amylase. *J. Food Process. Preserv.* **2016**, *41*, 12942. [CrossRef]
102. Tamargo, A.; Cueva, C.; Silva, M.; Molinero, N.; Miralles, B.; Bartolomé, B.; Moreno-Arribas, M.V. Gastrointestinal co-digestion of wine polyphenols with glucose/whey proteins affects their bioaccessibility and impact on colonic microbiota. *Food Res. Int.* **2022**, *155*, 111010. [CrossRef] [PubMed]
103. Shen, C.; Cheng, W.; Yu, P.; Wang, L.; Zhou, L.; Zeng, L.; Yang, Q. Resveratrol pretreatment attenuates injury and promotes proliferation of neural stem cells following oxygen-glucose deprivation/reoxygenation by upregulating the expression of Nrf2, HO-1 and NQO1 in vitro. *Mol. Med. Rep.* **2016**, *14*, 3646–3654. [CrossRef]
104. Son, Y.; Byun, S.J.; Pae, H.-O. Involvement of heme oxygenase-1 expression in neuroprotection by piceatannol, a natural analog and a metabolite of resveratrol, against glutamate-mediated oxidative injury in HT22 neuronal cells. *Amino Acids* **2013**, *45*, 393–401. [CrossRef]
105. Ren, J.; Fan, C.; Chen, N.; Huang, J.; Yang, Q. Resveratrol pretreatment attenuates cerebral ischemic injury by upregulating expression of transcription factor Nrf2 and HO-1 in rats. *Neurochem. Res.* **2011**, *36*, 2352–2362. [CrossRef] [PubMed]
106. Martínez-Huélamo, M.; Rodríguez-Morató, J.; Boronat, A.; De la Torre, R. Modulation of Nrf2 by Olive Oil and Wine Polyphenols and Neuroprotection. *Antioxidants* **2017**, *6*, 73. [CrossRef]
107. Rocha-Parra, D.; Chirife, J.; Zamora, C.; De Pascual-Teresa, S. Chemical Characterization of an Encapsulated Red Wine Powder and Its Effects on Neuronal Cells. *Molecules* **2018**, *23*, 842. [CrossRef] [PubMed]
108. Li, Y.; Peng, Y.; Shen, Y.; Zhang, Y.; Liu, L.; Yang, X. Dietary polyphenols: Regulate the advanced glycation end products-RAGE axis and the microbiota-gut-brain axis to prevent neurodegenerative diseases. *Crit. Rev. Food Sci. Nutr.* **2022**, *19*, 1–27. [CrossRef]
109. Singh, A.P.; Singh, R.; Verma, S.S.; Rai, V.; Kaschula, C.H.; Maiti, P.; Gupta, S.C. Health benefits of resveratrol: Evidence from clinical studies. *Med. Res. Rev.* **2019**, *39*, 1851–1891. [CrossRef]
110. de Vries, K.; Strydom, M.; Steenkamp, V. A Brief Updated Review of Advances to Enhance Resveratrol's Bioavailability. *Molecules* **2021**, *26*, 4367. [CrossRef]
111. Farzin, L.; Asghari, S.; Rafraf, M.; Asghari-Jafarabadi, M.; Shirmohammadi, M. No beneficial effects of resveratrol supplementation on atherogenic risk factors in patients with nonalcoholic fatty liver disease. *Int. J. Vitam. Nutr. Res.* **2020**, *90*, 279–289. [CrossRef] [PubMed]
112. Mansur, A.P.; Roggerio, A.; Goes, M.F.S.; Avakian, S.D.; Leal, D.P.; Maranhão, R.C.; Strunz, C.M.C. Serum concentrations and gene expression of sirtuin 1 in healthy and slightly overweight subjects after caloric restriction or resveratrol supplementation: A randomized trial. *Int. J. Cardiol.* **2017**, *227*, 788–794. [CrossRef]

113. Amato, B.; Compagna, R.; Amato, M.; Gallelli, L.; de Franciscis, S.; Serra, R. Aterofisiol® in carotid plaque evolution. *Drug Des. Dev. Ther.* **2015**, *9*, 3877–3884.
114. Hoseini, A.; Namazi, G.; Farrokhian, A.; Reiner, Ž.; Aghadavod, E.; Bahmani, F.; Asemi, Z. The effects of resveratrol on metabolic status in patients with type 2 diabetes mellitus and coronary heart disease. *Food Funct.* **2019**, *10*, 6042–6051. [CrossRef]
115. Diaz, M.; Avila, A.; Degens, H.; Coeckelberghs, E.; Vanhees, L.; Cornelissen, V.; Azzawi, M. Acute resveratrol supplementation in coronary artery disease: Towards patient stratification. *Scand. Cardiovasc. J.* **2020**, *54*, 14–19. [CrossRef]
116. Marques, B.; Trindade, M.; Aquino, J.C.F.; Cunha, A.R.; Gismondi, R.O.; Neves, M.F.; Oigman, W. Beneficial effects of acute trans-resveratrol supplementation in treated hypertensive patients with endothelial dysfunction. *Clin. Exp. Hypertens.* **2018**, *40*, 218–223. [CrossRef]
117. Biesinger, S.; Michaels, H.A.; Quadros, A.S.; Qian, Y.; Rabovsky, A.B.; Badger, R.S.; Jalili, T. A combination of isolated phytochemicals and botanical extracts lowers diastolic blood pressure in a randomized controlled trial of hypertensive subjects. *Eur. J. Clin. Nutr.* **2016**, *70*, 10–16. [CrossRef] [PubMed]
118. Albrecht, T.; Waliszewski, M.; Roca, C.; Redlich, U.; Tautenhahn, J.; Pech, M.; Halloul, Z.; Gögebakan, Ö.; Meyer, D.R.; Gemeinhardt, I.; et al. Two-Year Clinical Outcomes of the CONSEQUENT Trial: Can Femoropopliteal Lesions be Treated with Sustainable Clinical Results that are Economically Sound? *Cardiovasc. Interv. Radiol.* **2018**, *41*, 1008–1014. [CrossRef]
119. Bhatt, J.K.; Thomas, S.; Nanjan, M.J. Resveratrol supplementation improves glycemic control in type 2 diabetes mellitus. *Nutr. Res.* **2012**, *32*, 537–541. [CrossRef]
120. Abdollahi, S.; Salehi-Abargouei, A.; Toupchian, O.; Sheikhha, M.H.; Fallahzadeh, H.; Rahmanian, M.; Tabatabaie, M.; Mozaffari-Khosravi, H. The Effect of Resveratrol Supplementation on Cardio-Metabolic Risk Factors in Patients with Type 2 Diabetes: A Randomized, Double-Blind Controlled Trial. *Phytother. Res.* **2019**, *33*, 3153–3162. [CrossRef]
121. Brasnyo, P.; Molnar, G.A.; Mohas, M.; Marko, L.; Laczy, B.; Cseh, J.; Mikolas, E.; Szijarto, I.A.; Merei, A.; Halmai, R.; et al. Resveratrol improves insulin sensitivity, reduces oxidative stress and activates the akt pathway in type 2 diabetic patients. *Br. J. Nutr.* **2011**, *106*, 383–389. [CrossRef]
122. Poulsen, M.K.; Nellemann, B.; Bibby, B.M.; Stødkilde-Jørgensen, H.; Pedersen, S.B.; Grønbaek, H.; Nielsen, S. No effect of resveratrol on VLDL-TG kinetics and insulin sensitivity in obese men with nonalcoholic fatty liver disease. *Diabetes Obes. Metab.* **2018**, *20*, 2504–2509. [CrossRef]
123. Timmers, S.; de Ligt, M.; Phielix, E.; van de Weijer, T.; Hansen, J.; Moonen-Kornips, E.; Schaart, G.; Kunz, I.; Hesselink, M.K.; Schrauwen-Hinderling, V.B.; et al. Resveratrol as Add-on Therapy in Subjects with Well-Controlled Type 2 Diabetes: A Randomized Controlled Trial. *Diabetes Care* **2016**, *39*, 2211–2217. [CrossRef] [PubMed]
124. Thazhath, S.S.; Wu, T.; Bound, M.J.; Checklin, H.L.; Standfield, S.; Jones, K.L.; Horowitz, M.; Rayner, C.K. Administration of resveratrol for 5 wk has no effect on glucagon-like peptide 1 secretion, gastric emptying, or glycemic control in type 2 diabetes: A randomized controlled trial. *Am. J. Clin. Nutr.* **2016**, *103*, 66–70. [CrossRef]
125. Pollack, R.M.; Barzilai, N.; Anghel, V.; Kulkarni, A.S.; Golden, A.; O'Broin, P.; Sinclair, D.A.; Bonkowski, M.S.; Coleville, A.J.; Powell, D.; et al. Resveratrol Improves Vascular Function and Mitochondrial Number but Not Glucose Metabolism in Older Adults. *J. Gerontol. A Biol. Sci. Med. Sci.* **2017**, *72*, 1703–1709. [CrossRef] [PubMed]
126. Boswijk, E.; de Ligt, M.; Habets, M.J.; Mingels, A.M.A.; van Marken Lichtenbelt, W.D.; Mottaghy, F.M.; Schrauwen, P.; Wildberger, J.E.; Bucerius, J. Resveratrol treatment does not reduce arterial inflammation in males at risk of type 2 diabetes: A randomized crossover trial. *Nukl. Nucl. Med.* **2022**, *61*, 33–41. [CrossRef]
127. Pecoraro, L.; Zoller, T.; Atkinson, R.L.; Nisi, F.; Antoniazzi, F.; Cavarzere, P.; Piacentini, G.; Pietrobelli, A. Supportive treatment of vascular dysfunction in pediatric subjects with obesity: The OBELIX study. *Nutr. Diabetes* **2022**, *12*, 2. [CrossRef]
128. Vors, C.; Couillard, C.; Paradis, M.E.; Gigleux, I.; Marin, J.; Vohl, M.C.; Couture, P.; Lamarche, B. Supplementation with Resveratrol and Curcumin Does Not Affect the Inflammatory Response to a High-Fat Meal in Older Adults with Abdominal Obesity: A Randomized, Placebo-Controlled Crossover Trial. *J. Nutr.* **2018**, *148*, 379–388. [CrossRef] [PubMed]
129. Mankowski, R.T.; You, L.; Buford, T.W.; Leeuwenburgh, C.; Manini, T.M.; Schneider, S.; Qiu, P.; Anton, S.D. Higher dose of resveratrol elevated cardiovascular disease risk biomarker levels in overweight older adults—A pilot study. *Exp. Gerontol.* **2020**, *131*, 110821. [CrossRef] [PubMed]
130. Kung, H.-C.; Lin, K.-J.; Kung, C.-T.; Lin, T.-K. Oxidative Stress, Mitochondrial Dysfunction, and Neuroprotection of Polyphenols with Respect to Resveratrol in Parkinson's Disease. *Biomedicines* **2021**, *9*, 918. [CrossRef] [PubMed]
131. Turner, R.S.; Thomas, R.G.; Craft, S.; Van Dyck, C.H.; Mintzer, J.; Reynolds, B.A.; Brewer, J.B.; Rissman, R.A.; Raman, R.; Aisen, P.S.; et al. A randomized, double-blind, placebo-controlled trial of resveratrol for Alzheimer disease. *Neurology* **2015**, *85*, 1383–1391. [CrossRef]
132. Paller, C.J.; Rudek, M.A.; Zhou, X.C.; Wagner, W.D.; Hudson, T.S.; Anders, N.; Hammers, H.J.; Dowling, D.; King, S.; Antonarakis, E.S.; et al.; et al. A phase i study of muscadine grape skin extract in men with biochemically recurrent prostate cancer: Safety, tolerability, and dose determination. *Prostate* **2015**, *75*, 1518–1525. [CrossRef] [PubMed]
133. Kjaer, T.N.; Ornstrup, M.J.; Poulsen, M.M.; Jorgensen, J.O.; Hougaard, D.M.; Cohen, A.S.; Neghabat, S.; Richelsen, B.; Pedersen, S.B. Resveratrol reduces the levels of circulating androgen precursors but has no effect on, testosterone, dihydrotestosterone, psa levels or prostate volume. A 4-month randomised trial in middle-aged men. *Prostate* **2015**, *75*, 1255–1263. [CrossRef] [PubMed]

134. Howells, L.M.; Berry, D.P.; Elliott, P.J.; Jacobson, E.W.; Hoffmann, E.; Hegarty, B.; Brown, K.; Steward, W.P.; Gescher, A.J. Phase i randomized, double-blind pilot study of micronized resveratrol (srt501) in patients with hepatic metastases—Safety, pharmacokinetics, and pharmacodynamics. *Cancer Prev. Res.* **2011**, *4*, 1419–1425. [CrossRef] [PubMed]
135. Patel, K.R.; Brown, V.A.; Jones, D.J.; Britton, R.G.; Hemingway, D.; Miller, A.S.; West, K.P.; Booth, T.D.; Perloff, M.; Crowell, J.A.; et al. Clinical pharmacology of resveratrol and its metabolites in colorectal cancer patients. *Cancer Res.* **2010**, *70*, 7392–7399. [CrossRef] [PubMed]
136. Zhu, W.; Qin, W.; Zhang, K.; Rottinghaus, G.E.; Chen, Y.C.; Kliethermes, B.; Sauter, E.R. Trans-resveratrol alters mammary promoter hypermethylation in women at increased risk for breast cancer. *Nutr. Cancer* **2012**, *64*, 393–400. [CrossRef]
137. Uberti, F.; Morsanuto, V.; Aprile, S.; Ghirlanda, S.; Stoppa, I.; Cochis, A.; Grosa, G.; Rimondini, L.; Molinari, C. Biological effects of combined resveratrol and vitamin D3 on ovarian tissue. *J. Ovarian Res.* **2017**, *10*, 61. [CrossRef]
138. Feng, Y.; Jin, C.; Lv, S.; Zhang, H.; Ren, F.; Wang, J. Molecular Mechanisms and Applications of Polyphenol-Protein Complexes with Antioxidant Properties: A Review. *Antioxidants* **2023**, *12*, 1577. [CrossRef]
139. Gambini, J.; Inglés, M.; Olaso, G.; Lopez-Grueso, R.; Bonet-Costa, V.; Gimeno-Mallench, L.; Mas-Bargues, C.; Abdelaziz, K.M.; Gomez-Cabrera, M.C.; Vina, J.; et al. Properties of Resveratrol: In Vitro and In Vivo Studies about Metabolism, Bioavailability, and Biological Effects in Animal Models and Humans. *Oxidative Med. Cell Longev.* **2015**, *2015*, 837042. [CrossRef]
140. Maity, B.; Bora, M.; Sur, D.J.O.P.; Medicine, E. An effect of combination of resveratrol with vitamin D3 on modulation of proinflammatory cytokines in diabetic nephropathy induces rat. *Orient. Pharm. Exp. Med.* **2018**, *18*, 127–138. [CrossRef]
141. Vetvicka, V.; Vetvickova, J. Combination of glucan, resveratrol and vitamin C demonstrates strong anti-tumor potential. *Anticancer Res.* **2012**, *32*, 81–87.
142. Mukherjee, S.; Debata, P.R.; Hussaini, R.; Chatterjee, K.; Baidoo, J.N.E.; Sampat, P.; Szerszen, A.; Navarra, J.P.; Fata, J.; Severinova, E.; et al. Unique synergistic formulation of curcumin, epicatechin gallate and resveratrol, tricurin, suppresses HPV E6, eliminates HPV+ cancer cells, and inhibits tumor progression. *Oncotarget* **2017**, *8*, 60904–60916. [CrossRef]
143. Piao, L.; Mukherjee, S.; Chang, Q.; Xie, X.; Li, H.; Castellanos, M.R.; Banerjee, P.; Iqbal, H.; Ivancic, R.; Wang, X.; et al. TriCurin, a novel formulation of curcumin, epicatechin gallate, and resveratrol, inhibits the tumorigenicity of human papillomavirus-positive head and neck squamous cell carcinoma. *Oncotarget* **2017**, *8*, 60025–60035. [CrossRef]
144. Ahmad, K.A.; Harris, N.H.; Johnson, A.D.; Lindvall, H.C.; Wang, G.; Ahmed, K. Protein kinase CK2 modulates apoptosis induced by resveratrol and epigallocatechin-3-gallate in prostate cancer cells. *Mol. Cancer* **2007**, *6*, 1006–1012. [CrossRef] [PubMed]
145. Roomi, M.W.; Kalinovsky, T.; Roomi, N.W.; Niedzwiecki, A.; Rath, M. In vitro and in vivo inhibition of human Fanconi anemia head and neck squamous carcinoma by a phytonutrient combination. *Int. J. Oncol.* **2015**, *46*, 2261–2266. [CrossRef] [PubMed]
146. Intagliata, S.; Modica, M.N.; Santagati, L.M.; Montenegro, L. Strategies to Improve Resveratrol Systemic and Topical Bioavailability: An Update. *Antioxid* **2019**, *8*, 244. [CrossRef]
147. Wan, S.; Zhang, L.; Quan, Y.; Wei, K. Resveratrol-loaded PLGA nanoparticles: Enhanced stability, solubility and bioactivity of resveratrol for non-alcoholic fatty liver disease therapy. *R. Soc. Open Sci.* **2018**, *5*, 181457. [CrossRef]
148. Aatif, M. Current Understanding of Polyphenols to Enhance Bioavailability for Better Therapies. *Biomedicines* **2023**, *11*, 2078. [CrossRef] [PubMed]
149. Siu, F.Y.; Ye, S.; Lin, H.; Li, S. Galactosylated PLGA nanoparticles for the oral delivery of resveratrol: Enhanced bioavailability and in vitro anti-inflammatory activity. *Int. J. Nanomed.* **2018**, *13*, 4133–4144. [CrossRef] [PubMed]
150. Thipe, V.C.; Panjtan Amiri, K.; Bloebaum, P.; Raphael Karikachery, A.; Khoobchandani, M.; Katti, K.K.; Jurisson, S.S.; Katti, K.V. Development of resveratrol-conjugated gold nanoparticles: Interrelationship of increased resveratrol corona on anti-tumor efficacy against breast, pancreatic and prostate cancers. *Int. J. Nanomed.* **2019**, *14*, 4413–4428. [CrossRef]
151. Santos, A.C.; Pereira, I.; Magalhaes, M.; Pereira-Silva, M.; Caldas, M.; Ferreira, L.; Figueiras, A.; Ribeiro, A.J.; Veiga, F. Targeting Cancer Via Resveratrol-Loaded Nanoparticles Administration: Focusing on In Vivo Evidence. *Aaps J.* **2019**, *21*, 57. [CrossRef]
152. Kumar, A.; Kurmi, B.D.; Singh, A.; Singh, D. Potential role of resveratrol and its nano-formulation as anti-cancer agent. *Explor. Target. Anti-Tumor Ther.* **2022**, *3*, 643–658. [CrossRef]
153. Carlson, L.J.; Cote, B.; Alani, A.W.; Rao, D.A. Polymeric micellar co-delivery of resveratrol and curcumin to mitigate in vitro doxorubicin-induced cardiotoxicity. *J. Pharm. Sci.* **2014**, *103*, 2315–2322. [CrossRef]
154. Santos, J.L.; Choquette, M.; Bezerra, J.A. Cholestatic Liver Disease in Children. *Curr. Gastroenterol. Rep.* **2010**, *12*, 30–39. [CrossRef]
155. Yang, C.H.; Perumpail, B.J.; Yoo, E.R.; Ahmed, A.; Kerner, J.A., Jr. Nutritional Needs and Support for Children with Chronic Liver Disease. *Nutrients* **2017**, *9*, 1127. [CrossRef] [PubMed]
156. European Food Safety Agency (EFSA). Opinion of the Scientific Panel on food additives, flavourings, processing aids and materials in contact with food (AFC) related to D-alpha-tocopheryl polyethylene glycol 1000 succinate (TPGS) in use for food for particular nutritional purposes. *EFSA J.* **2007**, *490*, 1–20.
157. Thébaut, A.; Nemeth, A.; Le Mouhaër, J.; Scheenstra, R.; Baumann, U.; Koot, B.; Gottrand, F.; Houwen, R.; Monard, L.; de Micheaux, S.L.; et al. Oral Tocofersolan Corrects or Prevents Vitamin E Deficiency in Children with Chronic Cholestasis. *J. Pediatr. Gastroenterol. Nutr.* **2016**, *63*, 610–615. [CrossRef] [PubMed]
158. Chimento, A.; De Amicis, F.; Sirianni, R.; Sinicropi, M.S.; Puoci, F.; Casaburi, I.; Saturnino, C.; Pezzi, V. Progress to Improve Oral Bioavailability and Beneficial Effects of Resveratrol. *Int. J. Mol. Sci.* **2019**, *20*, 1381. [CrossRef]

159. Zuccari, G.; Alfei, S.; Zorzoli, A.; Marimpietri, D.; Turrini, F.; Baldassari, S.; Marchitto, L.; Caviglioli, G. Increased Water-Solubility and Maintained Antioxidant Power of Resveratrol by Its Encapsulation in Vitamin E TPGS Micelles: A Potential Nutritional Supplement for Chronic Liver Disease. *Pharmaceutics* **2021**, *13*, 1128. [CrossRef] [PubMed]
160. Soldatova, Y.V.; Faingold, I.I.; Poletaeva, D.A.; Kozlov, A.V.; Emel'yanova, N.S.; Khodos, I.I.; Chernyaev, D.A.; Kurmaz, S.V. Design and Investigation of New Water-Soluble Forms of α-Tocopherol with Antioxidant and Antiglycation Activity Using Amphiphilic Copolymers of N-Vinylpyrrolidone. *Pharmaceutics* **2023**, *15*, 1388. [CrossRef]
161. Vasconcelos, T.; Araújo, F.; Lopes, C.; Loureiro, A.; Das Neves, J.; Marques, S.; Sarmento, B. Multicomponent self-nano emulsifying delivery systems of resveratrol with enhanced pharmacokinetics profile. *Eur. J. Pharm. Sci.* **2019**, *137*, 105011. [CrossRef] [PubMed]
162. Calvo-Castro, L.A.; Schiborr, C.; David, F.; Ehrt, H.; Voggel, J.; Sus, N.; Behnam, D.; Bosy-Westphal, A.; Frank, J. The Oral Bioavailability of Trans-Resveratrol from a Grapevine-Shoot Extract in Healthy Humans is Significantly Increased by Micellar Solubilization. *Mol. Nutr. Food Res.* **2018**, *62*, e1701057. [CrossRef] [PubMed]
163. Santos, A.C.; Veiga, F.; Sequeira, J.A.D.; Fortuna, A.; Falcão, A.; Souto, E.B.; Pattekari, P.; Ribeiro, C.F.; Ribeiro, A.J. First-time oral administration of resveratrol-loaded layer-by-layer nanoparticles to rats—A pharmacokinetics study. *Analyst* **2019**, *144*, 2062–2079. [CrossRef]
164. Yang, C.; Wang, Y.; Xie, Y.; Liu, G.; Lu, Y.; Wu, W.; Chen, L. Oat protein-shellac nanoparticles as a delivery vehicle for resveratrol to improve bioavailability in vitro and in vivo. *Nanomedicine* **2019**, *14*, 2853–2871. [CrossRef]
165. Peñalva, R.; Morales, J.; González-Navarro, C.J.; Larrañeta, E.; Quincooces, G.; Peñuelas, I.; Irache, J.; Juan, M. Increased Oral Bioavailability of Resveratrol by Its Encapsulation in Casein Nanoparticles. *Int. J. Mol. Sci.* **2018**, *19*, 2816. [CrossRef]
166. Singh, S.K.; Makadia, V.; Sharma, S.; Rashid, M.; Shahi, S.; Mishra, P.R.; Wahajuddin, M.; Gayen, J.R. Preparation and in-vitro/in-vivo characterization of trans-resveratrol nanocrystals for oral administration. *Drug Deliv. Transl. Res.* **2017**, *7*, 395–407. [CrossRef] [PubMed]
167. Wu, M.; Zhong, C.; Deng, Y.; Zhang, Q.; Zhang, X.; Zhao, X. Resveratrol loaded glycyrrhizic acid-conjugated human serum albumin nanoparticles for tail vein injection II: Pharmacokinetics, tissue distribution and bioavailability. *Drug Deliv.* **2020**, *27*, 81–90. [CrossRef]
168. Katekar, R.; Thombre, G.; Riyazuddin, M.; Husain, A.; Rani, H.; Praveena, K.S.; Gayen, J.R. Pharmacokinetics and brain targeting of trans-resveratrol loaded mixed micelles in rats following intravenous administration. *Pharm. Dev. Technol.* **2019**, *25*, 300–307. [CrossRef]
169. Guo, L.; Peng, Y.; Yao, J.; Sui, L.; Gu, A.; Wang, J. Anticancer Activity and Molecular Mechanism of Resveratrol–Bovine Serum Albumin Nanoparticles on Subcutaneously Implanted Human Primary Ovarian Carcinoma Cells in Nude Mice. *Cancer Biother. Radiopharm.* **2010**, *25*, 471–477. [CrossRef]
170. Lian, B.; Wu, M.; Feng, Z.; Deng, Y.; Zhong, C.; Zhao, X. Folate-conjugated human serum albumin-encapsulated resveratrol nanoparticles: Preparation, characterization, bioavailability and targeting of liver tumors. *Artif. Cells Nanomed. Biotechnol.* **2019**, *47*, 154–165. [CrossRef]
171. Jadhav, P.; Bothiraja, C.; Pawar, A. Resveratrol-piperine loaded mixed micelles: Formulation, characterization, bioavailability, safety and in vitro anticancer activity. *RSC Adv.* **2016**, *6*, 112795–112805. [CrossRef]
172. Suktham, K.; Koobkokkruad, T.; Wutikhun, T.; Surassmo, S. Efficiency of resveratrol-loaded sericin nanoparticles: Promising bionanocarriers for drug delivery. *Int. J. Pharm.* **2018**, *537*, 48–56. [CrossRef]
173. Hao, J.; Tong, T.; Jin, K.; Zhuang, Q.; Han, T.; Bi, Y.; Wang, J.; Wang, X. Folic acid-functionalized drug delivery platform of resveratrol based on pluronic 127/d-alpha-tocopheryl polyethylene glycol 1000 succinate mixed micelles. *Int. J. Nanomed.* **2017**, *12*, 2279–2292. [CrossRef]
174. De la Lastra, C.A.; Villegas, I. Resveratrol as an antioxidant and pro-oxidant agent: Mechanisms and clinical implications. *Biochem. Soc. Trans.* **2007**, *35*, 1156–1160. [CrossRef]
175. Pervaiz, S.; Holme, A.L. Resveratrol: Its biologic targets and functional activity. *Antioxid. Redox Signal.* **2009**, *11*, 2851–2897. [CrossRef]
176. Martins, L.A.M.; Coelho, B.P.; Behr, G.; Pettenuzzo, L.F.; Souza, I.C.C.; Moreira, J.C.F.; Borojevic, R.; Gottfried, C.; Guma, F.C.R. Resveratrol induces pro-oxidant effects and time-dependent resistance to cytotoxicity in activated hepatic stellate cells. *Cell Biochem. Biophys.* **2014**, *68*, 247–257. [CrossRef]
177. Robb, E.L.; Winkelmolen, L.; Visanji, N.; Brotchie, J.; Stuart, J.A. Dietary resveratrol administration increases MnSOD expression and activity in mouse brain. *Biochem. Biophys. Res. Commun.* **2008**, *372*, 254–259. [CrossRef] [PubMed]
178. Rüweler, M.; Gülden, M.; Maser, E.; Murias, M.; Seibert, H. Cytotoxic, cytoprotective and antioxidant activities of resveratrol and analogues in c6 astroglioma cells in vitro. *Chem. Biol. Int.* **2009**, *182*, 128–135. [CrossRef]
179. Li, D.D.; Han, R.M.; Liang, R.; Chen, C.-H.; Lai, W.; Zhang, J.-P.; Skibsted, L.H. Hydroxyl radical reaction with trans-resveratrol: Initial carbon radical adduct formation followed by rearrangement to phenoxyl radical. *J. Phys. Chem. B* **2012**, *116*, 7154–7161. [CrossRef] [PubMed]
180. Yang, N.-C.; Lee, C.-H.; Song, T.-Y. Evaluation of resveratrol oxidation in vitro and the crucial role of bicarbonate ions. *Biosci. Biotechnol. Biochem.* **2010**, *74*, 63–68. [CrossRef] [PubMed]
181. Gadacha, W.; Ben-Attia, M.; Bonnefont-Rousselot, D.; Aouani, E.; Ghanem-Boughanmi, N.; Touitou, Y. Resveratrol opposite effects on rat tissue lipoperoxidation: Pro-oxidant during day-time and antioxidant at night. *Redox Rep.* **2009**, *14*, 154–158. [CrossRef] [PubMed]

182. Giordano, M.E.; Lionetto, M.G. Intracellular Redox Behavior of Quercetin and Resveratrol Singly and in Mixtures. *Molecules* **2023**, *28*, 4682. [CrossRef] [PubMed]
183. Nizami, Z.N.; Aburawi, H.E.; Semlali, A.; Muhammad, K.; Iratni, R. Oxidative Stress Inducers in Cancer Therapy: Preclinical and Clinical Evidence. *Antioxidants* **2023**, *12*, 1159. [CrossRef]
184. Szende, B.; Tyihak, E.; Kiraly-Veghely, Z. Dose-dependent effect of resveratrol on proliferation and apoptosis in endothelial and tumor cell cultures. *Exp. Mol. Med.* **2000**, *32*, 88. [CrossRef] [PubMed]
185. San Hipolito-Luengo, A.; Alcaide, A.; Ramos-Gonzalez, M.; Cercas, E.; Vallejo, S.; Romero, A.; Talero, E.; Sanchez-Ferrer, C.F.; Motilva, V.; Peiro, C. Dual effects of resveratrol on cell death and proliferation of colon cancer cells. *Nutr. Cancer* **2017**, *69*, 1019–1027. [CrossRef]
186. Mukherjee, S.; Dudley, J.I.; Das, D.K. Dose-dependency of resveratrol in providing health benefits. *Dose Response* **2010**, *8*, 478–500. [CrossRef]
187. Van Ginkel, P.R.; Sareen, D.; Subramanian, L.; Walker, Q.; Darjatmoko, S.R.; Lindstrom, M.J.; Kulkarni, A.; Albert, D.M.; Polans, A.S. Resveratrol inhibits tumor growth of human neuroblastoma and mediates apoptosis by directly targeting mitochondria. *Clin. Cancer Res.* **2007**, *13*, 5162–5169. [CrossRef]
188. Brown, V.A.; Patel, K.R.; Viskaduraki, M.; Crowell, J.A.; Perloff, M.; Booth, T.D.; Vasilinin, G.; Sen, A.; Schinas, A.M.; Piccirilli, G.; et al. Repeat dose study of the cancer chemopreventive agent resveratrol in healthy volunteers: Safety, pharmacokinetics and effect on the insulin-like growth factor axis. *Cancer Res.* **2010**, *70*, 9003–9011. [CrossRef]
189. Tomé-Carneiro, J.; Gonzálvez, M.; Larrosa, M.; Yáñez-Gascón, M.J.; García-Almagro, F.J.; Ruiz-Ros, J.A.; Tomás-Barberán, F.A.; García-Conesa, M.T.; Espín, J.C. Grape resveratrol increases serum adiponectin and downregulates inflammatory genes in peripheral blood mononuclear cells: A triple-blind, placebo-controlled, one-year clinical trial in patients with stable coronary artery disease. *Cardiovasc. Drugs Ther.* **2013**, *27*, 37–48. [CrossRef]
190. Patel, K.R.; Scott, E.; Brown, V.A.; Gescher, A.J.; Steward, W.P.; Brown, K. Clinical trials of resveratrol. *Ann. N. Y. Acad. Sci.* **2011**, *1215*, 161–169. [CrossRef]
191. Bode, L.M.; Bunzel, D.; Huch, M.; Cho, G.S.; Ruhland, D.; Bunzel, M.; Bub, A.; Franz, C.M.; Kulling, S.E. In vivo and in vitro metabolism of trans-resveratrol by human gut microbiota. *Am. J. Clin. Nutr.* **2013**, *97*, 295–309. [CrossRef]
192. Ferry-Dumazet, H.; Garnier, O.; Mamani-Matsuda, M.; Vercauteren, J.; Belloc, F.; Billiard, C.; Dupouy, M.; Thiolat, D.; Kolb, J.P.; Marit, G.; et al. Resveratrol inhibits the growth and induces the apoptosis of both normal and leukemic hematopoietic cells. *Carcinogenesis* **2002**, *23*, 1327–1333. [CrossRef] [PubMed]
193. Klinge, C.M.; Blankenship, K.A.; Risinger, K.E.; Bhatnagar, S.; Noisin, E.L.; Sumanasekera, W.K.; Zhao, L.; Brey, D.M.; Keynton, R.S. Resveratrol and estradiol rapidly activate MAPK signaling through estrogen receptors alpha and beta in endothelial cells. *J. Biol. Chem.* **2005**, *280*, 7460–7468. [CrossRef] [PubMed]
194. Pearson, K.J.; Baur, J.A.; Lewis, K.N.; Peshkin, L.; Price, N.L.; Labinskyy, N.; Swindell, W.R.; Kamara, D.; Minor, R.K.; Perez, E.; et al. Resveratrol delays age-related deterioration and mimics transcriptional aspects of dietary restriction without extending lifespan. *Cell Metab.* **2008**, *8*, 157–168. [CrossRef]
195. La Porte, C.; Voduc, N.; Zhang, G.; Seguin, I.; Tardiff, D.; Singhal, N.; Cameron, D.W. Steady-state pharmacokinetics and tolerability of trans-resveratrol 2000mg twice daily with food, quercetin and alcohol (ethanol) in healthy human subjects. *Clin. Pharmacokinet.* **2010**, *49*, 449–454. [CrossRef] [PubMed]
196. Baron, S.; Bedarida, T.; Cottart, C.H.; Vibert, F.; Vessieres, E.; Ayer, A.; Henrion, D.; Hommeril, B.; Paul, J.L.; Renault, G.; et al. Dual effects of resveratrol on arterial damage induced by insulin resistance in aged mice. *J. Gerontol. A Biol. Sci. Med. Sci.* **2014**, *69*, 260–269. [CrossRef] [PubMed]

Disclaimer/Publisher's Note: The statements, opinions and data contained in all publications are solely those of the individual author(s) and contributor(s) and not of MDPI and/or the editor(s). MDPI and/or the editor(s) disclaim responsibility for any injury to people or property resulting from any ideas, methods, instructions or products referred to in the content.

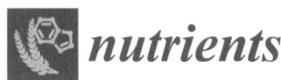

Review

Synergic Role of Dietary Bioactive Compounds in Breast Cancer Chemoprevention and Combination Therapies

Marisabel Mecca [1,*,†], Marzia Sichetti [1,*,†], Martina Giuseffi [1], Eugenia Giglio [1], Claudia Sabato [1], Francesca Sanseverino [2] and Graziella Marino [3]

[1] Laboratory of Preclinical and Translational Research, Centro di Riferimento Oncologico della Basilicata (IRCCS-CROB), 85028 Rionero in Vulture, Italy; martina.giuseffi@crob.it (M.G.); eugenia.giglio@crob.it (E.G.); claudia.sabato@crob.it (C.S.)
[2] Unit of Gynecologic Oncology, Centro di Riferimento Oncologico della Basilicata (IRCCS-CROB), 85028 Rionero in Vulture, Italy; francesca.sanseverino@crob.it
[3] Unit of Breast Cancer, Centro di Riferimento Oncologico della Basilicata (IRCCS-CROB), 85028 Rionero in Vulture, Italy; graziella.marino@crob.it
* Correspondence: marisabel.mecca@crob.it (M.M.); marzia.sichetti@crob.it (M.S.)
† These authors contributed equally to this work.

Abstract: Breast cancer is the most common tumor in women. Chemotherapy is the gold standard for cancer treatment; however, severe side effects and tumor resistance are the major obstacles to chemotherapy success. Numerous dietary components and phytochemicals have been found to inhibit the molecular and signaling pathways associated with different stages of breast cancer development. In particular, this review is focused on the antitumor effects of PUFAs, dietary enzymes, and glucosinolates against breast cancer. The major databases were consulted to search in vitro and preclinical studies; only those with solid scientific evidence and reporting protective effects on breast cancer treatment were included. A consistent number of studies highlighted that dietary components and phytochemicals can have remarkable therapeutic effects as single agents or in combination with other anticancer agents, administered at different concentrations and via different routes of administration. These provide a natural strategy for chemoprevention, reduce the risk of breast cancer recurrence, impair cell proliferation and viability, and induce apoptosis. Some of these bioactive compounds of dietary origin, however, show poor solubility and low bioavailability; hence, encapsulation in nanoformulations are promising tools able to increase clinical efficiency.

Keywords: phytochemicals; diet; breast cancer; cancer prevention; PUFA; bromelain; isothiocyanate; glucosinolates

1. Introduction

Breast cancer (BC) is the second most common cause of cancer death in women [1,2]. Clinical and demographic indicators of BC prognosis include large tumor size, lymph node involvement, hormone receptor-negative subtype, diagnosis at an early age, and low socio-economic status [3]. Both genetic and environmental factors play a pivotal role in the risk of BC development among women [4].

BC is well known as a heterogeneous, complex disease with a spectrum of histopathological patterns and molecular characteristics due to genetic, epigenetic, and transcriptomic changes [5,6]. All this has led to a wide range of clinical findings, treatment responses, and clinical outcomes. Traditional classification criteria are based on biological features such as tumor size, lymph nodes involved, histological grade, and patient age and have limited the development of tailored treatment strategies so far [6]. Tumors with similar clinical and pathological conditions can often show different behaviors. To date, the molecular classification of tumors through detailed analysis of genetic changes and biological events involved in the initiation and progression of cancer has been extensively studied. In particular, BC heterogeneity is associated with differences or losses in molecular biomarkers: the amplification or overexpression of progesterone receptor (PR), estrogen receptor (ER), and human epidermal growth factor receptor 2 oncogene (HER2) [6–10]. About two-thirds of BC cases are ER$^+$ and/or PR$^+$, which are hormonally sensitive and responsive to endocrine therapy. Overexpression of the tyrosine kinase receptor HER2 has been frequently reported in hormone receptor-negative (HR$^-$) compared to HR$^+$ cancers correlated with hyperproliferation, aggressive behavior, and serious illness. Additionally, triple-negative breast cancer (TNBC), which accounts for almost 15% to 20% of BC cases, is clinically negative for ER, PR, and HER2 expression. TNBC has a damaging clinical behavior, frequently metastasizes, is difficult to treat, and does not respond to hormonal therapy or HER2 receptor-targeted therapy. Surgical resection, radiation, endocrine/hormonal therapy, chemotherapy, targeted therapy, or a combination of these approaches is used to treat and manage BC [11]. However, chemotherapy always causes severe side effects and toxicity in non-targeted tissues, such as fatigue, nausea, vomiting, hair loss, etc. Another side to the coin is drug resistance, the most challenging aspect of chemotherapy success. Therefore, many in vitro and in vivo studies have focused on increasing the effectiveness of chemotherapy while reducing its dose and side effects.

There is increasing evidence of an association between certain foods (such as alcohol, fruits, vegetables, meat, and soy foods) and the development and treatment of BC. Lifestyle factors such as diet, weight, and physical activity can significantly influence BC outcomes [12–14]. Establishing a dietary pattern based on high intakes of fruits, vegetables, whole grains, poultry, and fish and low intakes of sugars and high-fat dairy products can help women experiencing BC. It has been shown that adopting a balanced diet, particularly during chemotherapy, is important to ensure an adequate intake of energy and nutrients. In addition, a healthy lifestyle may also reduce the toxicity of anti-cancer therapies, improving their effectiveness and promoting women's long-term health by reducing BC comorbidities (e.g., obesity, hypertension, hyperlipidemia, and diabetes) [15]. In this regard, over the past few years the co-use of chemotherapy and natural bioactive compounds has attracted great attention for the extraordinary antioxidant, anti-inflammatory, and antineoplastic properties of these compounds [16–19]. Phytochemicals are nutritional bioactive compounds found in different plant foods or dietary products and classified by their wide range of chemical and structural features, usually associated with diverse biological effects [20]. Some of these dietary compounds have been shown to have anti-angiogenic properties, specifically affecting molecular pathways and receptors involved in cell proliferation and restoring the tumor microenvironment [19]. Nevertheless, there are several challenges in phytochemical usage such as poor solubility, poor bioavailability, low stability, and sometimes the requirement of a high dosage. Phytochemicals differ in their solubility and heat resistance, impacting the quality of the products and their use in food and nutraceutical development [20]. For this reason, these compounds cannot be easily introduced through a balanced diet. Several studies, in fact, have been focused on different formulations to enhance the bioavailability and the therapeutic benefits of these dietary bioactive compounds. The most important advance in this research is the incorporation of these bioactive compounds into nanoformulations (characterized by low size with high surface/mass ratio and absorption), alone or together with conventional drugs, for more specific chemical delivery to cancer cells [21]. The origin of this nanotherapeutic approach was motivated by the enhanced permeability of the blood vessel endothelium in solid tumors and the ability of antitumor drugs and bioactive natural compounds with low molecular weights to cross this barrier in both directions, which prevents tumor tissues from efficiently accumulating these compounds. This feature of the cancer endothelium has inspired the research and creation of new drug delivery systems to target tumor cells effectively and passively [22–24]. In passive delivery systems, the drug gets encapsulated to protect it from being metabolized, which allows it to passively and slowly reach the target tumor tissue through the bloodstream. The active delivery systems instead exploit specific proteins, antibodies, and ligands on the surface of the delivery system. This system specifically binds to the surface antigen or receptor expressed by tumor tissue, triggering endocytosis in specific tumor cells. The most important and interesting aspect is that, while on the one hand, it is possible to enhance the antitumor effect of the drugs, on the other hand, it reduce the distribution of the drugs in normal tissues, limiting the possible onset of side effects. The last and most challenging drug delivery system is the physiochemical one based on the tumor microenvironment, mimicking biological responsiveness to control drug release at the target site.

In this review article, we will highlight some of the most significant dietary and phytochemical compounds that show significant anti-breast cancer activity both in vitro and in vivo.

A potential dietary strategy to reduce cancer risk is the use of polyunsaturated fatty acids (PUFAs), of which ω-3 and ω-6 are the two major classes. The terms ω-3 and ω-6 PUFAs refer to two groups of PUFAs that respectively contain a double carbon–carbon bond at the third carbon atom (n-3 position) and at the sixth (n-6 position) from the methyl end of the carbon chain. Historically, the intake of ω-3 and ω-6 PUFAs is estimated to be similar, but in recent years, the Western diet has led to a significant increase in ω-6 PUFA intake, leading to a growth in the ω-6/ω-3 PUFA ratio [25]. Excessive amounts of ω-6 or high ω-6/ω-3 ratios are linked to the development of various diseases, including cardiovascular, autoimmune, and some cancer diseases; on the other hand, increased amounts of ω-3 PUFA have been shown to have an inhibitory effect [25]. Previous studies have shown that ω-3 PUFAs competitively inhibit ω-6 fatty acids, thus lowering levels of inflammatory eicosanoids generated from ω-6 metabolism [14], and that higher ω-3 relative to ω-6 could reduce BC through inflammation, oxidative stress, and estrogen metabolism [26,27].

Another phytotherapeutic agent broadly used for its history of safe use is bromelain from pineapple extract. Bromelain has been used as a traditional folk medicine since ancient times as a treatment for severe wounds, edema, chronic rhinosinusitis, cardiovascular diseases, rheumatoid arthritis, and fibrinolytic affects, but only recently have its anticancer activity and immunomodulatory effects been highlighted [28]. Bromelain is a complex mixture of proteases, in particular thiol endopeptidases, able to interfere directly with cell surface receptors and several downstream pathways that support malignancy.

Isothiocyanate, also known as glucosinolate, is the most abundant naturally occurring dietary chemopreventive compound. Glucosinolates are abundant in cruciferous vegetables such as *Brassica oleracea*, watercress, Brussels sprouts, cabbage, Japanese radish, and cauliflower, and they significantly contribute to their cancer chemopreventive effect [29,30]. Upon consumption, glucosinolates are hydrolyzed by the plant enzyme myrosinase or in the colon through the actions of gut microorganisms in bioactive molecules such as indole-3 carbinol and sulforaphane [31]. Several studies have demonstrated that the ingestion of cruciferous vegetables may reduce overall tumor risk, especially for BC. In particular, several studies demonstrated that sulforaphane increases levels of detoxification enzymes and reduces cancer cell growth, inhibiting cell cycle, inducing apoptosis and autophagy, and removing cancer stem cells (CSCs) [32].

This review's primary objective is to provide a comprehensive report on the most up-to-date scientific and clinical evidence available for these five primary phytochemical classes, many of which are currently being used as adjuvant therapeutics or chemopreventive agents in BC therapies at our hospital research institute.

2. Materials and Methods

An updated review of the role of PUFAs, bromelain, and glucosinolates in the chemoprevention of breast cancer was performed. Published studies were searched in specialized databases such as PubMed/MedLine, Scopus, Science Direct, and Google Scholar using the following keywords: "breast cancer", "cancer prevention", "phytochemicals", "dietary bioactive compounds", "polyunsaturated fatty acids", "bromelain", "glucosinolates", "sulforaphane", "indole-3 carbinol", and "breast cancer cell lines" (Table 1). In particular, we focused on MCF-7 and T-47D as ER-positive cancer models, SK-BR-3 as HER2-positive cancer models, and MDA-MB-231 and MDA-MB-468 (PR-, ER-, and HER-2-negative cell lines) for triple-negative breast cancer (TNBC) studies. Lastly, MCF-10A cells are frequently used as a normal control in breast cancer studies.

Table 1. Summary of non−cancerous and malignant breast cancer cells lines and their molecular classification.

Cell Lines	Organism	Immunoprofile	Characteristics
BT−474	Human	ER$^-$, PR$^+$, HER2$^+$	Epithelial cell line from ductal carcinoma
BT−549	Human	ER$^-$, PR$^-$, HER2$^-$	Epithelial cell line from ductal carcinoma
GI−101A	Human	ER$^-$, PR$^-$, HER2$^+$ enriched	Epithelial cell line from a metastatic breast tumor
HCC70	Human	ER$^-$, PR$^-$, HER2$^-$	Epithelial cell line from ductal carcinoma
HCC1806	Human	ER$^-$, PR$^-$, HER2$^-$	Epithelial cell line from mammary gland
MCF−10A	Human	ER$^-$, PR$^-$, HER2$^-$ and EGFR$^+$	Non-tumorigenic epithelial cell line from mammary gland
MCF−10F	Human	ER$^-$, PR$^-$, HER2$^-$ and EGFR$^+$	Non-tumorigenic epithelial cell line from mammary gland
MCF−7	Human	ER$^+$, PR$^+$, HER2$^-$	Epithelial cell line from mammary adenocarcinoma
MDA−MB−231	Human	ER$^-$, PR$^-$, HER2$^-$ and EGFR$^+$	Epithelial cell line from mammary adenocarcinoma
MDA−MB−453	Human	ER$^-$, PR$^-$, HER2$^+$ enriched and AR$^+$	Epithelial cell line from metastatic mammary carcinoma
MDA−MB−468	Human	ER$^-$, PR$^-$, HER2$^-$ and EGFR$^+$	Epithelial cell line from mammary adenocarcinoma
SK−BR−3	Human	ER$^-$, PR$^-$, HER2$^+$ enriched	Epithelial cell line from mammary adenocarcinoma
SUM−159PT	Human	ER$^-$, PR$^-$, HER2$^-$	Epithelial cell line from mammary carcinoma
T−47D	Human	ER$^+$, PR$^+$, HER2$^-$	Epithelial cell line from infiltrating ductal carcinoma
ZR−75−1	Human	ER$^+$, PR$^+$, HER2$^-$	Epithelial cell line from ductal carcinoma

ER (estrogen receptor), PR (progesteron receptor), HER2 (human epidermal growth factor receptor 2), EGFR (epidermal growth factor receptor), and AR (androgen receptor).

Each article was published before May 2024 and written in English, and its significance was estimated by analyzing the title and abstract. Non-English text, lack of access to the full text, and publication in journals with no impact factor were considered exclusion criteria. Articles that met all search criteria were evaluated in the literature and included in this review.

3. Polyunsaturated Fatty Acids (PUFAs)

Clinical and preclinical studies have shown that there is a relationship between the quantity and quality of dietary fat intake and tumor incidence and progress [33]. In mammals, both ω-6 and ω-3 PUFAs are essential for health and must be included in the diet, as they cannot be synthesized endogenously. Data obtained from experiments conducted in previous trials demonstrate that optimum amounts of ω-6 and ω-3 PUFAs can prevent or inhibit cell proliferation and/or induce apoptosis in various tumors. PUFAs, mainly ω-3 and ω-6, exert their inhibitory effects by acting as precursors of various bioactive lipids with anticancer activity [34], interfering with the regulation of cell growth, differentiation, apoptosis, and metastasis by affecting gene expression or signaling transduction pathways. Indeed, they exert antitumor effects in the following ways:

- Reducing the expression of some growth factors such as HER2, EGFR, and insulin-like growth factor 1 (IGF-1R);
- Inhibiting cell proliferation by activating peroxisome proliferator-activated receptor gamma (PPARγ) or decreasing levels of fatty acid synthase (FAS) protein;
- promoting apoptosis by blocking phosphoinositide PI3K/Akt pathways, Akt phosphorylation, and NF-κB activity and reducing the B-cell lymphoma 2/B-cell lymphoma 2-like protein 4 (Bcl-2/Bax) ratio (Figure 1).

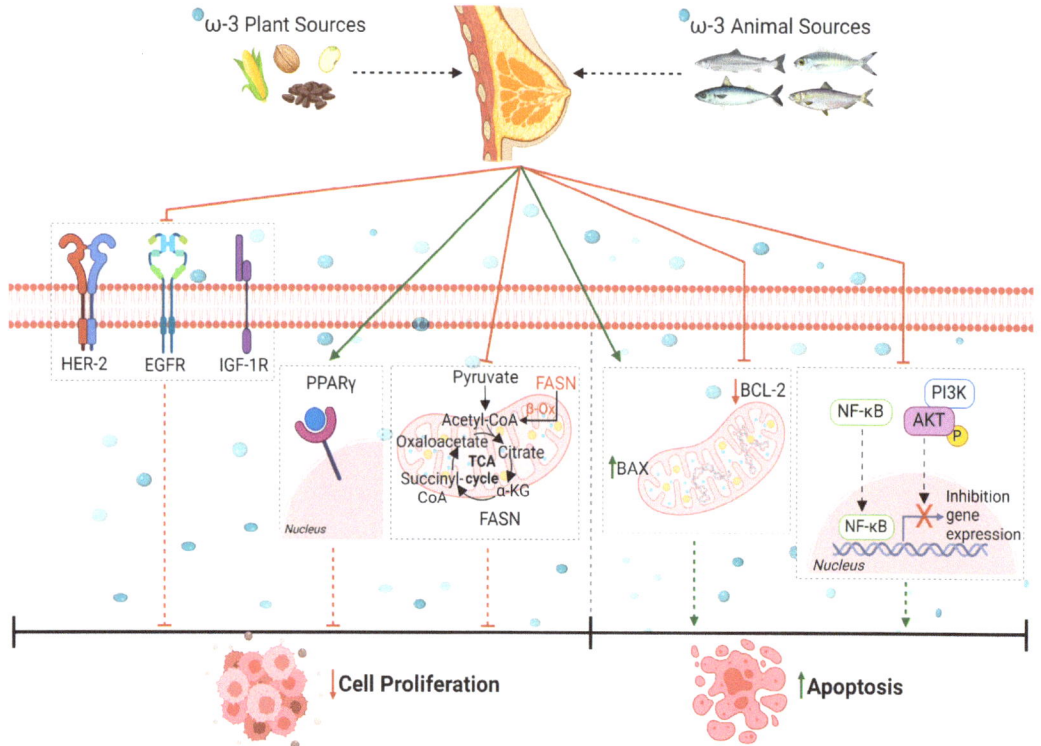

Figure 1. Scheme showing how ω-3 PUFAs inhibit (⊥) cell proliferation by reducing (↓) the expression of some growth factors, including human epidermal growth factor receptor-2 (HER2), epidermal growth factor receptor (EGFR), and insulin-like growth factor 1 (IGF-1R), by either activating (↑) peroxisome proliferator-activated receptor gamma (PPARγ) or decreasing levels of fatty acid synthase (FAS) protein. Furthermore, PUFAs promote cell apoptosis by blocking phosphoinositide 3-kinase/protein kinase B (PI3K/Akt) pathways, downregulating phosphorylated Akt, inhibiting nuclear factor-kappa B (NF-κB) activity, and lowering B-cell lymphoma 2/B-cell lymphoma 2-like protein 4 (Bcl-2/Bax ratio). Created with BioRender.com (https://app.biorender.com/illustrations/65fc51a4a6668e33e3bf3d89 (accessed on 9 April 2024)).

3.1. ω-3 PUFAs

Alpha-linolenic acid (ALA, 18:3*n*-3) is the precursor of ω-3 PUFAs such as docosahexaenoic acid (DHA, 22:6*n*-3) and eicosapentaenoic acid (EPA, 20:5*n*-3). Because the human body has a limited ability to produce EPA and DHA from ALA, these PUFAs should be consumed through food sources. The major sources of ALA are plant oils, while those of EPA and DHA are marine animal products such as fish oils and other marine animal fats. They have important roles in human physiology and also exert beneficial effects on some chronic degenerative diseases such as cardiovascular diseases [35], rheumatoid arthritis [36], diabetes [37], several autoimmune diseases [38], and cancer [39]. ω-3 PUFAs have demonstrated an ability to chemosensitize BC tumors and thus potentially improve treatment efficacy. Therefore, the consumption of ω-3 PUFAs, for which fish is the greatest dietary source, may provide an opportunity to increase survival in women with BC [40]. Altogether, ALA, EPA, and DHA have several effects against breast cancer development in vivo. Another interesting aspect of ω-3 PUFAs is their use as ideal components of nanoformulations designed to be delivered more precisely to tumor tissues; because tumor cells grow at abnormal rates and require large amounts of FA to form their cell membranes, they necessitate and incorporate high quantities of ALA, EPA, and DHA [41]. Additionally, they have many double bonds, making them highly susceptible to peroxidation. Therefore, their inclusion in nanoformulations may help to protect them from oxidative degradation and improve their bioavailability and tumor specificity [21]. Recent studies investigated nanoformulations containing both doxorubicin (DOX) and ω-3 PUFAs to improve DOX delivery in BC. Recently, DOX was included in a mixed PUFA nanoformulation (MPUFAs-DOX@liposomes) containing a high amount of ω-3 PUFA, which showed higher toxicity than free DOX or DOX@liposomes in MCF-7 cells [42]. The authors attributed the enhanced anticancer activity to the increased lipophilicity of the nanoformulations, increased release rate of DOX from the ω-3 nanosystem, and enhanced uptake of DOX when delivered to cancer cells through the nanosystem [42].

3.1.1. α-Linolenic Acid

ALA is a plant-derived ω-3 PUFA found in soybean oil (7.8%), canola oil (9.2%), and hemp oil (20%) [40], with important protective effects in BC. Dietary ALA supplementation inhibited the proliferation of breast cancer in xenograft rodent models with high levels of estrogen; indeed, ALA derived from flaxseed oil reduced MCF-7 cell proliferation and increased cell death [43] by downregulating tyrosine kinase receptors like EGFR and HER2, resulting in pAkt diminution. Further, in vitro studies also demonstrated that ALA reduced MCF-7 cell proliferation by 33% [43]. ALA from flaxseed oil showed a powerful ability to reduce the palpable tumor size when combined with tamoxifen, and it was also found to decrease HER2 expression and re-regulate growth factor signaling pathways by inhibiting IGF-1R and Bcl-2 [44]. A recent work showed that a nanoformulation made up of ALA and paclitaxel had a higher anti-BC effect in vitro and in vivo [45], since small hydrophobic molecules (like ALA) in nanoformulations allow for greater drug loading and for higher biocompatibility. So far, there are not many studies that support the inclusion of ALA in nanostructures because EPA and DHA show greater antitumor activity than ALA, but ALA advantages are often underestimated.

3.1.2. Eicosapentaenoic Acid

EPA is a long-chain ω-3 PUFA that has 20 carbon atoms and five double bonds (20:5), whereas DHA has a longer chain, with 22 carbon atoms and six double bounds (22:6). DHA and EPA make significant contributions to the physical properties of biological membranes, such as membrane organization, ion permeability, elasticity, and eicosanoid composition. Among oily fish species, mackerel (1.8–5.3% by weight), herring (1.2–3.1%) and salmon (1.0–1.4%) contain a lot of EPA and DHA [16]. A higher intake of marine ω-3 PUFAs (EPA and DHA) was related to reduced BC relapse and all-cause mortality rates [46], but it is still unclear if EPA and DHA have different or similar effects on BC. In support of the specific effect of EPA on BC, various in vitro studies showed that EPA can induce BC cell apoptosis by inhibiting anti-apoptotic regulatory proteins, e.g., Bcl-2 [47], and by reducing total and phosphorylated Akt content in MCF-7 cells; moreover, in the same cells, combined treatment with EPA and tamoxifen enhanced the reduction in cancer proliferation. EPA-rich foods have also been shown to hinder breast cancer growth in animal and human studies. These inhibitory effects have been attributed to the high absorption of EPA by cancer phospholipids and subsequently to the disruption of inflammatory eicosanoid biosynthesis from arachidonic acid [48]. Recently, it has been proven that EPA regulates tumor growth in MCF-7 xenografts via the inhibitory G-mediated signaling pathway [49]. In addition, a clinical study in humans showed that plasma concentrations of EPA correspond to high levels of PPARγ mRNA in adipose tissue [50]. Because PPARγ activators can inhibit cell growth, the overexpression of PPARγ induced by EPA could be a potential mechanism of action, suggesting that EPA may act individually to hinder the growth and progression of BC.

3.1.3. Docosahexaenoic Acid

Some studies have established the antitumor activity of DHA [51,52]. This activity involves influencing tumor proliferation, apoptosis, and differentiation and inhibiting angiogenesis [53], tumor cell invasion [54], and metastasis [55]. Barascu et al. [56] showed that EPA and DHA reduced MCF-7 and MDA-MB-231 cell growth and increased apoptosis, particularly for DHA, and specifically, they showed that ω-3 PUFA can hinder cell growth by blocking the cell cycle during the G2/M transition. HER2 signaling has an important role in many processes involved in cellular proliferation and survival [57]. In vitro studies have shown that DHA is able to disrupt lipid rafts in HER2-overexpressing cells, inhibiting the HER2 signaling pathway and therefore causing cell death [57]. Menéndez et al. [58] proved that DHA supplementation could downregulate the expression of the HER2/neu oncogene in SK-BR-3 and BT-474 cells, confirming the potential of DHA in HER2$^+$ BC treatment. They also demonstrated that pre-exposure to DHA synergistically enhanced the cytotoxic effect of conventional drugs such as taxane and Taxol on highly metastatic BC cells [58] due to the fusion of DHA with cellular lipids, altering membrane fluidity and function and improving drug absorption [58]. Accordingly, human clinical trials have shown that DHA supplementation with chemotherapy improves survival in patients with metastatic BC [59]. They observed that time to progression (TTP) was significantly higher in patients with high DHA incorporation compared to patients with low DHA incorporation (8.7 months vs. 2.8 months). Moreover, they found that the overall survival (OS) was almost doubled in patients with high DHA incorporation (33 months vs. 17 months) [59]. It has also been hypothesized increased intracellular DHA levels induce the activation of apoptotic effector enzymes, e.g., caspase-8 and caspase-3, and the downregulation of Bcl-2, thereby causing apoptosis [60,61]. In vivo studies have also shown that DHA decreases the incidence of BC, coinciding with an increase in BRCA1 at the transcriptional and protein synthesis levels, which is an important sign of tumor suppression [62,63]. Nevertheless, recent studies have shown that DHA alone was not capable of reducing EGFR levels in MDA-MB-231 cells but enhanced EGFR inhibitors, indicating its potential in combined treatment [64]. DHA is also involved in the regulation of transcription factors such as NF-κB [65], activator protein 1 (AP-1) [66], c-myc [19], p53 [59,67], and PPARs. Taking a new perspective, it is thought that ω-3 PUFA can regulate microRNA expression in BC, e.g., miR-21. In this work, in fact, it was demonstrated that DHA reduces miR-21 levels, related to proliferation and metastasis development [68]. Metabolic dysfunction is one of the hallmarks of a tumor: cancer cells have altered energy production and rely heavily on aerobic glycolysis; thus, some of the main effectors of glycolysis can be used as tumor therapeutic targets [69]. Several studies have demonstrated that DHA can modulate various metabolic pathways in tumor cells by metabolic reprogramming, suggesting its potential implementation for the modulation of aerobic glycolysis and the Warburg effect [70]. Both parameters, the extracellular acidification rate (ECAR) and the oxygen consumption rate (OCR), which respectively indicate glycolysis and oxidative phosphorylation, significantly decreased in BT-474 and MDA-MB-231 cells due to DHA addition compared to those in untreated cells and non-tumorigenic control MCF-10A cells. These results indicate that, regardless of tumor cell types, DHA can alter the biological profile of tumor cells selectively by modifying mitochondrial structure and function, by activating AMPK protein, by decreasing ATP levels, by activating the LKB1 kinase protein, and by inhibiting hypoxia-inducible factor 1 (HIF1-α) [70,71]. One greatly researched nanoapproach for BC treatment regarding the combination of ω-3 PUFA and conventional drugs is the incorporation of DHA and DOX in nanostructures. DHA is often used to enhance the antitumor effects of DOX because it is deemed the most powerful ω-3 PUFA and is capable of enhancing induced cytotoxicity in cancer cells [72]. These nanostructures were used also in a BC spheroid model for the first time, showing an increase in cytotoxicity and a better penetration of doxorubicin [73]. Indeed, in a population-based follow-up study of women affected by BC, Khankari et al. [74] found that high intakes of DHA reduced all-cause mortality risk by 16% to 34% after 15 years of follow-up.

3.1.3.1. ω-6 PUFAs

Linoleic acid (LA) and arachidonic acid (AA) are the two most common ω-6 PUFAs in typical Western diets. LA is found in some vegetable oils such as corn and safflower oils, while AA is usually derived from animal food sources or can be synthesized from LA [75]. ω-3 PUFAs are known to compete with LA, which is also known to be a main nutrient for tumors [41]. The ratio of these two PUFA classes are important because ω-3 and ω-6 have similar biological pathways and can compete with each other, creating an imbalance [76]. ALA represents a key molecule involved in the anti-inflammatory response. LA is associated with pro-inflammatory responses. Cancer development appears to be directly influenced by the dietary ω-3/ω-6 PUFA ratio. High levels of ω-6 PUFAs in Western countries have been associated with several types of tumor [41,77].

To quantitatively ascertain the relationship between the risk of BC and high intake of ω-3/ω-6 PUFAs, a meta-analysis of five cohort studies and six prospective nested case-control studies was performed [78]. According to reports, people with a higher intake of ω-3/ω-6 PUFAs had a lower risk of BC. Moreover, with an increment of about 1/10 in the ω-3/ω-6 PUFA ratio, a further 6% reduction in BC risk was observed. More importantly, a subgroup analysis has revealed that individuals with a higher adsorption of ω-3/ω-6 PUFAs in serum phospholipids had a 38% reduction in BC risk. Since EPA and DHA cannot be synthesized in mammals and conversion between ω-3 and ω-6 PUFAs does not occur in humans, serum phospholipid levels of ω-3/ω-6 PUFAs reflect their food absorption [79].

4. Bromelain

Pineapple (*Ananas comosus*) has been used since ancient times as medicine because of its anti-inflammatory and immunomodulatory effects (Figure 2). However, only recently has it been highlighted that the plant's therapeutic qualities are primarily due to bromelain. Bromelain extract is a complex mixture of proteinase (commonly known as thiol proteinase or cysteine endopeptidase) and a smaller portion of non-protease components (such as phosphatases, glucosidases, peroxides, celluloses, glycoproteins, and carbohydrates) [80–84]. In biochemical terms, bromelain is a non-toxic compound with therapeutic values, classified as a protein-digesting enzyme protease [28]. Both the stem and the fruit of pineapple plants contain bromelain, yet the inedible stem contains a far higher amount of bromelain (around 80%) than the fruit (10%) [81–84]. Indeed, typically, stems are used to produce commercial bromelain using centrifugation, lyophilization, and ultrafiltration [80,84–86]. The stable secondary structure of stem bromelain has an optimal pH near neutrality and a maximal enzymatic activity at 30 °C [86]. The human body effectively absorbs its active form in the gastrointestinal tract, reaching a concentration of about 12 gm/day [83,87–89]. Bromelain is a good option for the development of future oral enzyme treatments in oncology because of all these qualities without any major side effects. Since its discovery, numerous in vitro and in vivo studies have shown that bromelain has various phytomedical activities: anti-inflammatory, fibrinolytic, anti-coagulative, antithrombotic, drug absorption-enhancing, and, most interestingly, anticancer actions [81,83,85,89]. Even though the anticancer effect is mainly due to enzymatic activity, some studies have highlighted that the non-enzymatic components of bromelain (polysaccharides, glycoproteins, vitamin C, β-carotene, and flavonoids) have a synergistic impact on the complex network involved [82,90]. Numerous studies have shown that, depending on the milieu, bromelain modulates the immune response in different ways. [28,83,91]. This is especially relevant in tumor development, where a network of secreted factors, infiltrating cells, stromal cells, fibroblasts, and inflammatory immune cells shape the tumor microenvironment (TME) [92,93]. The TME is a complex and continuously evolving entity where pro-tumorigenic inflammation and antitumor immunity promote cancer.

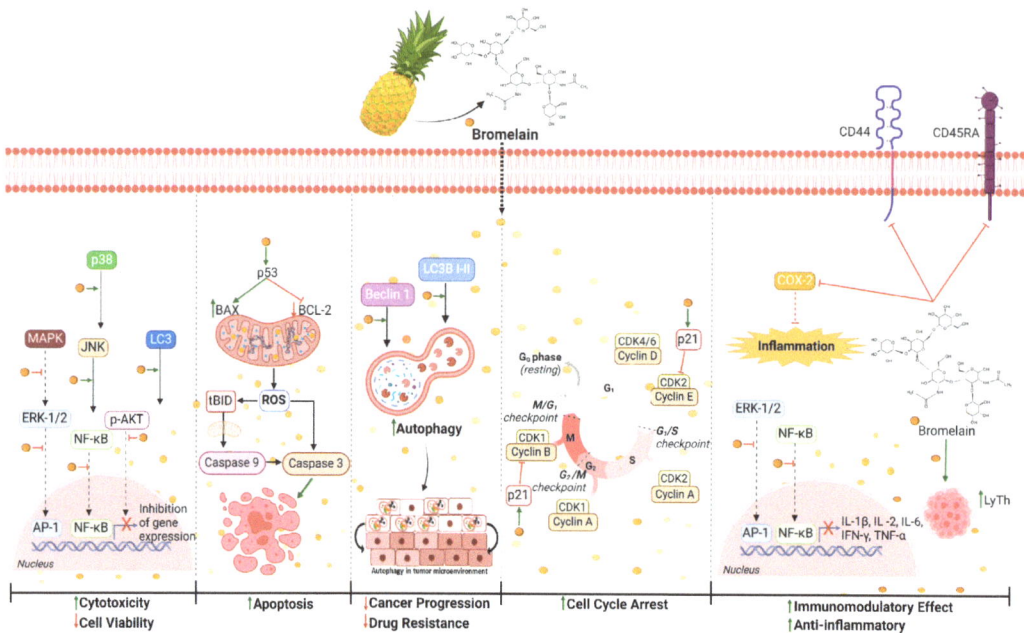

Figure 2. Suggested anticancer molecular mechanisms of bromelain. It induces (↑) cytotoxicity and reduces (↓) cancer cell proliferation primarily by (I) modulating the expression of genes crucial for cell differentiation and proliferation via the mitogen-activated protein kinase (MAPK) signaling pathway, extracellular signal-related kinase (ERK), nuclear factor-kappa B (NF-κB), c-Jun N-terminal kinase (JNK), serine/threonine protein kinase (Akt), microtubule-associated protein B-light chain 3 (LC3), and p38; (II) inducing cell death by apoptosis/autophagy via Bcl-2-associated X (BAX), B-cell lymphoma 2 (Bcl-2), caspases-3 and -9, reactive oxygen species (ROS), p53, LC3, and BECLIN 1; (III) blocking (⊥) the cell cycle by inhibiting cyclins B and E through the activation of p21; (IV) having an immunomodulatory effect by reducing the production of IL-1β, IL-2, IL-6 (interleukin), interferon-gamma (IFN-γ), and tumor necrosis factor (TNF-α) by stimulating T helper cells (LyTh), and via the proteolytic cleavage of clusters of differentiation 44 (CD44) and CD45RA; and (V) reducing inflammation by influencing cyclooxygenase-2 (COX-2). Created with BioRender.com. https://app.biorender.com/illustrations/6613c5688fba6222e90aa178 (accessed on 10 April 2024).

Various in vitro research models showed that bromelain caused a dose-dependent suppression of pro-inflammatory interleukin IL-6, IL-1β, and tumor necrosis factor alpha (TNF-α) production [94,95]. Bromelain treatment inhibited both NF-κB and MAPK pathways, resulting in a decrease in cyclooxygenases-2 (COX-2) and prostaglandin E2 (PGE2), two significant inflammatory mediators linked to the survival, invasion, proliferation, and immune escape of tumor cells [96–98]. A comparable anti-inflammatory impact of bromelain has additionally been noted, as decreasing extracellular signaling regulates kinase (ERK), c-Jun NH2-terminal kinase (JNK), p38 activation, and AP-1 transcription factor activity [99]. p38, JNK, and ERK pathways work together to phosphorylate and activate transcription factors, which in turn causes the expression of particular target genes in response to inflammatory stimuli [100,101]. However, environmental stress preferentially stimulates the p38 and JNK pathways, while mitogen stimuli primarily activate the ERK pathway. Extremely relevant is the effect of bromelain enzyme activity on immune superficial molecules/receptors. Immune cells treated with bromelain showed decreased expression of a vast array of superficial marker (cluster domain, CD) essential for adhesion, migration, and activation during inflammation [102–104]. In particular, the pro-inflammatory CD44 receptor expressed both in cancer cells and in immune cells is removed by bromelain action [94]. The downregulation of CD44 regulates lymphocyte homing and migration to the site of inflammation and is directly linked to tumor proliferation and progression. Furthermore, the presence of a proteinase inhibitor caused notable reduction in the proteolytic reactivity of bromelain against immune cell CDs [28]. Considerable evidence demonstrated the capability of bromelain to arrest cell proliferation or drive apoptosis or autophagy in GI-101A, MCF-7, and MDA-MB-231 triple-negative cells. Fouz et al. [105] have highlighted the antiproliferative effect of bromelain on MCF-7 cells. Interestingly, even when bromelain was encapsulated into lipid-core nanocapsules, the proteolytic and antiproliferative activities were preserved, producing a significantly greater impact than the bromelain solution [106]. Some years later, in two different studies by Raesi et al. [99,107] demonstrated dose-dependent antiproliferative and growth inhibition effects. MCF-7 cells seemed to be more resistant to lower concentrations of bromelain, with a growing sensitivity from an IC_{50} of 65 µg/mL [99] to a maximum of 100 µg/mL [108]. Significant results about how bromelain and cisplatin work together to synergistically improve the induction of death in MDA-MB-231 and MCF-7 cells were provided by Raesi et al. [107] and Pauzi et al. [109]. Referring to the study of Bhui et al. [110], it is important to highlight how bromelain drives both autophagy and apoptosis mechanisms. Bromelain induced autophagy and delayed apoptosis by phosphorylating JNK and p38 MAPKs, by reducing the phosphorylation of ERK1/2, and by suppressing autophagy marker levels (microtubule-associated protein 1A/1B-light chain 3 (LC3B II) and beclin-1) [110]. A similar effect was evaluated based on levels of pro-apoptotic proteins p53, p21, and Bax, which appeared upregulated, and anti-apoptotic proteins Bcl2, Bcl-x, and COX-2, which instead were downregulated [109,111,112]. The data provided by Dhandayuthapani et al. [113] are intriguing since they provides crucial details regarding the apoptosis promotion seen in GI-101A cells treated with bromelain. The findings of this investigation have shown that bromelain strongly increased the activity of caspase-3 and activated pro-caspase-9 to its active form [113]. Because ROS have multiple biological activities in numerous cellular processes and tumor development, it is challenging to attribute anticancer activity to ROS. Bhatnagar et al. carried out one of the earliest investigations on the pro-oxidative characteristics of bromelain on MCF-7 cells [111]. Bromelain increased ROS production, which caused oxidative stress and apoptosis. Additional studies revealed that bromelain increased ROS content, causing the mitochondrial membrane to depolarize, crucial in autophagy and cell apoptosis [114,115].

5. Glucosinolates

The scientific community's interest in vegetables has been focused on preventing and reducing the risk of developing a tumor. Vegetables are a widely available and crucial components of the human diet, representing a significant proportion of nutritional intake in most countries, except for Western countries. Their high per capita consumption makes them a great source of vitamins, minerals, dietary fibers, and especially phytochemicals [116]. Numerous studies have shown that consuming cruciferous vegetables (broccoli, cabbage, cauliflower, and Brussels sprouts), which contain phytochemicals, might reduce the risk of developing cancer [117,118]. Cruciferous vegetables have many beneficial effects that can be attributed to the high content of sulforaphane (1-isothiocyanato-4-(methylsulfinyl)-butane) and indole glucosinolates. These compounds are metabolites derived from glucosinolates and play pivotal roles in various biological processes such as apoptosis, cell cycle arrest, autophagy, angiogenesis, and antioxidant and anti-inflammatory related signaling pathways and genes [117,118]. Glucosinolates derive from glucose and amino acids, and their side chains contain various modifications. In light of the chemical structure of the side chain, glucosinolates are divided into aliphatic (methionine, isoleucine, leucine, valine), aromatic (phenylalanine, tyrosine), and indole (tryptophan) groups. Glucosinolates are sulfur- and nitrogen-rich compounds, which upon hydrolysis by endogenous myrosinases enzymes that co-exist in the plant, generate a range of bioactive metabolites (e.g., isothiocyanates, thiocyanates, and nitriles) [119]. Glucosinolates, in particular glucoraphanin and glucobrassicin, are stored in vacuoles, protecting them from myrosinase degradation [119,120]. Indeed, glucoraphanin and myrosinase are located in different compartments of the plant. When the plant tissue is damaged, it triggers sulforaphane production [121]. Hence, in nature, the glucosinolate/isothiocyanate system serves a defensive mechanism against insects, pathogens, and herbivores [122]. Several factors, both endogenous and exogenous, can influence the concentration of glucosinolates. These include environmental temperature, radiation, soil fertility, water availability, tissue damage, and the type of tissue. Notably, higher glucosinolate concentrations are found in roots and seeds of younger tissue than in late vegetative tissue, whereas foliage displays moderate concentrations. Glucoraphanin can be found in all parts of broccoli plants, but it is primarily concentrated in the aerial sections, developing florets (flower buds), and seeds [123]. The level of glucoraphanin in broccoli seeds is largely influenced by genetic factors and the environment in which plants are grown, including location, year, drought, pollution, and disease pressure [124].

Cruciferae's high content of glucosinolates is responsible for chemopreventive effects compared to other vegetables. However, when broccoli is cooked or blanched, the water-soluble glucosinolates are released into the water, affecting their content [122,125–127]. Hence, cooking methods that use less water, such as steaming or microwaving, may result in the retention of maximum sulforaphane content, in contrast to boiling [125–127]. For this reason, it is preferred to consume raw or freshly harvested broccoli. Even myrosinase is destroyed during meal preparation, being particularly sensitive to high temperatures and pH [128]. Unlike raw sprouts, many commercially available supplements lack myrosinase, which cannot be encapsulated because it requires freshness [129]. Bricker et al. [130] performed an in vivo study to observe how various cooking methods for broccoli sprouts or purified sulforaphane impact the conversion of glucoraphane to sulforaphane. The concentrations of sulforaphane metabolites in steamed broccoli sprouts were found to be significantly lower than those in non-heated sprouts. However, mild heating at 60 °C was observed to further increase sulforaphane metabolites in most tissues. The analysis of metabolite distribution in all tissues indicates the potential for systemic benefits of consuming cruciferous vegetable. Overall, this is an interesting finding that highlights the importance of proper cooking methods to maximize the nutritional value of vegetables. Atwell et al. [131] demonstrated that the consumption of myrosinase-treated broccoli sprout extract containing sulforaphane resulted in three times higher levels of sulforaphane metabolites in the plasma and urine of sprout consumers.

Isothiocyanate formation does not solely depend on plant myrosinase; enzymatic hydrolysis can also occur in the human upper digestive tract during the consumption of raw plants. Several studies have found that certain specific microbial strains, like cecal microbiota, possess myrosinase-like activity and glucoraphanin hydrolysis capabilities [132].

5.1. Sulforaphane

Sulforaphane is characterized by an electrophilic central carbon, which is part of the isothiocyanate group and can react with cysteine residues from other molecules and facilitate interactions with important signaling mediators [133] such as Nrf2, NF-κB, and inflammasome complexes.

Sulforaphane's major target is Nrf2, a transcription factor that, after being activated, migrates into the nucleus and binds to antioxidant response elements (AREs), resulting in the enhanced expression of antioxidant and cytoprotective enzymes (e.g., NQO1, HO-1, glutamate-cysteine ligase catalytic subunit (GCLC), CAT, and SOD) (Figure 3). Licznerska et al. [134] found that Nrf2 expression increased after sulforaphane treatment, showing the highest increase in MCF-7 cells relative to MDA-MB-231 and MCF10-A control cells. Nrf2 antioxidant signaling, induced by sulforaphane, reportedly disrupts the NF-κB pathway [135]. Kim et al. [136] evaluated the synergistic effect of paclitaxel and sulforaphane treatment on MDA-MB-231 and MCF-7 cells. Sulforaphane's presence in MDA-MB-231 cells prevented paclitaxel from activating NF-κB, expressing Bcl-2, and phosphorylating AKT. According to the authors, paclitaxel activates NF-κB through the classic signaling pathway, which involves IKK activation and IκBα degradation. The activation of IKK caused by paclitaxel was suppressed by sulforaphane treatment, which in turn suppressed the activation of NF-κB. In addition, sulforaphane and paclitaxel co-administration resulted in an improvement in paclitaxel-induced apoptosis through caspase-3, -8, and -9 while reducing Bcl-2 expression [136] (Figure 3). The regulation of inflammatory mediators, which are crucial for BC growth and progression, is a widely recognized function of NF-κB. Hunakova et al. [137] showed that sulforaphane inhibited the synthesis of pro-inflammatory cytokines (e.g., IL-1β, IL-6, TNF-α, IFN-γ), immunomodulatory cytokines (e.g., IL-4), and growth factors involved in angiogenesis (PDGF and VEGF) in a manner dependent on dosage.

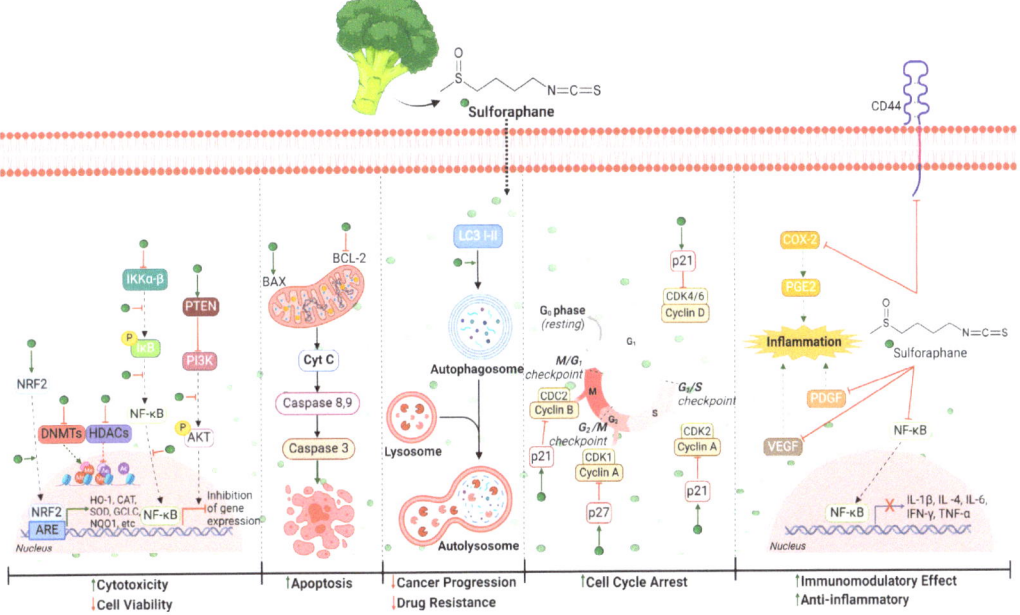

Figure 3. Suggested anticancer molecular mechanisms of sulforaphane. It induces (↑) cytotoxicity and reduces (↓) cancer cells proliferation primarily by (I) modulating the expression of genes crucial for cell differentiation and proliferation via the phosphatase and tensin homolog (PTEN), phosphoinositide 3-kinases (PI3K), and serine/threonine protein kinase (AKT) signaling pathways; via inhibitors of nuclear factor-kappa-B kinase subunit alpha and beta (IKK-α,β) and nuclear factor-kappa-B (NF-κB), inhibiting (⊥) DNA methyltransferases (DNMTs) and histone deacetylases (HDACs); and via nuclear factor erythroid 2-related factor 2 (NRF2) by binding antioxidant response elements (AREs); (II) inducing cell death by apoptosis via Bcl-2-associated X (Bax); B-cell lymphoma 2 (Bcl-2); cytochrome complex (Cyt C); caspases 8, 9, and 3; and by autophagy via microtubule-associated protein light chain 3 I,II (LC3 I,II); (III) blocking the cell cycle by inhibiting cyclins D, A, and B through the activation of p21 and p27; (IV) having an immunomodulatory effect by reducing the production of IL-1β, IL-4, IL-6 (interleukin), interferon-gamma (IFN-γ), and tumor necrosis factor (TNF-α) and via the proteolytic cleavage of clusters of differentiation 44 (CD44); and (V) reducing inflammation by inhibiting cyclooxygenase-2 (COX-2), prostaglandin E2 (PGE2), vascular endothelial growth factor (VEGF), and platelet-derived growth factor (PDGF). Created with BioRender.com. "https://app.biorender.com/illustrations/661e36e12bb8f001aab26646 (accessed on 16 April 2024)".

To date, it has demonstrated that sulforaphanes in combination with classic chemotherapy drugs increase their effectiveness and safety. Xu et al. [138] showed that nanoparticles loaded with a mixture of cisplatin and sulforaphane decrease intracellular levels of glutathione via indirect sulforaphane Nrf2-activation. The significant reduction in glutathione was accompanied by a large rise in DNA-bound cisplatin and in death brought on by damage to DNA, restoring cisplatin chemosensitivity [138]. The effects of doxorubicin and sulforaphane were investigated by Rong et al. [139] using in vitro and in vivo studies. Usually, the tumor microenvironment is characterized by high levels of PGE2 (Figure 3). BC cells that are resistant to doxorubicin produce PGE2, which creates an immunosuppressive environment. Sulforaphane treatment can enhance the anticancer effects of chemotherapy drugs by blocking NF-κB and inhibiting the COX-2 level. Keshandehghan et al. [140] looked at the co-effects of sulforaphane and metformin on MCF-10A, MCF-7, and BT-474 cells. Although each compound has its own impact on cell progression and proliferation, when combined, their impact may be greater. The sulforaphane and metformin co-treatment had a greater impact on cell viability if there was an higher expression of HER2 mRNA; in particular, the co-treatment specifically impacted the Bcl-2/Bax ratio, cancer stem cell (CSC) genes, and CD44 expression. The development of drug carriers is aimed at improving the therapeutic success and preventing the systemic toxicity of chemotherapy. Pogorzelska et al. [141] developed a liposomal formulation combining doxorubicin and sulforaphane. Liposomes efficiently delivered both compounds into MDA-MB-231 and MCF-10A cells. Surprisingly, sulforaphane increased the amount of doxorubicin in the tumor cell nuclei. The co-treatment, in particular, caused a two-fold reduction in main cancer development, and doxorubicin concentration could be reduced by four times.

Besides its function in modulating the Nrf2/NF-κB signaling pathway, many studies have demonstrated that sulforaphane is a highly effective cell proliferation inhibitor, leading to apoptosis and cell cycle blocking. Kanematsu et al. [142] showed that different sulforaphane concentrations (1–100 μM) induced apoptosis in a manner dependent on dosage and timing in MCF-7 and MDA-MB-231 cells. In particular, sulforaphane caused S and G2/M cell cycle blocking linked to elevated p21 and p27 levels and lowered levels of cyclin A, cyclin B1, and CDC2 (Figure 3). In addition, an increase in caspase-3 and LC3-I and -II proteins, as well as the presence of autophagic vacuoles, triggered cell death. Lewinska et al. [143] in an interesting study demonstrated that sulforaphane (5–10 μM) promoted cell cycle arrest via p21 and p27 upregulation, while apoptosis was triggered at 20 μM. Sulforaphane caused accumulation at in the G2/M phase in MCF-7 and MDA-MB-231 cells, whereas it promoted arrest in the G0/G1 phase in SK-BR-3 cells. These data were subsequently confirmed by Cao et al. [144], who demonstrated that different concentrations of sulforaphane (0, 1, 2, 5, and 10 μM) hindered the viability of MCF-7 cells depending on dosage. In particular, sulforaphane decreased cyclin D1, involved in the cell cycle transition from the G1 to S phase, while it increased p21 and PTEN levels. Cancer cells rely on PTEN and PI3K/AKT pathways to regulate apoptosis and cell proliferation [145]. In particular, by phosphorylating p21, AKT stops the cell cycle at the G0/G1 phase [144]. Additionally, sulforaphane treatment reduced the expression of Bcl-2; upregulated Bax and cleaved caspase-3, -8, and -9; and significantly decreased CSC markers and CD44 [144] (Figure 3). Data consistent with those were obtained by Castro et al. [146], who tested sulforaphane's effectiveness on mammosphere formation and the maintenance of breast cancer stem cells (BCSCs) isolated from MDA-MB-231-Luc-D3H1 cells. The ability of BCSC cells to form mammospheres decreased significantly after being administered sulforaphane, as indicated by their superficial markers CD44+/CD24−/CD49f+. This indicates a decreased capacity for these stem/progenitor cells to self-renew. Thus, phytochemicals are becoming new BCSC-eliminating agents, as well as future leads for drug development.

There is a widespread belief that sulforaphane is involved in epigenetic modulation, specifically by controlling the activation or silencing of specific genes and by attaching to DNA methyltransferases (DNMTs) and histone deacetylases (HDACs) [147,148] (Figure 3). Meeran et al. [149] demonstrated a considerable reduction in DNMT1 and DNMT3 levels by sulforaphane in MCF-7 and MDA-MB-231 cells but not in normal MCF-10A cells. Sulforaphane is a potent HDAC inhibitor, which suppresses the human telomerase reverse transcriptase (hTERT). This can lead to phenotypic changes in ER-negative cells, which become "ER enriched" [149]. Lewinska et al. [143] confirmed this epigenetic mechanism by detecting the upregulation of histone deacetylase 5 (HDAC5) mRNA levels in MCF-7, MDA-MB-231, and SK-BR-3 cells. However, the sulforaphane-treated MDA-MB-231 cells showed a reduction in HDAC3, HDAC4, HDAC6, HDAC7, HDAC8, HDAC9, and HDAC10 mRNA levels. The anticancer activity of sulforaphane is promoted by DNA hypomethylation, as shown by the reduced expression of DNMT1 and DNMT3B [143]. Li et al. [150] conducted a novel in vivo experiment that involved a prenatal/maternal mouse model to gain insight into how environmental factors, such as diet, can impact epigenetic programming and predict disease risk later in life. The data indicated that sulforaphane intake before birth shows a significant benefit in preventing the development of BC compared to treatment after birth. Prenatal and maternal sulforaphane intake had a significant impact on the levels and enzymatic activity of HDAC1, resulting in an active chromatin status and changing newborns gene expression profiles, possibly resulting in an increased risk of disease later in life. How early a person is introduced to dietary sulforaphane can have a major impact on how effective it is at preventing BC [150].

5.2. Indole-3 Carbinol

Among the glucosinolates, indole glucosinolates represent a major category. The breakdown of indole-3-methyl glucosinolate, also known as glucobrassicin, by myrosinase leads to the unstable intermediate form indole-3-methyl isothiocyanate, which is subsequently decomposed into indole-3-acetonitrile and indole-3-carbinol (I3C). I3C undergoes acid condensation in the gastric environment into dimers (3,3'-diindolymethane—sDIM), trimers, and tetramers [151,152]. A substantial body of evidence has been published on the healthful effects of I3C, including anti-inflammatory [153–156], neuroprotective [157–159], and anticancer activities [160–164]. Its proficiency in interfering with distinctive signaling pathways that regulate angiogenesis, apoptosis, cell cycle progression, estrogen signaling, and estrogen metabolism leads to its antitumor activity. In addition, the beneficial effects of I3C include its capacity to neutralize free radicals and inhibit lipid peroxidation, thereby reducing both hepatotoxicity and carcinogenesis [165–167]. These findings support the hypothesis that I3C may be also used as a chemopreventive and therapeutic agent in breast cancer.

According to a recent study, it was found that administering I3C at a concentration of 10 µM for 48 h effectively hampered cell growth in human breast cancer cells (MCF-7, MDA-MB-231) by triggering the apoptotic pathway (Caspase 3-4-8) [168]. The activation of the apoptotic pathway was attributed to the suppression of the Akt and NF-kB signaling pathways by I3C [169,170]. Moreover, there is strong evidence to suggest that I3C has antiproliferative properties that target specific components and regulators of the cell cycle. In a study conducted by Cover et al. [171], it was found that I3C can inhibit the growth of human MCF-7 cells via G1 cell cycle arrest by selectively inhibiting cyclin-dependent kinase 6 (CDK6) activity at both the transcriptomic and protein levels. Additionally, this reduction is associated with a decrease in endogenous retinoblastoma (Rb) phosphorylation. The expression of CDK2 and CDK4 was not affected by I3C treatment. Analogously, I3C signaling also suppressed breast cancer cell growth and reduced CDK6 production in estrogen-dependent and estrogen-independent ways [171]. The selective downregulation of CDK6 expression following indole I3C treatment was further confirmed at the mechanistic level: it was demonstrated that I3C interacts with the Sp1 transcription factor binding sites within the CDK6 gene promoter region, resulting in a loss of cellular CDK6 activity [172]. Furthermore, the upregulation of the p21Waf1/Cip1 CDK inhibitor was also reported to be a significant effect of I3C [173]. The findings of cell growth suppression were further confirmed in MCF7 cells, where I3C treatment (100 µM) was efficient in suppressing cell growth and causing a cell cycle shift to G1. The antiproliferative effect was further enhanced when I3C was used in combination with tamoxifen (1 µM), a well-known estrogen receptor antagonist, providing evidence of its potential use for the management of estrogen-responsive breast cancer subtypes. The protein levels of CDK6 and the p21 CDK inhibitor were found to be decreased and increased, respectively, following IC3 treatment. In contrast, tamoxifen did not affect the levels of these cell cycle proteins [174]. The effectiveness of I3C was also investigated in vivo in mouse models. A study conducted by Hajra et al. [175] assessed the antitumor activity of I3C monotherapy (20 mg/kg b.w.) and its ability to enhance the effect of doxorubicin (5 mg/kg b.w. i.p.), an anthracycline drug, in an animal model of breast adenocarcinoma (Erlich ascites carcinoma). The treatment was administered by feeding mice on two schedules: a concomitant treatment schedule (10 days of treatment after cell inoculation) and a pretreatment schedule (10 days of treatment after cell inoculation preceded by pretreatment for 15 days). The study revealed that the co-administration of I3C and doxorubicin on both treatment schedules resulted in the highest tumor growth inhibition (59.74% and 69.48%, respectively, in comparison to the tumor control group); moreover, increased levels of oxidative stress markers (ROS, NOS, lipid peroxidation), apoptotic index, and DNA damage in tumor cells were also reported. Additionally, I3C exhibited a cardioprotective effect by reducing doxorubicin-induced cardiotoxicity (ROS, NOS, LPO) and decreasing the expression of pro-inflammatory mediators (COX-2, iNOS, IL-6). The cardioprotective effect was also demonstrated in creatine phosphokinase and creatine kinase MB decreases. Furthermore, I3C also promoted the activity of antioxidant enzymes and inhibited peritoneal neovascularization by downregulating VEGF-A and MMP-9 [175]. A study conducted by Wang X. et al. [176] also evaluated the effect of a pairwise combination screening of two phytochemicals, I3C and luteolin (3′,4′,5,7-tetrahydroxyflavone), on breast cancer proliferation [176]. The biological assessment of I3C and luteolin, both individually and in combination, was conducted on ERα+ cells (MCF-7 and T-47D) and TNBC cells (MDA-MB-231 and BT-549). Individual agents inhibited BC cell proliferation in a dose-dependent manner. However, the inhibitory concentration was a higher molar concentration, whereas their combination (L30I40) demonstrated a synergistic antiproliferative effect on ER+ cells at a lower molar concentration of 30 µM and 40 µM, respectively. The biological effect was achieved via the downregulation of CDK4/6 and the induction of apoptosis. Furthermore, the combination treatment was further assessed in an animal model of MCF-7 cell-derived xenograft mice. A significantly lower tumor weight and tumor size were reported in the combination group with LUT and I3C (LUT10 mg + I3C10 mg/kg/day) compared to those in the control treatment (vehicle, alone treatments), suggesting L30I40 treatment as a chemotherapeutic approach for the treatment of ER+ BC subtypes [176]. The therapeutic potential of I3C against breast cancer was revealed by Rahman et al. [177] in a study conducted on non-tumorigenic and tumorigenic breast epithelial cells, MCF-10A and MCF-10CA1a, respectively, which revealed that I3C selectively induced apoptosis in the breast cancer cells by upregulating the Bax/Bcl-2 ratio and downregulating Bcl-XL expression [177]. According to Caruso et al. [178] a wide range of ER-α+ cells (MCF-7, ZR-75-1, T-47D) were more sensitive to I3C's antitumor effects than ER-α-negative breast cancer cells (MDA-MB-231, MDA-MB-157, MDA-MB-436) and immortalized human mammary epithelial cells (HMECs). The study also found that I3C impacts several molecular mechanisms, including hormone receptor signaling (ERα, PR, GATA3, AR), increased apoptosis (cleaved caspase 3, SMAC, IAP), p53-signaling, and oxidative stress (ATF-3), as well as the arrest of cell proliferation (p21, c-myc, Rb pS807/S81) in ERα-sensitive cells compared to ER-α-negative cells [178]. In addition to the above, among the cellular signaling pathways that were also modulated by I3C supplementation was that of aryl hydrocarbon receptor (AhR) [179–181]. AhR belongs to the nuclear receptor superfamily and is a ligand-activated receptor that, upon translocation into the nucleus, activates genes linked to inflammation, detoxification, and cancer [179,182]. The anticancer activity of IC3, including mammosphere formation inhibition, has been evaluated in cancer stem cells derived from breast cancer MCF-7 cells in vitro [183]. The molecular mechanistic model of AhR activation was evaluated for several structurally diverse AhR agonists, including 3-methylcholanthrene (3MC), benzo[a]pyrene (BaP), 7,12-dimethylbenz[a]anthracene (DMBA), kynurenine (KYN), 6-formylindolo [3,2-b]carbazole (FICZ), indole-3-acetic acid (IAA), and indole derivatives such as indole-3-carbinol (I3C) and indirubin, in MCF-7 cells genetically engineered for the AhR gene (AhR-wild type/knockout in MCF-7 cells) [183]. Each AhR agonist demonstrated a characteristic suppression of mammosphere formation, which was observed to be dose- and AhR-dependent. Moreover, at a higher concentration (100 µM) of I3C and IAA, similar suppression levels of mammosphere formation were observed in AhR-WT and in AhR-KO cells, without impaired cytotoxicity [183]. Additionally, the activation of xenobiotic transcription factors was also evaluated at the transcriptional level. The upregulation of genes associated with xenobiotic metabolism was assessed in [183,184] after I3C treatment and suggests that I3C can modify drug efficacy and safety. Moreover, further evidence has been provided to support the hypothesis that the AhR signaling pathway plays a role in promoting the anticancer effect of I3C in ER-α^+ cell lines [178]. Several AhR target genes (CYP1A1, CYP1A2, ALDH1A3, ALDH3A1) were upregulated in ER-α^+ cells (MCF-7) after I3C administration, compared to expression in ER-α-negative cells at the transcriptomic level (microarray). Furthermore, the sensitivity to I3C was found to be reduced following the AhR knockdown of MCF-7 cells [178]. Numerous studies have revealed that I3C has the capability to reduce the growth of BC cells by regulating microRNA expression (miRNA) [185,186] and by modulating the epigenetic mechanism [187]. Hargraves et al. [185] discovered that I3C's antitumor effects are closely associated with raised levels of miR-34a expression, which rely on the existence of the p53 protein. In particular, in human breast cancer cells (MCF-7) possessing wild-type p53, I3C triggered a dose-dependent surge in miR-34a expression, as well as the activation of the phosphorylated form of p53 at serine-15. However, the induction of miR-34a expression by I3C was blocked when mammary epithelial cells (MCF-10A) were transfected with a dominant negative p53. Furthermore, I3C was found to restrain the proliferation of MCF-7 cells by arresting the cell cycle at the G1 phase when used at a concentration of 200 µM [185]. According to research conducted by El-Daly et al. [186], the use of I3C in MCF-7 cells can influence the epigenetic network of tumor suppressor microRNAs and oncogenic microRNAs. This, in turn, impacts critical signaling pathways that control cell cycle progression (CDK4, CDK6) and the anti-apoptotic pathway (Bcl-2, survivin) via their suppression. The study discovered that after 72 h of I3C treatment, tumor suppressor microRNAs' expression levels increased (let-7a-e, miR-17-5p, miR-19a, miR-20a). Conversely, there was a decrease in the expression of oncogenic microRNAs (miR-181a/b, miR-210, miR-221, and miR-106a) observed both at 48 h and 72 h [186]. Similarly, the interaction between epigenetic modulation, predominantly acetylation-based, and the administration of the dietary bioactive compound has been also evaluated in TNBC (MDA-MB-231, BT-549, HCC70, HCC1806), which lacks effective treatment options. The administration of an epigenetic modifier, vorinostat, and the dietary bioactive compound I3C, both used as single agents, was found to induce a re-expression of the ER-α and PR receptors. Furthermore, I3C was demonstrated to enhance the anticancer effect of vorinostat, inhibiting cell growth and invasion through an estrogen-independent mechanism in HCC70 and HCC1806 breast cancer cells [187]. Due to its instability in an acid milieu, such as the gastric juice, and its consequent rapid oligomerization in 3,3'-diindolylmethane (DIM), encapsulation technology has been proposed as a promising approach to increase its stability and prevent its degradation [188,189]. Among such approaches, Gehrcke et al. [190] proved the cytotoxic effect of free I3C and I3C embedded in nanocapsules of poly-(ϵ-caprolactone), prepared using rosehip oil (RHO), on the breast adenocarcinoma MCF-7 cell line. A higher cytotoxic effect was reported for I3C embedded in nanocapsules (85%) than for free I3C (50%) by using a sulforhodamine B assay. Furthermore, the encapsulation technology also increased I3C photostability [190]. The aforementioned findings elucidate the therapeutic potentiality of I3C, either alone or in combination with chemotherapeutic or epigenetic drugs, as supported by experimental in vitro and in vivo evidence.

Among the condensation products of I3C, DIM is the primary bioactive in vivo compound [188]. The analysis of plasma samples from a female population at elevated risk of breast cancer following the oral administration of I3C revealed the presence of DIM at all tested doses of I3C, ranging from 400 mg to 1200 mg. Conversely, due to its high instability, I3C was undetectable in plasma samples regardless of the I3C dose. Therefore, DIM was the sole condensation product detected in human plasma [191]. The antitumor effectiveness of DIM was also evaluated in breast cancer cell lines. In human MCF-7 and T47-D cell lines, DIM was found to induce apoptosis [192,193] and inhibit breast cancer cell growth. Specifically, DIM was effective in MCF-7 and MDA-MB-231 cell lines in a concentration- and time-dependent manner [193,194]. Several lines of evidence support its ability to impair breast cancer proliferation through the inhibition of multiple signaling pathways [195–200]. Furthermore, the modulatory effect of DIM on miRNA expression was investigated in human breast cancer cells [186,201,202] and in breast cancer organoids [203]. Moreover, to enhance the bioavailability of DIM, nanoformulations of DIM were examined. These included DIM nanoparticles coated with PEG/chitosan [204] and DIM-chitosan [205]. The results demonstrated enhanced in vitro antitumor activity against breast cancer cells, as evidenced by a significant reduction in cell migration and angiogenesis and a marked increase in apoptosis [204].

6. Conclusions and Future Prospects

Cancer remains a global challenge. Common treatment for BC includes hormonal therapy, surgery, targeted therapy, radiation therapy, and chemotherapy. Researchers have been motivated to find an alternative treatment, as standard therapies are correlated with the onset of side effects and poor surgical healing. Moreover, cancer cells gradually have started to exhibit drug resistance, hindering the therapeutic effect. To overcome these multiple obstacles of conventional treatments, there is a pressing need for new therapeutic, adjuvant, or chemopreventive compounds.

In recent decades, the use of medicinal plants, herbs, and dietary products with pharmacological significance has been rediscovered. What is especially intriguing are plant-derived small molecules (phytochemicals) used in traditional medicine for decades, which have been demonstrated to have remarkable antitumor activity. The protective action of certain dietary micronutrients, namely PUFAs, bromelain, sulforaphane, and indole-3-carbinol, against BC by inhibiting proliferation, invasion, angiogenesis, and metastasis has been well documented.

BC is now largely understood to be a heterogenous disease that is characterized by mutations in different sets of genes and pathways. Dietary bioactive compounds have shown multi-targeted "pleiotropic" effects with the ability to interfere with multiple oncogenic signaling pathways involved in the regulation of different stages of breast cancer development, such as PI3K/Akt/mTOR, JAK/STAT, MAPK, and NF-κB pathways; cell cycle and apoptosis; proliferation; metastasis; and angiogenesis. A thorough understanding of its multiple antitumor effects could lay the foundation for future research and comprehension to improve its clinical utility as well as applications in primary (preventing cancer), secondary (preventing potential metastasis growth), and tertiary (for cascading problems) care.

Unfortunately, the poor solubility and low bioavailability of these compounds limit their direct use in clinical applications. However, technological advancements and alternative therapeutic approaches have overcome these challenges. A variety of nanoformulations are now being used in a great range of biomedical applications, including large-scale production, stability, bioavailability, and quality control of drug loading and release.

Bromelain, ω-3 PUFAs, sulforaphane, and indole-3-carbinol are considered promising approaches to treating BC because of their reduced toxicity and side effects, making them ideal co-adjuvant supplements for traditional drugs and breast cancer chemoprevention tools. In conclusion, the use of dietary compounds and phytochemicals as part of standard treatment for BC requires further investigation.

Author Contributions: Conceptualization, M.M. and M.S.; software, M.M.; data curation, M.M. and M.S.; writing—original draft preparation, M.M., M.S., M.G., E.G. and C.S.; writing—review and editing, M.M. and M.S.; supervision, M.M., M.S., F.S. and G.M.; funding acquisition, G.M. All authors have read and agreed to the published version of the manuscript.

Funding: This work was supported by 2023 current research project funds (2779753), Italian Ministry of Health, to IRCCS-CROB, Rionero in Vulture, Potenza, Italy.

Conflicts of Interest: The authors declare no conflicts of interest.

References

1. World Health Organization (WHO). Breast Cancer. 2024. Available online: https://www.who.int/news-room/fact-sheets/detail/breast-cancer (accessed on 13 March 2024).
2. National Cancer Institute. Hormone Therapy for Breast Cancer. 2022. Available online: https://www.cancer.gov/types/breast/breast-hormone-therapy-fact-sheet (accessed on 13 March 2024).
3. Arzanova, E.; Mayrovitz, H.N. The Epidemiology of Breast Cancer. In *Breast Cancer*, 1st ed.; Mayrovitz, H.N., Ed.; Exon Publications: Brisbane, Australia, 2022; Chapter 1; pp. 1–19.
4. Admoun, C.; Mayrovitz, H.N. The Etiology of Breast Cancer. In *Breast Cancer*, 1st ed.; Mayrovitz, H.N., Ed.; Exon Publications: Brisbane, Australia, 2022; Chapter 2; pp. 21–30.
5. Orrantia-Borunda, E.; Anchondo-Nuñez, P.; Acuña-Aguilar, L.E.; Gómez-Valles, F.O.; Ramírez-Valdespino, C.A. Subtypes of Breast Cancer. In *Breast Cancer*, 1st ed.; Mayrovitz, H.N., Ed.; Exon Publications: Brisbane, Australia, 2022; Chapter 3; pp. 31–42.
6. Yersal, O.; Barutca, S. Biological subtypes of breast cancer: Prognostic and therapeutic implications. *World J. Clin. Oncol.* 2014, 5, 412–424. [CrossRef] [PubMed]
7. Dai, X.; Xiang, L.; Li, T.; Bai, Z. Cancer Hallmarks, Biomarkers and Breast Cancer Molecular Subtypes. *J. Cancer* 2016, 7, 1281–1294. [CrossRef] [PubMed]
8. Baliu-Piqué, M.; Pandiella, A.; Ocana, A. Breast Cancer Heterogeneity and Response to Novel Therapeutics. *Cancers* 2020, 12, 3271. [CrossRef] [PubMed]
9. Zubair, M.; Wang, S.; Ali, N. Advanced Approaches to Breast Cancer Classification and Diagnosis. *Front. Pharmacol.* 2021, 11, 632079. [CrossRef]
10. Clusan, L.; Ferrière, F.; Flouriot, G.; Pakdel, F. A Basic Review on Estrogen Receptor Signaling Pathways in Breast Cancer. *Int. J. Mol. Sci.* 2023, 24, 6834. [CrossRef] [PubMed]
11. Iacopetta, D.; Ceramella, J.; Baldino, N.; Sinicropi, M.S.; Catalano, A. Targeting Breast Cancer: An Overlook on Current Strategies. *Int. J. Mol. Sci.* 2023, 24, 3643. [CrossRef] [PubMed]
12. Dominguez, L.J.; Veronese, N.; Di Bella, G.; Cusumano, C.; Parisi, A.; Tagliaferri, F.; Ciriminna, S.; Barbagallo, M. Mediterranean diet in the management and prevention of obesity. *Exp. Gerontol.* 2023, 174, 112121. [CrossRef] [PubMed]
13. Bradshaw, P.T.; Ibrahim, J.G.; Stevens, J.; Cleveland, R.; Abrahamson, P.E.; Satia, J.A.; Teitelbaum, S.L.; Neugut, A.I.; Gammon, M.D. Post diagnosis change in bodyweight and survival after breast cancer diagnosis. *Epidemiology* 2012, 23, 320–327. [CrossRef] [PubMed]
14. Divella, R.; Marino, G.; Infusino, S.; Lanotte, L.; Gadaleta-Caldarola, G.; Gadaleta-Caldarola, G. The Mediterranean Lifestyle to Contrast Low-Grade Inflammation Behavior in Cancer. *Nutrients* 2023, 15, 1667. [CrossRef]
15. De Cicco, P.; Catani, M.V.; Gasperi, V.; Sibilano, M.; Quaglietta, M.; Savini, I. Nutrition and Breast Cancer: A Literature Review on Prevention, Treatment and Recurrence. *Nutrients* 2019, 11, 1514. [CrossRef]
16. Mazurakova, A.; Koklesova, L.; Samec, M.; Kudela, E.; Kajo, K.; Skuciova, V.; Csizmár, S.H.; Mestanova, V.; Pec, M.; Adamkov, M.; et al. Anti-breast cancer effects of phytochemicals: Primary, secondary, and tertiary care. *EPMA J.* 2022, 13, 315–334. [CrossRef] [PubMed]
17. Iqbal, J.; Abbasi, B.A.; Batool, R.; Mahmood, T.; Ali, B.; Khalil, A.T.; Kanwal, S.; Shah, S.A.; Ahmad, R. Potential phytocompounds for developing breast cancer therapeutics: Nature's healing touch. *Eur. J. Pharmacol.* 2018, 827, 125–148. [CrossRef]
18. Choudhari, A.S.; Mandave, P.C.; Deshpande, M.; Ranjekar, P.; Prakash, O. Phytochemicals in Cancer Treatment: From Preclinical Studies to Clinical Practice. *Front. Pharmacol.* 2020, 10, 1614. [CrossRef]
19. Augimeri, G.; Montalto, F.I.; Giordano, C.; Barone, I.; Lanzino, M.; Catalano, S.; Andò, S.; De Amicis, F.; Bonofiglio, D. Nutraceuticals in the Mediterranean Diet: Potential Avenues for Breast Cancer Treatment. *Nutrients* 2021, 13, 2557. [CrossRef] [PubMed]
20. Kumar, A.P.N.; Kumar, M.; Jose, A.; Tomer, V.; Oz, E.; Proestos, C.; Zeng, M.; Elobeid, T.K.S.; Oz, F. Major Phytochemicals: Recent Advances in Health Benefits and Extraction Method. *Molecules* 2023, 28, 887. [CrossRef]
21. Fernandes, R.S.; Silva, J.O.; Mussi, S.V.; Lopes, S.C.A.; Leite, E.A.; Cassali, G.D.; Cardoso, V.N.; Townsend, D.M.; Colletti, P.M.; Ferreira, L.A.M.; et al. Nanostructured Lipid Carrier Co-loaded with Doxorubicin and Docosahexaenoic Acid as a Theranostic Agent: Evaluation of Biodistribution and Antitumor Activity in Experimental Model. *Mol. Imaging Biol.* 2018, 20, 437–447. [CrossRef] [PubMed]
22. Fang, J. EPR Effect-Based Tumor Targeted Nanomedicine: A Promising Approach for Controlling Cancer. *J. Pers. Med.* 2022, 12, 95. [CrossRef] [PubMed]

23. Patra, J.K.; Das, G.; Fraceto, L.F.; Campos, E.V.R.; Rodriguez-Torres, M.D.P.; Acosta-Torres, L.S.; Diaz-Torres, L.A.; Grillo, R.; Swamy, M.K.; Sharma, S.; et al. Nano based drug delivery systems: Recent developments and future prospects. *J. Nanobiotechnol.* **2018**, *16*, 71. [CrossRef]
24. Huang, M.; Zhai, B.T.; Fan, Y.; Sun, J.; Shi, Y.J.; Zhang, X.F.; Zou, J.B.; Wang, J.W.; Guo, D.Y. Targeted drug delivery systems for curcumin in breast cancer therapy. *Int. J. Nanomed.* **2023**, *18*, 4275–4311. [CrossRef]
25. Simopoulos, A.P. The importance of the ratio of omega-6/omega-3 essential fatty acids. *Biomed. Pharmacother.* **2002**, *56*, 365–379. [CrossRef]
26. Chénais, B.; Blanckaert, V. The janus face of lipids in human breast cancer: How polyunsaturated Fatty acids affect tumor cell hallmarks. *Int. J. Breast Cancer* **2012**, *2012*, 712536. [CrossRef] [PubMed]
27. Bougnoux, P.; Hajjaji, N.; Maheo, K.; Couet, C.; Chevalier, S. Fatty acids and breast cancer: Sensitization to treatments and prevention of metastatic re-growth. *Prog. Lipid Res.* **2010**, *49*, 76–86. [CrossRef] [PubMed]
28. Hikisz, P.; Bernasinska-Slomczewska, J. Beneficial Properties of Bromelain. *Nutrients* **2021**, *13*, 4313. [CrossRef] [PubMed]
29. Wu, X.; Zhou, Q.H.; Xu, K. Are isothiocyanates potential anti-cancer drugs? *Acta Pharmacol. Sin.* **2009**, *30*, 501–512. [CrossRef] [PubMed]
30. Vanduchova, A.; Anzenbacher, P.; Anzenbacherova, E. Isothiocyanate from Broccoli, Sulforaphane, and Its Properties. *J. Med. Food* **2019**, *22*, 121–126. [CrossRef] [PubMed]
31. Fahey, J.W.; Holtzclaw, W.D.; Wehage, S.L.; Wade, K.L.; Stephenson, K.K.; Talalay, P. Sulforaphane Bioavailability from Glucoraphanin-Rich Broccoli: Control by Active Endogenous Myrosinase. *PLoS ONE* **2015**, *10*, e0140963. [CrossRef] [PubMed]
32. Kuran, D.; Pogorzelska, A.; Wiktorska, K. Breast Cancer Prevention-Is there a Future for Sulforaphane and Its Analogs? *Nutrients* **2020**, *12*, 1559. [CrossRef] [PubMed]
33. Xin, W.; Wei, W.; Li, X. Effects of fish oil supplementation on cardiac function in chronic heart failure: A meta-analysis of randomised controlled trials. *Heart* **2012**, *98*, 1620–1625. [CrossRef] [PubMed]
34. Liu, J.; Ma, D.W. The role of n-3 polyunsaturated fatty acids in the prevention and treatment of breast cancer. *Nutrients* **2014**, *6*, 5184–5223. [CrossRef]
35. Kar, S.; Webel, R. Fish oil supplementation & coronary artery disease: Does it help? *Mo Med.* **2012**, *109*, 142.
36. Miles, E.A.; Calder, P.C. Influence of marine n-3 polyunsaturated fatty acids on immune function and a systematic review of their effects on clinical outcomes in rheumatoid arthritis. *Br. J. Nutr.* **2012**, *107*, S171–S184. [CrossRef] [PubMed]
37. Rudkowska, I. Fish oils for cardiovascular disease: Impact on diabetes. *Maturitas* **2010**, *67*, 25–28. [CrossRef] [PubMed]
38. Chapkin, R.S.; Kim, W.; Lupton, J.R.; McMurray, D.N. Dietary docosahexaenoic and eicosapentaenoic acid: Emerging mediators of inflammation. *Prostaglandins Leukot Essent Fat. Acids* **2009**, *81*, 187–191. [CrossRef] [PubMed]
39. Vaughan, V.C.; Hassing, M.R.; Lewandowski, P.A. Marine polyunsaturated fatty acids and cancer therapy. *Br. J. Cancer* **2013**, *108*, 486–492. [CrossRef] [PubMed]
40. Racine, R.A.; Deckelbaum, R.J. Sources of the very-long-chain unsaturated omega-3 fatty acids: Eicosapentaenoic acid and docosahexaenoic acid. *Curr. Opin. Clin. Nutr. Metab. Care* **2007**, *10*, 123–128. [CrossRef] [PubMed]
41. Grammatikos, S.I.; Subbaiah, P.V.; Victor, T.A.; Miller, W.M. n-3 and n-6 fatty acid processing and growth effects in neoplastic and non-cancerous human mammary epithelial cell lines. *Br. J. Cancer* **1994**, *70*, 219–227. [CrossRef] [PubMed]
42. Wang, Y.; Fan, P.; Zhu, L.; Zhuang, W.; Jiang, L.; Zhang, H.; Huang, H. Enhanced in vitro antitumor efficacy of a polyunsaturated fatty acid-conjugated pH-responsive self-assembled ion-pairing liposome-encapsulated prodrug. *Nanotechnology* **2020**, *31*, 155101. [CrossRef]
43. Truan, J.S.; Chen, J.M.; Thompson, L.U. Flaxseed oil reduces the growth of human breast tumors (MCF-7) at high levels of circulating estrogen. *Mol. Nutr. Food Res.* **2010**, *54*, 1414–1421. [CrossRef]
44. Saggar, J.K.; Chen, J.; Corey, P.; Thompson, L.U. Dietary flaxseed lignan or oil combined with tamoxifen treatment affects MCF-7 tumor growth through estrogen receptor-and growth factor-signalling pathways. *Mol. Nutr. Food Res.* **2010**, *54*, 415–425. [CrossRef]
45. Xu, M.Q.; Hao, Y.L.; Wang, J.R.; Li, Z.Y.; Li, H.; Feng, Z.H.; Wang, H.; Wang, J.W.; Zhang, X. Antitumor activity of α-linolenic acid-paclitaxel conjugate nanoparticles: In vitro and in vivo. *Int. J. Nanomed.* **2021**, *16*, 7269–7281. [CrossRef]
46. Patterson, R.E.; Flatt, S.W.; Newman, V.A.; Natarajan, L.; Rock, C.L.; Thomson, C.A.; Caan, B.J.; Parker, B.A.; Pierce, J.P. Marine fatty acid intake is associated with breast cancer prognosis. *J. Nutr.* **2011**, *141*, 201–206. [CrossRef]
47. DeGraffenried, L.A.; Friedrichs, W.E.; Fulcher, L.; Fernandes, G.; Silva, J.M.; Peralba, J.M.; Hidalgo, M. Eicosapentaenoic acid restores tamoxifen sensitivity in breast cancer cells with high Akt activity. *Ann. Oncol.* **2003**, *14*, 1051–1056. [CrossRef]
48. Rose, D.P.; Connolly, J.M.; Rayburn, J.; Coleman, M. Influence of diets containing eicosapentaenoic or docosahexaenoic acid on growth and metastasis of breast cancer cells in nude mice. *J. Natl. Cancer Inst.* **1995**, *87*, 587–592. [CrossRef]
49. Sauer, L.A.; Dauchy, R.T.; Blask, D.E.; Krause, J.A.; Davidson, L.K.; Dauchy, E.M. Eicosapentaenoic acid suppresses cell proliferation in MCF-7 human breast cancer xenografts in nude rats via a pertussis toxin–sensitive signal transduction pathway. *J. Nutr.* **2005**, *135*, 2124–2129. [CrossRef] [PubMed]
50. Chambrier, C.; Bastard, J.P.; Rieusset, J.; Chevillotte, E.; Bonnefont-Rousselot, D.; Therond, P.; Hainque, B.; Riou, J.P.; Laville, M.; Vidal, H. Eicosapentaenoic acid induces mRNA expression of peroxisome proliferator-activated receptor γ. *Obes. Res.* **2002**, *10*, 518–525. [CrossRef]

51. Merendino, N.; Costantini, L.; Manzi, L.; Molinari, R.; D'Eliseo, D.; Velotti, F. Dietary ω-3 polyunsaturated fatty acid DHA: A potential adjuvant in the treatment of cancer. *Biomed. Res. Int.* **2013**, *2013*, 310186. [CrossRef] [PubMed]
52. Chamras, H.; Ardashian, A.; Heber, D.; Glaspy, J.A. Fatty acid modulation of MCF-7 human breast cancer cell proliferation, apoptosis and differentiation. *J. Nutr. Biochem.* **2002**, *13*, 711–716. [CrossRef]
53. Spencer, L.; Mann, C.; Metcalfe, M.; Webb, M.B.; Pollard, C.; Spencer, D.; Berry, D.; Steward, W.; Dennison, A. The effect of omega-3 FAs on tumour angiogenesis and their therapeutic potential. *Eur. J. Cancer* **2009**, *45*, 2077–2086. [CrossRef] [PubMed]
54. D'Eliseo, D.; Manzi, L.; Merendino, N.; Velotti, F. Docosahexaenoic acid inhibits invasion of human RT112 urinary bladder and PT45 pancreatic carcinoma cells via down-modulation of granzyme B expression. *J. Nutr. Biochem.* **2012**, *23*, 452–457. [CrossRef]
55. Horia, E.; Watkins, B.A. Complementary actions of docosahexaenoic acid and genistein on COX-2, PGE 2 and invasiveness in MDA-MB-231 breast cancer cells. *Carcinogenesis* **2007**, *28*, 809–815. [CrossRef]
56. Barascu, A.; Besson, P.; Le Floch, O.; Bougnoux, P.; Jourdan, M.L. CDK1-cyclin B1 mediates the inhibition of proliferation induced by omega-3 fatty acids in MDA-MB-231 breast cancer cells. *Int. J. Biochem. Cell Biol.* **2006**, *38*, 196–208. [CrossRef]
57. Ravacci, G.R.; Brentani, M.M.; Tortelli, T., Jr.; Torrinhas, R.S.M.; Saldanha, T.; Torres, E.A.F.; Waitzberg, D.L. Lipid raft disruption by docosahexaenoic acid induces apoptosis in transformed human mammary luminal epithelial cells harboring HER-2 overexpression. *J. Nutr. Biochem.* **2013**, *24*, 505–515. [CrossRef] [PubMed]
58. Menendez, J.A.; Lupu, R.; Colomer, R. Exogenous supplementation with ω-3 polyunsaturated fatty acid docosahexaenoic acid (DHA; 22, 6n-3) synergistically enhances taxane cytotoxicity and downregulates Her-2/neu (c-erbB-2) oncogene expression in human breast cancer cells. *Eur. J. Cancer Prev.* **2005**, *14*, 263–270. [CrossRef] [PubMed]
59. Bougnoux, P.; Hajjaji, N.; Ferrasson, M.N. Improving outcome of chemotherapy of metastatic breast cancer by docosahexaenoic acid: A phase II trial. *Altern. Med. Rev.* **2010**, *15*, 91–92. [CrossRef] [PubMed]
60. Kang, K.S.; Wang, P.; Yamabe, N.; Fukui, M.; Jay, T.; Zhu, B.T. Docosahexaenoic acid induces apoptosis in MCF-7 cells in vitro and in vivo via reactive oxygen species formation and caspase 8 activation. *PLoS ONE* **2010**, *5*, e10296. [CrossRef] [PubMed]
61. Chiu, L.C.M.; Wong, E.Y.L.; Ooi, V.E. Docosahexaenoic Acid from a Cultured Microalga Inhibits Cell Growth and Induces Apoptosis by Upregulating Bax/Bcl-2 Ratio in Human Breast Carcinoma MCF-7 Cells. *Ann. N. Y. Acad. Sci.* **2004**, *1030*, 361–368. [CrossRef] [PubMed]
62. Jourdan, M.L.; Mahéo, K.; Barascu, A.; Goupille, C.; De Latour, M.P.; Bougnoux, P.; Rio, P.G. Increased BRCA1 protein in mammary tumours of rats fed marine ω-3 fatty acids. *Oncol. Rep.* **2007**, *17*, 713–719. [CrossRef]
63. Bernard-Gallon, D.J.; Vissac-Sabatier, C.; Antoine-Vincent, D.; Rio, P.G.; Maurizis, J.C.; Fustier, P.; Bignon, Y.J. Differential effects of n-3 and n-6 polyunsaturated fatty acids on BRCA1 and BRCA2 gene expression in breast cell lines. *Br. J. Nutr.* **2002**, *87*, 281–289. [CrossRef] [PubMed]
64. Rogers, K.R.; Kikawa, K.D.; Mouradian, M.; Hernandez, K.; McKinnon, K.M.; Ahwah, S.M.; Pardini, R.S. Docosahexaenoic acid alters epidermal growth factor receptor-related signaling by disrupting its lipid raft association. *Carcinogenesis* **2010**, *31*, 1523–1530. [CrossRef]
65. Colas, S.; Mahéo, K.; Denis, F.; Goupille, C.; Hoinard, C.; Champeroux, P.; Tranquart, F.; Bougnoux, P. Sensitization by dietary docosahexaenoic acid of rat mammary carcinoma to anthracycline: A role for tumor vascularization. *Clin. Cancer Res.* **2006**, *12*, 5879–5886. [CrossRef]
66. Signori, C.; DuBrock, C.; Richie, J.P.; Prokopczyk, B.; Demers, L.M.; Hamilton, C.; Hartman, T.J.; Liao, J.; El-Bayoumy, K.; Manni, A. Administration of omega-3 fatty acids and Raloxifene to women at high risk of breast cancer: Interim feasibility and biomarkers analysis from a clinical trial. *Eur. J. Clin. Nutr.* **2012**, *66*, 878–884. [CrossRef] [PubMed]
67. Freitas, R.D.; Campos, M.M. Protective effects of omega-3 fatty acids in cancer-related complications. *Nutrients* **2019**, *11*, 945. [CrossRef] [PubMed]
68. Mandal, C.C.; Ghosh-Choudhury, T.; Dey, N.; Choudhury, G.G.; Ghosh-Choudhury, N. miR-21 is targeted by omega-3 polyunsaturated fatty acid to regulate breast tumor CSF-1 expression. *Carcinogenesis* **2012**, *33*, 1897–1908. [CrossRef] [PubMed]
69. Chen, J.Q.; Russo, J. Dysregulation of glucose transport, glycolysis, TCA cycle and glutaminolysis by oncogenes and tumor suppressors in cancer cells. *Biochim. Biophys. Acta* **2012**, *1826*, 370–384. [CrossRef] [PubMed]
70. Mouradian, M.; Kikawa, K.D.; Dranka, B.P.; Komas, S.M.; Kalyanaraman, B.; Pardini, R.S. Docosahexaenoic acid attenuates breast cancer cell metabolism and the Warburg phenotype by targeting bioenergetic function. *Mol. Carcinog.* **2015**, *54*, 810–820. [CrossRef]
71. Manzi, L.; Costantini, L.; Molinari, R.; Merendino, N. Effect of dietary ω-3 polyunsaturated fatty acid DHA on glycolytic enzymes and warburg phenotypes in cancer. *Biomed. Res. Int.* **2015**, *2015*, 137097. [CrossRef] [PubMed]
72. Zhu, L.; Lin, M. The synthesis of nano-doxorubicin and its anticancer effect. *Anticancer. Agents Med. Chem.* **2021**, *21*, 2466–2477. [CrossRef]
73. Mussi, S.V.; Sawant, R.; Perche, F.; Oliveira, M.C.; Azevedo, R.B.; Ferreira, L.A.; Torchilin, V.P. Novel nanostructured lipid carrier co-loaded with doxorubicin and docosahexaenoic acid demonstrates enhanced in vitro activity and overcomes drug resistance in MCF-7/Adr cells. *Pharm. Res.* **2014**, *31*, 1882–1892. [CrossRef]
74. Khankari, N.K.; Bradshaw, P.T.; Steck, S.E.; He, K.; Olshan, A.F.; Shen, J.; Ahn, J.; Chen, Y.; Ahsan, H.; Terry, M.B.; et al. Dietary intake of fish, polyunsaturated fatty acids, and survival after breast cancer: A population-based follow-up study on Long Island, New York. *Cancer* **2015**, *121*, 2244–2252. [CrossRef]

75. Zou, Z.; Bidu, C.; Bellenger, S.; Narce, M.; Bellenger, J. n-3 polyunsaturated fatty acids and HER2-positive breast cancer: Interest of the fat-1 transgenic mouse model over conventional dietary supplementation. *Biochimie* **2014**, *96*, 22–27. [CrossRef]
76. Russo, G.L. Dietary n-6 and n-3 polyunsaturated fatty acids: From biochemistry to clinical implications in cardiovascular prevention. *Biochem. Pharmacol.* **2009**, *77*, 937–946. [CrossRef] [PubMed]
77. Gerber, M. Omega-3 fatty acids and cancers: A systematic update review of epidemiological studies. *Br. J. Nutr.* **2012**, *107*, S228–S239. [CrossRef] [PubMed]
78. Mokbel, K.; Mokbel, K. Chemoprevention of breast cancer with vitamins and micronutrients: A concise review. *In Vivo* **2019**, *33*, 983–997. [CrossRef] [PubMed]
79. Yang, B.; Ren, X.L.; Fu, Y.Q.; Gao, J.L.; Li, D. Ratio of n-3/n-6 PUFAs and risk of breast cancer: A meta-analysis of 274135 adult females from 11 independent prospective studies. *BMC Cancer* **2014**, *14*, 105. [CrossRef] [PubMed]
80. Colletti, A.; Li, S.; Marengo, M.; Adinolfi, S.; Cravotto, G. Recent Advances and Insights into Bromelain Processing, Pharmacokinetics and Therapeutic Uses. *Appl. Sci.* **2021**, *11*, 8428. [CrossRef]
81. Agrawal, P.; Nikhade, P.; Patel, A.; Mankar, N.; Sedani, S. Bromelain: A Potent Phytomedicine. *Cureus* **2022**, *14*, e27876. [CrossRef] [PubMed]
82. Pezzani, R.; Jiménez-Garcia, M.; Capó, X.; Sönmez Gürer, E.; Sharopov, F.; Rachel, T.Y.L.; Ntieche Woutouoba, D.; Rescigno, A.; Peddio, S.; Zucca, P.; et al. Anticancer properties of bromelain: State-of-the-art and recent trends. *Front. Oncol.* **2023**, *12*, 1068778. [CrossRef] [PubMed]
83. Chobotova, K.; Vernallis, A.B.; Majid, F.A. Bromelain's activity and potential as an anti-cancer agent: Current evidence and perspectives. *Cancer Lett.* **2010**, *290*, 148–156. [CrossRef]
84. Ramli, A.N.; Aznan, T.N.; Illias, R.M. Bromelain: From production to commercialisation. *J. Sci. Food Agric.* **2017**, *97*, 1386–1395. [CrossRef]
85. Chakraborty, A.J.; Mitra, S.; Tallei, T.E.; Tareq, A.M.; Nainu, F.; Cicia, D.; Dhama, K.; Emran, T.B.; Simal-Gandara, J.; Capasso, R. Bromelain a Potential Bioactive Compound: A Comprehensive Overview from a Pharmacological Perspective. *Life* **2021**, *11*, 317. [CrossRef]
86. De Lencastre Novaes, L.C.; Jozala, A.F.; Lopes, A.M.; de Carvalho Santos-Ebinuma, V.; Mazzola, P.G.; Pessoa Junior, A. Stability, purification, and applications of bromelain: A review. *Biotechnol. Prog.* **2016**, *32*, 5–13. [CrossRef] [PubMed]
87. Pavan, R.; Jain, S.; Shraddha Kumar, A. Properties and therapeutic application of bromelain: A review. *Biotechnol. Res. Int.* **2012**, *2012*, 976203. [CrossRef] [PubMed]
88. Varilla, C.; Marcone, M.; Paiva, L.; Baptista, J. Bromelain, a Group of Pineapple Proteolytic Complex Enzymes (*Ananas comosus*) and Their Possible Therapeutic and Clinical Effects. A Summary. *Foods* **2021**, *10*, 2249. [CrossRef] [PubMed]
89. Rajan, P.K.; Dunna, N.R.; Venkatabalasubramanian, S. A comprehensive overview on the anti-inflammatory, antitumor, and ferroptosis functions of bromelain: An emerging cysteine protease. *Expert. Opin. Biol. Ther.* **2022**, *22*, 615–625. [CrossRef] [PubMed]
90. Kumar, V.; Mangla, B.; Javed, S.; Ahsan, W.; Kumar, P.; Garg, V.; Dureja, H. Bromelain: A review of its mechanisms, pharmacological effects and potential applications. *Food Funct.* **2023**, *14*, 8101–8128. [CrossRef] [PubMed]
91. Rathnavelu, V.; Alitheen, N.B.; Sohila, S.; Kanagesan, S.; Ramesh, R. Potential role of bromelain in clinical and therapeutic applications. *Biomed. Rep.* **2016**, *5*, 283–288. [CrossRef] [PubMed]
92. Greten, F.R.; Grivennikov, S.I. Inflammation and Cancer: Triggers, Mechanisms, and Consequences. *Immunity* **2019**, *51*, 27–41. [CrossRef] [PubMed]
93. Anderson, N.M.; Simon, M.C. The tumor microenvironment. *Curr. Biol.* **2020**, *30*, R921–R925. [CrossRef]
94. Engwerda, C.R.; Andrew, D.; Ladhams, A.; Mynott, T.L. Bromelain modulates T cell and B cell immune responses in vitro and in vivo. *Cell Immunol.* **2001**, *210*, 66–75. [CrossRef]
95. Huang, J.R.; Wu, C.C.; Hou, R.C.; Jeng, K.C. Bromelain inhibits lipopolysaccharide-induced cytokine production in human THP-1 monocytes via the removal of CD14. *Immunol. Investig.* **2008**, *37*, 263–277. [CrossRef]
96. Bhui, K.; Prasad, S.; George, J.; Shukla, Y. Bromelain inhibits COX-2 expression by blocking the activation of MAPK regulated NF-kappa B against skin tumor-initiation triggering mitochondrial death pathway. *Cancer Lett.* **2009**, *282*, 167–176. [CrossRef]
97. Lee, J.-H.; Lee, J.-B.; Lee, J.-T.; Park, H.-R.; Kim, J.-B. Medicinal Effects of Bromelain (*Ananas comosus*) Targeting Oral Environment as an Anti-oxidant and Anti-inflammatory Agent. *J. Food Nutr. Res.* **2018**, *6*, 773–784. [CrossRef]
98. Kasemsuk, T.; Vivithanaporn, P.; Unchern, S. Anti-inflammatory effects of bromelain in Lps-induced human U937 macrophages. *Chiang Mai J. Sci.* **2018**, *45*, 299–307.
99. Raeisi, F.; Raeisi, E.; Heidarian, E.; Shahbazi-Gahroui, D.; Lemoigne, Y. Bromelain inhibitory effect on colony formation: An in vitro study on human AGS, PC3, and MCF7 cancer cells. *J. Med. Signals Sens.* **2019**, *9*, 267–273. [CrossRef]
100. Yin, Y.; Wang, S.; Sun, Y.; Matt, Y.; Colburn, N.H.; Shu, Y.; Han, X. JNK/AP-1 pathway is involved in tumor necrosis factor-alpha induced expression of vascular endothelial growth factor in MCF7 cells. *Biomed. Pharmacother.* **2009**, *63*, 429–435. [CrossRef] [PubMed]
101. Jin, K.; Qian, C.; Lin, J.; Liu, B. Cyclooxygenase-2-Prostaglandin E2 pathway: A key player in tumor-associated immune cells. *Front. Oncol.* **2023**, *13*, 1099811. [CrossRef] [PubMed]
102. Hale, L.P.; Greer, P.K.; Sempowski, G.D. Bromelain treatment alters leukocyte expression of cell surface molecules involved in cellular adhesion and activation. *Clin. Immunol.* **2002**, *104*, 183–190. [CrossRef] [PubMed]

103. Fitzhugh, D.J.; Shan, S.; Dewhirst, M.W.; Hale, L.P. Bromelain treatment decreases neutrophil migration to sites of inflammation. *Clin. Immunol.* **2008**, *128*, 66–74. [CrossRef] [PubMed]
104. Secor, E.R., Jr.; Singh, A.; Guernsey, L.A.; McNamara, J.T.; Zhan, L.; Maulik, N.; Thrall, R.S. Bromelain treatment reduces CD25 expression on activated CD4+ T cells in vitro. *Int. Immunopharmacol.* **2009**, *9*, 340–346. [CrossRef]
105. Fouz, N.; Amid, A.; Hashim, Y.Z. Cytokinetic study of MCF-7 cells treated with commercial and recombinant bromelain. *Asian Pac. J. Cancer Prev.* **2014**, *14*, 6709–6714. [CrossRef]
106. Oliveira, C.P.; Prado, W.A.; Lavayen, V.; Büttenbender, S.L.; Beckenkamp, A.; Martins, B.S.; Lüdtke, D.S.; Campo, L.F.; Rodembusch, F.S.; Buffon, A.; et al. Bromelainfunctionalized multiple-wall lipid-core nanocapsules: Formulation, chemical structure and antiproliferative effect against human breast cancer cells (MCF-7). *Pharm. Res.* **2017**, *34*, 438–452. [CrossRef] [PubMed]
107. Raeisi, E.; Aazami, M.H.; Aghamiri, S.M.; Satari, A.; Hosseinzadeh, S.; Lemoigne, Y.; Esfandiar, H. Bromelain-based chemo-herbal combination effect on human cancer cells: In-vitro study on AGS and MCF7 proliferation and apoptosis. *Curr. Issues Pharm. Med. Sci.* **2020**, *33*, 155–161. [CrossRef]
108. Karimian Rad, F.; Ramezani, M.; Mohammadgholi, A. Physicochemical properties of bromelain adsorption on magnetic carbon nanoparticles and in vitro cytotoxicity on breast cancer cells. *Herb. Med. J.* **2020**, *5*, 153–162.
109. Pauzi, A.Z.; Yeap, S.K.; Abu, N.; Lim, K.L.; Omar, A.R.; Aziz, S.A.; Chow, A.L.; Subramani, T.; Tan, S.G.; Alitheen, N.B. Combination of cisplatin and bromelain exerts synergistic cytotoxic effects against breast cancer cell line MDA-MB-231 in vitro. *Chin. Med.* **2016**, *11*, 46. [CrossRef]
110. Bhui, K.; Tyagi, S.; Prakash, B.; Shukla, Y. Pineapple bromelain induces autophagy, facilitating apoptotic response in mammary carcinoma cells. *Biofactors* **2010**, *36*, 474–482. [CrossRef] [PubMed]
111. Bhatnagar, P.; Patnaik, S.; Srivastava, A.K.; Mudiam, M.K.; Shukla, Y.; Panda, A.K.; Pant, A.B.; Kumar, P.; Gupta, K.C. Anti-cancer activity of bromelain nanoparticles by oral administration. *J. Biomed. Nanotechnol.* **2014**, *10*, 3558–3575. [CrossRef] [PubMed]
112. Haiyan, S.; Funing, M.; Keming, L.; Wei, S.; Guiying, X.; Rulin, Z.; Shenghe, C. Growth of breast cancer cells inhibited by bromelains extracted from the different tissues of pineapple. *Folia Biol.* **2020**, *68*, 81–88. [CrossRef]
113. Dhandayuthapani, S.; Perez, H.D.; Paroulek, A.; Chinnakkannu, P.; Kandalam, U.; Jaffe, M.; Rathinavelu, A. Bromelain-induced apoptosis in GI-101A breast cancer cells. *J. Med. Food* **2012**, *15*, 344–349. [CrossRef] [PubMed]
114. Mekkawy, M.H.; Fahmy, H.A.; Nada, A.S.; Ali, O.S. Radiosensitizing effect of bromelain using tumor mice model via Ki-67 and PARP-1 inhibition. *Integr. Cancer Ther.* **2021**, *20*, 15347354211060369. [CrossRef]
115. Gao, L.; Loveless, J.; Shay, C.; Teng, Y. Targeting ROS-Mediated Crosstalk Between Autophagy and Apoptosis in Cancer. *Adv. Exp. Med. Biol.* **2020**, *1260*, 1–12.
116. Slavin, J.L.; Lloyd, B. Health benefits of fruits and vegetables. *Adv. Nutr.* **2012**, *3*, 506–516. [CrossRef] [PubMed]
117. Saavedra-Leos, M.Z.; Jordan-Alejandre, E.; Puente-Rivera, J.; Silva-Cázares, M.B. Molecular pathways related to sulforaphane as adjuvant treatment: A nanomedicine perspective in breast cancer. *Medicina* **2022**, *58*, 1377. [CrossRef] [PubMed]
118. Kaboli, P.J.; Khoshkbejari, M.A.; Mohammadi, M.; Abiri, A.; Mokhtarian, R.; Vazifemand, R.; Xiao, Z. Targets and mechanisms of sulforaphane derivatives obtained from cruciferous plants with special focus on breast cancer–contradictory effects and future perspectives. *Biomed. Pharmacother.* **2020**, *121*, 109635.
119. Halkier, B.A.; Gershenzon, J. Biology and biochemistry of glucosinolates. *Annu. Rev. Plant Biol.* **2006**, *57*, 303–333. [CrossRef] [PubMed]
120. Kissen, R.; Rossiter, J.T.; Bones, A.M. The 'mustard oil bomb': Not so easy to assemble? Localization, expression and distribution of the components of the myrosinase enzyme system. *Phytochem. Rev.* **2009**, *8*, 69–86. [CrossRef]
121. Zhang, S.; Ying, D.Y.; Cheng, L.J.; Bayrak, M.; Jegasothy, H.; Sanguansri, L.; Augustin, M.A. Sulforaphane in broccoli-based matrices: Effects of heat treatment and addition of oil. *LWT* **2020**, *128*, 109443. [CrossRef]
122. Hopkins, R.J.; van Dam, N.M.; van Loon, J.J. Role of glucosinolates in insect-plant relationships and multitrophic interactions. *Annu. Rev. Entomol.* **2009**, *54*, 57–83. [CrossRef] [PubMed]
123. Yagishita, Y.; Fahey, J.W.; Dinkova-Kostova, A.T.; Kensler, T.W. Broccoli or sulforaphane: Is it the source or dose that matters? *Molecules* **2019**, *24*, 3593. [CrossRef]
124. Farnham, M.W.; Stephenson, K.K.; Fahey, J.W. Glucoraphanin level in broccoli seed is largely determined by genotype. *Hortic. Sci.* **2005**, *40*, 50–53. [CrossRef]
125. Conaway, C.C.; Getahun, S.M.; Liebes, L.L.; Pusateri, D.J.; Topham, D.K.; Botero-Omary, M.; Chung, F.L. Disposition of glucosinolates and sulforaphane in humans after ingestion of steamed and fresh broccoli. *Nutr. Cancer* **2000**, *38*, 168–178. [CrossRef]
126. Vermeulen, M.; Klöpping-Ketelaars, I.W.; van den Berg, R.; Vaes, W.H. Bioavailability and kinetics of sulforaphane in humans after consumption of cooked versus raw broccoli. *J. Agric. Food Chem.* **2008**, *56*, 10505–10509. [CrossRef] [PubMed]
127. Wang, Z.; Kwan, M.L.; Pratt, R.; Roh, J.M.; Kushi, L.H.; Danforth, K.N.; Zhang, Y.; Ambrosone, C.B.; Tang, L. Effects of cooking methods on total isothiocyanate yield from cruciferous vegetables. *Food Sci. Nutr.* **2020**, *8*, 5673–5682. [CrossRef] [PubMed]
128. Oloyede, O.O.; Wagstaff, C.; Methven, L. The impact of domestic cooking methods on myrosinase stability, glucosinolates and their hydrolysis products in different cabbage (*Brassica oleracea*) accessions. *Foods* **2021**, *10*, 2908. [CrossRef]
129. Dosz, E.B.; Jeffery, E.H. Commercially produced frozen broccoli lacks the ability to form sulforaphane. *J. Funct. Foods* **2013**, *5*, 987–990. [CrossRef]

130. Bricker, G.V.; Riedl, K.M.; Ralston, R.A.; Tober, K.L.; Oberyszyn, T.M.; Schwartz, S.J. Isothiocyanate metabolism, distribution, and interconversion in mice following consumption of thermally processed broccoli sprouts or purified sulforaphane. *Mol. Nutr. Food Res.* **2014**, *58*, 1991–2000. [CrossRef] [PubMed]
131. Atwell, L.L.; Hsu, A.; Wong, C.P.; Stevens, J.F.; Bella, D.; Yu, T.W.; Ho, E. Absorption and chemopreventive targets of sulforaphane in humans following consumption of broccoli sprouts or a myrosinase-treated broccoli sprout extract. *Mol. Nutr. Food Res.* **2015**, *59*, 424–433. [CrossRef]
132. Sikorska-Zimny, K.; Beneduce, L. The Metabolism of Glucosinolates by Gut Microbiota. *Nutrients* **2021**, *13*, 2750. [CrossRef]
133. Treasure, K.; Harris, J.; Williamson, G. Exploring the anti-inflammatory activity of sulforaphane. *Immunol. Cell Biol.* **2023**, *101*, 805–828. [CrossRef]
134. Licznerska, B.; Szaefer, H.; Krajka-Kuźniak, V. R-sulforaphane modulates the expression profile of AhR, ERα, Nrf2, NQO1, and GSTP in human breast cell lines. *Mol. Cell Biochem.* **2021**, *476*, 525–533. [CrossRef]
135. Soundararajan, P.; Kim, J.S. Anti-carcinogenic glucosinolates in cruciferous vegetables and their antagonistic effects on prevention of cancers. *Molecules* **2018**, *23*, 2983. [CrossRef]
136. Kim, S.H.; Park, H.J.; Moon, D.O. Sulforaphane sensitizes human breast cancer cells to paclitaxel-induced apoptosis by downregulating the NF-κB signaling pathway. *Oncol. Lett.* **2017**, *13*, 4427–4432. [CrossRef] [PubMed]
137. Hunakova, L.; Sedlakova, O.; Cholujova, D.; Gronesova, P.; Duraj, J.; Sedlak, J. Modulation of markers associated with aggressive phenotype in MDA-MB-231 breast carcinoma cells by sulforaphane. *Neoplasma* **2009**, *56*, 548. [CrossRef] [PubMed]
138. Xu, Y.; Han, X.; Li, Y.; Min, H.; Zhao, X.; Zhang, Y.; Qi, Y.; Shi, J.; Qi, S.; Bao, Y.; et al. Sulforaphane Mediates Glutathione Depletion via Polymeric Nanoparticles to Restore Cisplatin Chemosensitivity. *ACS Nano.* **2019**, *13*, 13445–13455. [CrossRef] [PubMed]
139. Rong, Y.; Huang, L.; Yi, K.; Chen, H.; Liu, S.; Zhang, W.; Wang, F. Co-administration of sulforaphane and doxorubicin attenuates breast cancer growth by preventing the accumulation of myeloid-derived suppressor cells. *Cancer Lett.* **2020**, *493*, 189–196. [CrossRef] [PubMed]
140. Keshandehghan, A.; Nikkhah, S.; Tahermansouri, H.; Heidari-Keshel, S.; Gardaneh, M. Co-treatment with sulforaphane and nano-metformin molecules accelerates apoptosis in HER2+ breast cancer cells by inhibiting key molecules. *Nutr. Cancer* **2020**, *72*, 835–848. [CrossRef] [PubMed]
141. Pogorzelska, A.; Mazur, M.; Światalska, M.; Wietrzyk, J.; Sigorski, D.; Fronczyk, K.; Wiktorska, K. Anticancer effect and safety of doxorubicin and nutraceutical sulforaphane liposomal formulation in triple-negative breast cancer (TNBC) animal model. *Biomed. Pharmacother.* **2023**, *161*, 114490. [CrossRef]
142. Kanematsu, S.; Uehara, N.; Miki, H.; Yoshizawa, K.; Kawanaka, A.; Yuri, T.; Tsubura, A. Autophagy inhibition enhances sulforaphane-induced apoptosis in human breast cancer cells. *Anticancer. Res.* **2010**, *30*, 3381–3390. [PubMed]
143. Lewinska, A.; Adamczyk-Grochala, J.; Deregowska, A.; Wnuk, M. Sulforaphane-Induced Cell Cycle Arrest and Senescence are accompanied by DNA Hypomethylation and Changes in microRNA Profile in Breast Cancer Cells. *Theranostics* **2017**, *7*, 3461–3477. [CrossRef]
144. Cao, W.; Lu, X.; Zhong, C.; Wu, J. Sulforaphane suppresses MCF-7 breast cancer cells growth via miR-19/PTEN axis to antagonize the effect of butyl benzyl phthalate. *Nutr. Cancer* **2023**, *75*, 980–991. [CrossRef]
145. Carnero, A.; Blanco-Aparicio, C.; Renner, O.; Link, W.; Leal, J.F. The PTEN/PI3K/AKT signalling pathway in cancer, therapeutic implications. *Curr. Cancer Drug Targets* **2008**, *8*, 187–198. [CrossRef]
146. Castro, N.P.; Rangel, M.C.; Merchant, A.S.; MacKinnon, G.; Cuttitta, F.; Salomon, D.S.; Kim, Y.S. Sulforaphane suppresses the growth of triple-negative breast cancer stem-like cells in vitro and in vivo. *Cancer Prev. Res.* **2019**, *12*, 147–158. [CrossRef] [PubMed]
147. Su, X.; Jiang, X.; Meng, L.; Dong, X.; Shen, Y.; Xin, Y. Anticancer activity of sulforaphane: The epigenetic mechanisms and the Nrf2 signaling pathway. *Oxid. Med. Cell Longev.* **2018**, *2018*, 5438179. [CrossRef]
148. Nandini, D.B.; Rao, R.S.; Deepak, B.S.; Reddy, P.B. Sulforaphane in broccoli: The green chemoprevention!! Role in cancer prevention and therapy. *J. Oral Maxillofac. Pathol.* **2020**, *24*, 405. [CrossRef]
149. Meeran, S.M.; Patel, S.N.; Tollefsbol, T.O. Sulforaphane causes epigenetic repression of hTERT expression in human breast cancer cell lines. *PLoS ONE* **2010**, *5*, e11457. [CrossRef]
150. Li, Y.; Buckhaults, P.; Li, S.; Tollefsbol, T. Temporal Efficacy of a Sulforaphane-Based Broccoli Sprout Diet in Prevention of Breast Cancer through Modulation of Epigenetic Mechanisms. *Cancer Prev. Res.* **2018**, *11*, 451–464. [CrossRef]
151. Amarakoon, D.; Lee, W.J.; Tamia, G.; Lee, S.H. Indole-3-Carbinol: Occurrence, Health-Beneficial Properties, and Cellular/Molecular Mechanisms. *Annu. Rev. Food Sci. Technol.* **2023**, *14*, 347–366. [CrossRef] [PubMed]
152. Williams, D.E. Indoles Derived from Glucobrassicin: Cancer Chemoprevention by Indole-3-Carbinol and 3,3′-Diindolylmethane. *Front. Nutr.* **2021**, *8*, 734334. [CrossRef] [PubMed]
153. Ampofo, E.; Lachnitt, N.; Rudzitis-Auth, J.; Schmitt, B.M.; Menger, M.D.; Laschke, M.W. Indole-3-carbinol is a potent inhibitor of ischemia-reperfusion-induced inflammation. *J. Surg. Res.* **2017**, *215*, 34–46. [CrossRef]
154. Khan, A.S.; Langmann, T. Indole-3-carbinol regulates microglia homeostasis and protects the retina from degeneration. *J. Neuroinflamm.* **2020**, *17*, 327. [CrossRef]
155. Prado, N.J.; Ramirez, D.; Mazzei, L.; Parra, M.; Casarotto, M.; Calvo, J.P.; Cuello Carrión, D.; Ponce Zumino, A.Z.; Diez, E.R.; Camargo, A.; et al. Anti-inflammatory, antioxidant, anti-hypertensive, and antiarrhythmic effect of indole-3-carbinol, a phytochemical derived from cruciferous vegetables. *Heliyon* **2022**, *8*, e08989. [CrossRef]

156. Peng, C.; Wu, C.; Xu, X.; Pan, L.; Lou, Z.; Zhao, Y.; Jiang, H.; He, Z.; Ruan, B. Indole-3-carbinol ameliorates necroptosis and inflammation of intestinal epithelial cells in mice with ulcerative colitis by activating aryl hydrocarbon receptor. *Exp. Cell Res.* **2021**, *404*, 112638. [CrossRef] [PubMed]
157. Qian, C.; Yang, C.; Lu, M.; Bao, J.; Shen, H.; Deng, B.; Li, S.; Li, W.; Zhang, M.; Cao, C. Activating AhR alleviates cognitive deficits of Alzheimer's disease model mice by upregulating endogenous Aβ catabolic enzyme neprilysin. *Theranostics* **2021**, *11*, 8797–8812. [CrossRef] [PubMed]
158. Mohamad, K.A.; El-Naga, R.N.; Wahdan, S.A. Neuroprotective effects of indole-3-carbinol on the rotenone rat model of Parkinson's disease: Impact of the SIRT1-AMPK signaling pathway. *Toxicol. Appl. Pharmacol.* **2022**, *435*, 115853. [CrossRef] [PubMed]
159. Saini, N.; Akhtar, A.; Chauhan, M.; Dhingra, N.; Pilkhwal Sah, S. Protective effect of indole-3-carbinol, an NF-κB inhibitor in experimental paradigm of Parkinson's disease: In silico and in vivo studies. *Brain Behav. Immun.* **2020**, *90*, 108–137. [CrossRef] [PubMed]
160. Lian, J.P.; Word, B.; Taylor, S.; Hammons, G.J.; Lyn-Cook, B.D. Modulation of the constitutive activated STAT3 transcription factor in pancreatic cancer prevention: Effects of indole-3-carbinol (I3C) and genistein. *Anticancer. Res.* **2004**, *24*, 133–137. [PubMed]
161. Adler, S.; Rashid, G.; Klein, A. Indole-3-carbinol inhibits telomerase activity and gene expression in prostate cancer cell lines. *Anticancer. Res.* **2011**, *31*, 3733–3737. [PubMed]
162. Megna, B.W.; Carney, P.R.; Nukaya, M.; Geiger, P.; Kennedy, G.D. Indole-3-carbinol induces tumor cell death: Function follows form. *J. Surg. Res.* **2016**, *204*, 47–54. [CrossRef] [PubMed]
163. Lee, C.M.; Lee, J.; Nam, M.J.; Park, S.H. Indole-3-carbinol induces apoptosis in human osteosarcoma MG-63 and U2OS cells. *Biomed. Res. Int.* **2018**, *2018*, 7970618. [CrossRef] [PubMed]
164. Lee, C.M.; Park, S.H.; Nam, M.J. Anticarcinogenic effect of indole-3-carbinol (I3C) on human hepatocellular carcinoma SNU449 cells. *Hum. Exp. Toxicol.* **2019**, *38*, 136–147. [CrossRef]
165. Shertzer, H.G.; Berger, M.L.; Tabor, M.W. Intervention in free radical mediated hepatotoxicity and lipid peroxidation by indole-3-carbinol. *Biochem. Pharmacol.* **1988**, *37*, 333–338. [CrossRef]
166. Choi, Y.; Abdelmegeed, M.A.; Song, B.J. Preventive effects of indole-3-carbinol against alcohol-induced liver injury in mice via antioxidant, anti-inflammatory, and anti-apoptotic mechanisms: Role of gut-liver-adipose tissue axis. *J. Nutr. Biochem.* **2018**, *55*, 12–25. [CrossRef] [PubMed]
167. Lim, H.M.; Park, S.H.; Nam, M.J. Induction of apoptosis in indole-3-carbinol-treated lung cancer H1299 cells via ROS level elevation. *Hum. Exp. Toxicol.* **2021**, *40*, 812–825. [CrossRef] [PubMed]
168. Baez-Gonzalez, A.S.; Carrazco-Carrillo, J.A.; Figueroa-Gonzalez, G.; Quintas-Granados, L.I.; Padilla-Benavides, T.; Reyes-Hernandez, O.D. Functional effect of indole-3 carbinol in the viability and invasive properties of cultured cancer cells. *Biochem. Biophys. Rep.* **2023**, *35*, 101492. [CrossRef] [PubMed]
169. Rahman, K.M.; Li, Y.; Sarkar, F.H. Inactivation of akt and NF-kappaB play important roles during indole-3-carbinol-induced apoptosis in breast cancer cells. *Nutr. Cancer* **2004**, *48*, 84–94. [CrossRef] [PubMed]
170. Howells, L.M.; Gallacher-Horley, B.; Houghton, C.E.; Manson, M.M.; Hudson, E.A. Indole-3-carbinol inhibits protein kinase B/Akt and induces apoptosis in the human breast tumor cell line MDA MB468 but not in the nontumorigenic HBL100 line. *Mol. Cancer Ther.* **2002**, *1*, 1161–1172.
171. Cover, C.M.; Hsieh, S.J.; Tran, S.H.; Hallden, G.; Kim, G.S.; Bjeldanes, L.F.; Firestone, G.L. Indole-3-carbinol inhibits the expression of cyclin-dependent kinase-6 and induces a G1 cell cycle arrest of human breast cancer cells independent of estrogen receptor signaling. *J. Biol. Chem.* **1998**, *273*, 3838–3847. [CrossRef] [PubMed]
172. Cram, E.J.; Liu, B.D.; Bjeldanes, L.F.; Firestone, G.L. Indole-3-carbinol inhibits CDK6 expression in human MCF-7 breast cancer cells by disrupting Sp1 transcription factor interactions with a composite element in the CDK6 gene promoter. *J. Biol. Chem.* **2001**, *276*, 22332–22340. [CrossRef] [PubMed]
173. Firestone, G.L.; Bjeldanes, L.F. Indole-3-carbinol and 3-3′-diindolylmethane antiproliferative signaling pathways control cell-cycle gene transcription in human breast cancer cells by regulating promoter-Sp1 transcription factor interactions. *J. Nutr.* **2003**, *133* (Suppl. 7), 2448S–2455S. [CrossRef]
174. Cover, C.M.; Hsieh, S.J.; Cram, E.J.; Hong, C.; Riby, J.E.; Bjeldanes, L.F.; Firestone, G.L. Indole-3-carbinol and tamoxifen cooperate to arrest the cell cycle of MCF-7 human breast cancer cells. *Cancer Res.* **1999**, *59*, 1244–1251.
175. Hajra, S.; Patra, A.R.; Basu, A.; Saha, P.; Bhattacharya, S. Indole-3-Carbinol (I3C) enhances the sensitivity of murine breast adenocarcinoma cells to doxorubicin (DOX) through inhibition of NF-κβ, blocking angiogenesis and regulation of mitochondrial apoptotic pathway. *Chem. Biol. Interact.* **2018**, *290*, 19–36. [CrossRef]
176. Wang, X.; Zhang, L.; Dai, Q.; Si, H.; Zhang, L.; Eltom, S.E.; Si, H. Combined Luteolin and Indole-3-Carbinol Synergistically Constrains ERα-Positive Breast Cancer by Dual Inhibiting Estrogen Receptor Alpha and Cyclin-Dependent Kinase 4/6 Pathway in Cultured Cells and Xenograft Mice. *Cancers* **2021**, *13*, 2116. [CrossRef] [PubMed]
177. Rahman, K.M.; Aranha, O.; Sarkar, F.H. Indole-3-carbinol (I3C) induces apoptosis in tumorigenic but not in nontumorigenic breast epithelial cells. *Nutr. Cancer* **2003**, *45*, 101–112. [CrossRef] [PubMed]
178. Caruso, J.A.; Campana, R.; Wei, C.; Su, C.H.; Hanks, A.M.; Bornmann, W.G.; Keyomarsi, K. Indole-3-carbinol and its N-alkoxy derivatives preferentially target ERα-positive breast cancer cells. *Cell Cycle* **2014**, *13*, 2587–2599. [CrossRef] [PubMed]
179. Safe, S. Molecular biology of the Ah receptor and its role in carcinogenesis. *Toxicol. Lett.* **2001**, *120*, 1–7. [CrossRef] [PubMed]

180. Chen, I.; McDougal, A.; Wang, F.; Safe, S. Aryl hydrocarbon receptor-mediated antiestrogenic and antitumorigenic activity of diindolylmethane. *Carcinogenesis* **1998**, *19*, 1631–1639. [CrossRef] [PubMed]
181. Weng, J.R.; Tsai, C.H.; Kulp, S.K.; Chen, C.S. Indole-3-carbinol as a chemopreventive and anti-cancer agent. *Cancer Lett.* **2008**, *262*, 153–163. [CrossRef] [PubMed]
182. Larigot, L.; Juricek, L.; Dairou, J.; Coumoul, X. AhR signaling pathways and regulatory functions. *Biochim. Open* **2018**, *7*, 1–9. [CrossRef] [PubMed]
183. Saito, N.; Kanno, Y.; Yamashita, N.; Degawa, M.; Yoshinari, K.; Nemoto, K. The Differential Selectivity of Aryl Hydrocarbon Receptor (AHR) Agonists towards AHR-Dependent Suppression of Mammosphere Formation and Gene Transcription in Human Breast Cancer Cells. *Biol. Pharm. Bull.* **2021**, *44*, 571–578. [CrossRef] [PubMed]
184. National Toxicology Program. Toxicology studies of indole-3-carbinol in F344/N rats and B6C3F1/N mice and toxicology and carcinogenesis studies of indole-3-carbinol in Harlan Sprague Dawley rats and B6C3F1/N mice (gavage studies). *Natl. Toxicol. Program. Tech. Rep. Ser.* **2017**, *584*, NTP-TR-584.
185. Hargraves, K.G.; He, L.; Firestone, G.L. Phytochemical regulation of the tumor suppressive microRNA, miR-34a, by p53-dependent and independent responses in human breast cancer cells. *Mol. Carcinog.* **2016**, *55*, 486–498. [CrossRef]
186. El-Daly, S.M.; Gamal-Eldeen, A.M.; Gouhar, S.A.; Abo-Elfadl, M.T.; El-Saeed, G. Modulatory Effect of Indoles on the Expression of miRNAs Regulating G1/S Cell Cycle Phase in Breast Cancer Cells. *Appl. Biochem. Biotechnol.* **2020**, *192*, 1208–1223. [CrossRef] [PubMed]
187. Nouri Emamzadeh, F.; Word, B.; Cotton, E.; Hawkins, A.; Littlejohn, K.; Moore, R.; Miranda-Carbon, G.; Orish, C.N.; Lyn-Cook, B. Modulation of Estrogen α and Progesterone Receptors in Triple Negative Breast Cancer Cell Lines: The Effects of Vorinostat and Indole-3-Carbinol In Vitro. *Anticancer. Res.* **2020**, *40*, 3669–3683. [CrossRef] [PubMed]
188. Grose, K.R.; Bjeldanes, L.F. Oligomerization of indole-3-carbinol in aqueous acid. *Chem. Res. Toxicol.* **1992**, *5*, 188–193. [CrossRef] [PubMed]
189. Luo, Y.; Wang, T.T.; Teng, Z.; Chen, P.; Sun, J.; Wang, Q. Encapsulation of indole-3-carbinol and 3,3′-diindolylmethane in zein/carboxymethyl chitosan nanoparticles with controlled release property and improved stability. *Food Chem.* **2013**, *139*, 224–230. [CrossRef] [PubMed]
190. Gehrcke, M.; Giuliani, L.M.; Ferreira, L.M.; Barbieri, A.V.; Sari, M.H.M.; da Silveira, E.F.; Azambuja, J.H.; Nogueira, C.W.; Braganhol, E.; Cruz, L. Enhanced photostability, radical scavenging and antitumor activity of indole-3-carbinol-loaded rose hip oil nanocapsules. *Mat. Sci. Eng. C-Mater* **2017**, *74*, 279–286. [CrossRef] [PubMed]
191. Reed, G.A.; Arneson, D.W.; Putnam, W.C.; Smith, H.J.; Gray, J.C.; Sullivan, D.K.; Mayo, M.S.; Crowell, J.A.; Hurwitz, A. Single-dose and multiple-dose administration of indole-3-carbinol to women: Pharmacokinetics based on 3,3′-diindolylmethan. *Cancer Epidemiol. Biomark. Prev.* **2006**, *15*, 2477–2481. [CrossRef] [PubMed]
192. Ge, X.; Yannai, S.; Rennert, G.; Gruener, N.; Fares, F.A. 3,3′-Diindolylmethane induces apoptosis in human cancer cells. *Biochem. Biophys. Res. Commun.* **1996**, *228*, 153–158. [CrossRef] [PubMed]
193. Hong, C.; Kim, H.A.; Firestone, G.L.; Bjeldanes, L.F. 3,3′-Diindolylmethane (DIM) induces a G(1) cell cycle arrest in human breast cancer cells that is accompanied by Sp1-mediated activation of p21(WAF1/CIP1) expression. *Carcinogenesis* **2002**, *23*, 1297–1305. [CrossRef] [PubMed]
194. Hong, C.; Firestone, G.L.; Bjeldanes, L.F. Bcl-2 family-mediated apoptotic effects of 3,3′-diindolylmethane (DIM) in human breast cancer cells. *Biochem. Pharmacol.* **2002**, *63*, 1085–1097. [CrossRef]
195. Rahman, K.W.; Sarkar, F.H. Inhibition of nuclear translocation of nuclear factor-{kappa}B contributes to 3,3′-diindolylmethane-induced apoptosis in breast cancer cells. *Cancer Res.* **2005**, *65*, 364–371. [CrossRef]
196. Ahmad, A.; Ali, S.; Wang, Z.; Ali, A.S.; Sethi, S.; Sakr, W.A.; Raz, A.; Rahman, K.M. 3,3′-Diindolylmethane enhances taxotere-induced growth inhibition of breast cancer cells through downregulation of FoxM1. *Int. J. Cancer* **2011**, *129*, 1781–1791. [CrossRef]
197. Hsu, E.L.; Chen, N.; Westbrook, A.; Wang, F.; Zhang, R.; Taylor, R.T.; Hankinson, O. CXCR4 and CXCL12 down-regulation: A novel mechanism for the chemoprotection of 3,3′-diindolylmethane for breast and ovarian cancers. *Cancer Lett.* **2008**, *265*, 113–123. [CrossRef] [PubMed]
198. Lee, J. 3,3′-Diindolylmethane Inhibits TNF-α- and TGF-β-Induced Epithelial-Mesenchymal Transition in Breast Cancer Cells. *Nutr. Cancer* **2019**, *71*, 992–1006. [CrossRef] [PubMed]
199. Gong, Y.; Sohn, H.; Xue, L.; Firestone, G.L.; Bjeldanes, L.F. 3,3′-Diindolylmethane is a novel mitochondrial H(+)-ATP synthase inhibitor that can induce p21(Cip1/Waf1) expression by induction of oxidative stress in human breast cancer cells. *Cancer Res.* **2006**, *66*, 4880–4887. [CrossRef] [PubMed]
200. Xue, L.; Firestone, G.L.; Bjeldanes, L.F. DIM stimulates IFNgamma gene expression in human breast cancer cells via the specific activation of JNK and p38 pathways. *Oncogene* **2005**, *24*, 2343–2353. [CrossRef] [PubMed]
201. Hanieh, H. Aryl hydrocarbon receptor-microRNA-212/132 axis in human breast cancer suppresses metastasis by targeting SOX4. *Mol. Cancer* **2015**, *14*, 172. [CrossRef] [PubMed]
202. Jin, Y. 3,3′-Diindolylmethane inhibits breast cancer cell growth via miR-21-mediated Cdc25A degradation. *Mol. Cell Biochem.* **2011**, *358*, 345–354. [CrossRef] [PubMed]
203. Nikulin, S.V.; Alekseev, B.Y.; Sergeeva, N.S.; Karalkin, P.A.; Nezhurina, E.K.; Kirsanova, V.A.; Sviridova, I.K.; Akhmedova, S.A.; Volchenko, N.N.; Bolotina, L.V.; et al. Breast cancer organoid model allowed to reveal potentially beneficial combinations of 3,3′-diindolylmethane and chemotherapy drugs. *Biochimie* **2020**, *179*, 217–227. [CrossRef]

204. Harakeh, S.; Akefe, I.O.; Saber, S.H.; Alamri, T.; Al-Raddadi, R.; Al-Jaouni, S.; Tashkandi, H.; Qari, M.; Moulay, M.; Aldahlawi, A.; et al. Nanoformulated 3′-diindolylmethane modulates apoptosis, migration, and angiogenesis in breast cancer cells. *Heliyon* **2023**, *10*, e23553. [CrossRef]
205. Isabella, S.; Mirunalini, S. 3,3′-Diindolylmethane-encapsulated chitosan nanoparticles accelerate molecular events during chemical carcinogen-induced mammary cancer in Sprague Dawley rats. *Breast Cancer* **2019**, *26*, 499–509. [CrossRef]

Disclaimer/Publisher's Note: The statements, opinions and data contained in all publications are solely those of the individual author(s) and contributor(s) and not of MDPI and/or the editor(s). MDPI and/or the editor(s) disclaim responsibility for any injury to people or property resulting from any ideas, methods, instructions or products referred to in the content.

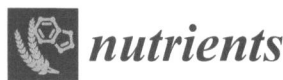

Article

Yacon (*Smallanthus sonchifolius*) Flour Reduces Inflammation and Had No Effects on Oxidative Stress and Endotoxemia in Wistar Rats with Induced Colorectal Carcinogenesis

Mariana Grancieri, Mirelle Lomar Viana, Daniela Furtado de Oliveira, Maria das Graças Vaz Tostes, Mariana Drummond Costa Ignacchiti, André Gustavo Vasconcelos Costa and Neuza Maria Brunoro Costa *

Department of Pharmacy and Nutrition, Center for Exact, Natural and Health Sciences, Federal University of Espirito Santo, Alto Universitário, S/N Guararema, Alegre 29500-000, ES, Brazil; marianagrancieri@gmail.com (M.G.); mirellelomar@gmail.com (M.L.V.); danielafdo@hotmail.com (D.F.d.O.); mgvaztostes@gmail.com (M.d.G.V.T.); marianadci@gmail.com (M.D.C.I.); agvcosta@gmail.com (A.G.V.C.)
* Correspondence: neuzambc@gmail.com

Abstract: Colorectal cancer has a high worldwide incidence. The aim of this study was to determine the effect of yacon flour (YF) on oxidative stress, inflammation, and endotoxemia in rats with induced colorectal cancer (CRC). The Wistar male rats were divided and kept for 8 weeks in four groups: S (basal diet, n = 10), Y (YF flour + basal diet, n = 10), C (CRC-induced control + basal diet, n = 12), CY (CRC-induced animals + YF, n = 12). CRC was induced by intraperitoneal injections of 1,2-dimethylhydrazine (25 mg/kg body weight). Groups Y and CY received 7.5% of the prebiotic FOS from YF. The treatment with YF increased fecal secretory immunoglobulin A levels and decreased lipopolysaccharides, tumor necrosis factor alpha and interleukin-12. However, no effect was observed on the oxidative stress by the total antioxidant capacity of plasma, anion superoxide, and nitric oxide analysis of the animals (p < 0.05). The short-chain fatty acids acetate, propionate, and butyrate showed interactions with NF-κB, TLR4, iNOS, and NADPH oxidase by in silico analysis and had a correlation (by the Person analysis) with CRC markers. The yacon flour treatment reduced the inflammation in rats with induced CRC, and could be a promising food to reduce the damages caused by colorectal cancer.

Keywords: prebiotics; yacon; endotoxemia; immune system; in silico; TNF-α

Citation: Grancieri, M.; Viana, M.L.; de Oliveira, D.F.; Vaz Tostes, M.d.G.; Costa Ignacchiti, M.D.; Costa, A.G.V.; Brunoro Costa, N.M. Yacon (*Smallanthus sonchifolius*) Flour Reduces Inflammation and Had No Effects on Oxidative Stress and Endotoxemia in Wistar Rats with Induced Colorectal Carcinogenesis. *Nutrients* **2023**, *15*, 3281. https://doi.org/10.3390/nu15143281

Academic Editor: Jacqueline Isaura Alvarez-Leite

Received: 12 June 2023
Revised: 17 July 2023
Accepted: 19 July 2023
Published: 24 July 2023

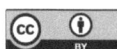

Copyright: © 2023 by the authors. Licensee MDPI, Basel, Switzerland. This article is an open access article distributed under the terms and conditions of the Creative Commons Attribution (CC BY) license (https://creativecommons.org/licenses/by/4.0/).

1. Introduction

Colorectal cancer (CRC) has been associated with increased cancer-related mortality, since it the second cause of cancer-related death in the world [1]. Most cases of CRC are classified as sporadic, which involves mutations in the adenomatous polyposis gene, DNA hypomethylation, and multiple epigenetic changes. However, besides genetic factors, environmental and lifestyle risk factors are also involved [2]. Furthermore, genetic, pharmacological, and epidemiological data information showed an association between inflammation and CRC, contributing to its progression and development [3,4].

The intestine is constituted by some physical and immunological barriers that protect its integrity, which include epithelial cells that isolate the intestinal microbiota from the deeper gut tissue, as well as mucus, and immunoglobulin A (IgA). These factors prevent pathogens from translocating to blood circulation, which could start an inflammatory cascade, leading to chronic inflammation and the development of diseases, such as CRC [5]. However, in the presence of cancer cells, when the CRC has already taken hold, the inflamed colorectal epithelial cells do not constitute an effective barrier, allowing for the entrance of bacteria and their derivatives, such as lipopolysaccharides (LPS). LPS is the main constituent of the cell membrane of Gram-negative bacteria and acts as an endotoxin. LPS can bind with the Toll-like receptor 4 (TLR4), which leads to the activation of many downstream Mitogen-Activated Protein Kinases (MAPK), of which can induce cell proliferation, apoptosis, and adhesion, and induce the activation of the nuclear factor-kappa B (NF-κB) signal pathway [6]. NF-κB acts as a transcription factor responsible for the production of many pro-inflammatory cytokines, such as tumor necrosis factor alpha (TNF-α), interleukin-12 (IL-12), and IL-6 [2,6]; these increase the inflammatory process that increases and feeds the carcinogenesis process, forming a loop.

Together with the high inflammation levels, cancer cells generate more reactive oxygen species (ROS), such as superoxide (O_2^-), hydroxyl radical (·OH), and hydrogen peroxide (H_2O_2), than normal cells. In general, a higher ROS level occurs in most cancer cells and their overproduction can intensify inflammation and intestinal barrier dysfunction, allowing for the translocation of bacteria and toxins. Furthermore, ROS production can drive cell injury and apoptosis by alterations in lipids, proteins, and DNA, and is a major cause of tumorigenesis [1,7].

The oxidative stress, as well as inflammation, may be regulated by some nutritional components [8]. Furthermore, there is a large amount of evidence stating that dairy products, whole grains, and dietary fiber consumption have a protective effect against CRC development [9]. Yacon (*Smallanthus sonchifolius*) is an Andean root that contains 40% to 70% of fructooligosaccharides (FOS) (dry matter), which is considered a prebiotic and is associated with CRC prevention [10,11].

It has been demonstrated that treatment with yacon flour increases the short-chain fatty acid (SCFA) levels, improves the intestine architecture, reduces aberrant crypts focus in rats with CRC [11–13] and also reduces the intestinal permeability and luminal pH [11,14]. Furthermore, rats with CRC treated with yacon flour for 2 weeks were able to increase their fecal IgA levels [15]. Therefore, the use of rats in this experimental model is well established; the immunological benefits of yacon intake have been demonstrated in other studies, in which serum anti-inflammatory cytokines, such as interleukin (IL)-10 and IL-4, were increased [16,17], and pro-inflammatory cytokines, such as interferon γ (IFNγ), were decreased. In addition, yacon consumption increased antioxidant enzymes [18].

Therefore, considering the positive feedback between CRC, oxidative stress and inflammation and its relationship with the malefic effects of CRC, it is necessary to establish new food alternatives to combat cancer and its complications. The aim of this study was to determine the effect of yacon flour (YF) on oxidative stress, inflammation, and endotoxemia in rats with induced colorectal cancer (CRC). Our hypothesis is that yacon flour, as a rich source of prebiotic fructooligosaccharide, can reduce inflammation, endotoxemia, and oxidative stress caused by colorectal cancer.

2. Methods and Materials

2.1. Animals and Experimental Diet

The male Wistar rats (n = 46) were from the Central Animal Breeding of the Universidade Federal do Espírito Santo, with 207 ± 5 g of initial body weight. The animals were kept in a room with control conditions (22 ± 2 °C, 12 h light–dark cycle) and water ad libitum. All the experimental procedures were performed in compliance with the ethical principles for animal experimentation, in accordance with Directive 86/609/EEC of 24 November 1986. The "Ethics Committee of Animals Use" from Universidade Federal do Espírito Santo (No. 004/2014) approved the study.

2.2. Yacon Flour Preparation and Experimental Diet

The yacon roots from Santa Maria de Jetibá, ES, Brazil, were from the same lot and prepared according to Vaz Tostes et al. [16]. All chemical analyses were performed in triplicate using the AOAC methods [19]. Moisture was determined using an oven (Nova Ética®, model 400/6 ND, São Paulo, Brazil) at 105 °C, ash by a muffle furnace (Quimis, Q320 M model, Diadema, SP, Brazil) at 550 °C, protein content by the Kjeldhal method, and lipid content through the Soxhlet method. Total dietary fiber was determined by the gravimetric–enzymatic method using a commercial kit (total dietary fiber assay kit, Sigma®,

Sigma-Aldrich, Barueri, SP, Brazil). The yacon flour calories were determined using a numerical calculation based on the macromolecule composition.

The content of FOS, inulin, and simple carbohydrates (glucose, fructose, and sucrose) in the yacon flour were identified and quantified by High Performance Liquid Chromatography (HPLC); column HPX-87p (BIO-RAD Laboratories, Santo Amaro, SP, Brazil); mobile phase: purified water [11]. The yacon flour composition is shown in Table 1.

Table 1. Composition of yacon flour (in the dry basis).

Components	Amount (g)
Non-digestible carbohydrates	
Fructooligosaccharide	52.20 ± 0.01
Inulin	6.61 ± 0.00
Other Fibers	10.68 ± 0.08
Macronutrients	
Simple Carbohydrates	
Fructose	8.16 ± 0.01
Glucose	3.76 ± 0.00
Sucrose	7.25 ± 0.01
Proteins	4.52 ± 0.25
Moisture	3.72 ± 0.51
Ash	2.94 ± 0.03
Lipids	0.33 ± 0.01

Data are presented as means ± standard deviation.

The experimental diet was based on the AIN-93M diet [20]. The diet of groups Y and CY was supplemented with 7.5% of FOS from yacon flour (14.37 g of YF/100 g of diet). Considering the yacon composition, all diets were adjusted to present analogous amounts of proteins, fibers, simple carbohydrates, and calories, so that the only additional nutrient was FOS from yacon flour (Table 2). Diets were stored (4 °C) for 15 days (maximum) to avoid FOS degradation.

Table 2. Composition of the AIN-93M diet with and without supplementation with yacon flour.

Ingredients (per kg of Diet)	S and C Groups AIN-93M	Y and CY Groups AIN-93M + YF
Casein (g)	140.0	130.14
Dextrinized starch (g)	150.5	150.5
Sucrose (g)	100.0	70.24
Soybean oil (mL)	40.0	40.0
Microcrystalline cellulose (g)	50.0	0
Minerals Mix (g)	30.5	30.5
Vitamin Mix (g)	10.0	10.0
L-cystine (g)	1.80	1.80
Choline bitartrate (g)	2.50	2.50
Corn starch (g)	474.7	423.95
Yacon flour (g)	0	140.37
Nutrition composition		
Caloric Density (kcal/g)	3.72	3.54

S = group without colon cancer induction and without yacon flour; C = group with colon cancer induction and without yacon flour; Y = group without colon cancer induction and with yacon flour; CY = group with colon cancer induction and yacon flour. YF = yacon flour.

2.3. Experimental Design

Out of 46 animals, 20 were kept healthy and 26 animals were induced to CRC through a subcutaneous injection (25 mg/kg body) of DMH (1,2-dimethylhydrazine, Sigma®) once a week for five weeks. DMH (pH 6.5) was prepared immediately before use by dissolution in NaCl (0.9%) and EDTA (15%) [21]. The subsequent 8 weeks consisted of an interval for CRC development.

At the end of the CRC induction period, in the 13th week of the experiment, two animals with CRC induction were euthanized for confirmation of aberrant crypt foci (ACF) development [22]. The other 24 animals with induced CRC were randomly divided by weight into groups C and CY, and the 20 animals without induced CRC (healthy) were randomly divided by weight into groups S and Y. Then, each group received their respective diets:

- Group S: animals without colorectal cancer induction and without yacon flour; $n = 10$
- Group Y: animals without colorectal cancer induction and with yacon flour; $n = 10$
- Group C: animals with colorectal cancer induction and without yacon flour; $n = 12$
- Group CY: animals with colorectal cancer induction and with yacon flour; $n = 12$

During the first 13 weeks (CRC-induction), all animals were fed with a basal and commercial diet (Brand: In Vivo™). In the 8 following weeks, the animals of groups S and C received the AIN-93M diet, and Y and CY groups received the AIN-93M diet with an addition of yacon flour to provide 7.5% of FOS (Grancieri et al. 2017). Each animal remained in an individual cage; they were properly identified to avoid errors between groups and animals, and all the researchers knew the identification of the animals.

At the end of experiment (22nd week), the animals were anesthetized (0.2 mL/100 g body weight) with a solution containing 37.5% ketamine, 25% xylazine, and 37.5% of the saline solution by intraperitoneal administration, and then the blood was collected by a cardiac puncture. The blood was placed in tubes with sodium heparin to obtain plasma, and in polypropylene tubes (Falcon, Fisher Scientific®, São Paulo, SP, Brazil) to evaluate the whole blood for immune analysis. The plasma was obtained by centrifugation of the blood (200× g, 10 min, 4 °C), separated from the erythrocyte part, and frozen at −80 °C. In addition, the luminal contents of the large intestines of the animals were collected and frozen at −80 °C (Figure 1).

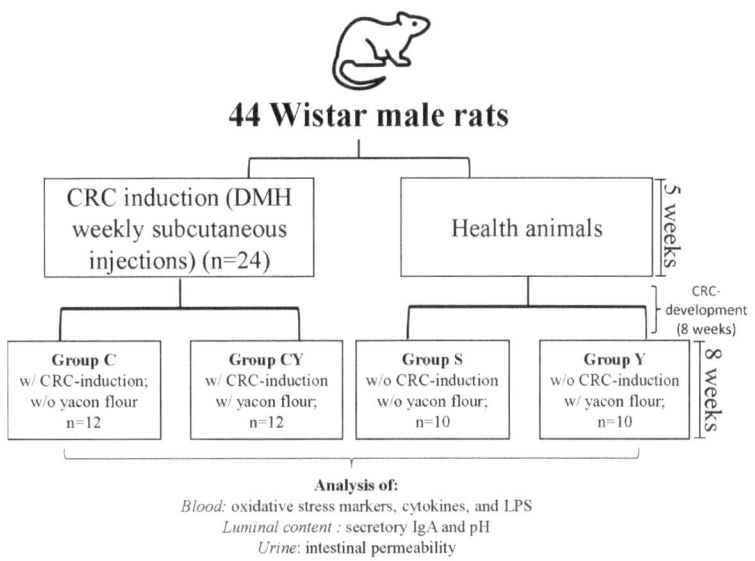

Figure 1. Experimental designer of experiment. DMH: 1,2-dimethilhydrazine; CRC: colorectal cancer; w/: with; w/o: without.

2.4. Oxidative Stress Markers

The preparation of opsonized zymozan-A and isolation of neutrophils was carried out according to Henson [23] using zymozan-A from Saccharomyces cerevisiae, which was resuspended in rat serum (from extra animals), and the concentration was adjusted to 10 mg/mL with Hanks Hepes.

The neutrophils were isolated from blood with 2.5% gelatin in PBS. The final cell concentration was adjusted to 5×10^5 cells/mL in Hanks Hepes (15 mM, pH 7.2, 0.1% gelatin). The extracellular release of superoxide anion (O_2^-) was measured by the ferrocytochrome C reduction method, considering only the inhibitory reduction by superoxide dismutase (SOD), as previously described [24]. The final suspension was read at 550 nm in length, and the resulting optical density was converted to reduced ferrocytochrome C using $\Delta E550$ nm = 2.1×10^4 $M^{-1} \cdot cm^{-1}$.

Regarding the nitric oxide production determination, 100 µL of the culture supernatant was mixed with the same volume of the Griess reagent (ref#G4410, Sigma®) and incubated at room temperature for 10–15 min [25]. Absorbance was determined at 540 nm. The NO_2^- concentration was determined using a standard curve (0.2–100 µM) of sodium nitrite ($NaNO_2$).

2.5. Secretory IgA, Endotoxemia and Total Antioxidant Capacity of Plasma

The concentration of sIgA was determined in the luminal contents of the animals' colons by the ELISA method, following the commercial kit instructions (Sigma-Aldrich®, St. Louis, MO, USA). The concentration of IgA in the samples was determined from a standard curve (0–200 µg/dL), and the results were given in µg/dL.

Endotoxemia was measured by the lipopolysaccharide (LPS) levels in the plasma. The analyses were carried out using the Limulus amoebocyte lysate (LAL) test by a commercial kit (Hycult Biotech®, HIT302, Hycult Biotech, Uden, The Netherlands) and standard LAL curve (0.04–10 EU/mL), following the manufacturer's recommendation. The results were expressed in EU/mL (endotoxin unit per mL plasma).

The TAC (total antioxidant capacity of plasma) was performed using a colorimetric kit (Cayman Chemical Companyl®, Ann Arbor, MI, USA), with Trolox (6-hydroxy-2,5,7,8-tetramethylchroman-2-carboxylic acid) as a standard. The results were expressed as millimoles (mM) of the Trolox equivalent (TE).

2.6. Cytokines Release

The blood was centrifuged ($3000 \times g$, 10 min, 4 °C) and the obtained plasma was analyzed for cytokine determination. Commercial kits were used to quantify IL-10 and IL-12 cytokines (Milliplex® Map) and TNF-α (EMD Millipore®, São Paulo, SP, Brazil) by the ELISA methods. The results were expressed in pg/mL from a standard curve of IL-12 (0–50,000 pg/mL), IL-10 (0–30,000 pg/mL), and TNF-α (0–30,000 pg/mL).

2.7. Aberrant Crypt Foci (ACF) Analysis

The colon of animals was fixed in formalin and stained with 1% methylene blue. The ACF on the mucosal surface of the large intestine were counted by two independent and trained researchers in a blind manner, using an optical microscope (4× objective).

2.8. Intestinal Permeability and Fecal Short-Chain Fatty Acids (SCFAs) Analysis

In the last week of experiment, the animals were fasted for 12 h and then received, by gavage, 2 mL of the solution (200 mg of lactulose and 100 mg of mannitol); samples of their urine were collected for 24 h. At the end, the collected urine volume was measured, recorded and stored at −80 °C [26]. Then, for the analysis, the urine was diluted 1:2 with distilled water, filtered (0.45 µm) and analyzed by the HPLC method.

Furthermore, the colonic feces of animals were quantified for their levels of SCFA, acetate, propionate, and butyrate. The extraction of the SCFA was performed by mixing

100 mg of luminal contents with 2 mL of perchloric acid (10%) and centrifuged (9000× g, 10 min, 25 °C). The supernatant was filtered (0.45 µm) and analyzed by HPLC [27].

The HPLC conditions for the analyses of lactulose, mannitol and SCFA were a Shimadzu HPLC system (Kyoto, Japan) with a degasses (Model DGU-14A), pump (Model LC-10AT), auto-sampler (Model SIL-20A), column oven (Model CTO-10AS), UV–vis detector (Model SPD-10AV), and a refractive index detector (Model RID-10A). The column used was Aminex HPX-87H (300 cm × 8.7 mm; BIO-RAD) in 55 °C with a pressure of 1920 psi, using H2SO4 0.005 mM as a mobile phase under isocratic conditions [28]. Lactulose, mannitol and SCFA levels (mg/g of feces) were determined by standard curves using commercial standards (Sigma-Aldrich).

2.9. Intraluminal pH of the Colon

The cecal luminal contents were removed, weighed, and 4 mg was diluted in 400 mL of distilled water. After the complete homogenization by vortex, the pH was read using a pH meter (Kasvi®, São José dos Pinhais, PR, Brazil) [11].

2.10. In Silico Analysis

The structural interaction between short-chain fatty acids (SCFAs) acetate, propionate, and butyrate, and p65-NF-κB, TLR4, inducible Nitric Oxide Synthase (iNOS), and Nicotinamide Adenine Dinucleotide Phosphate Oxidase (NADPH oxidase) was evaluated by molecular docking. The SCFAs were designed using Instant MarvinSketch (ChemAxon Ltd., Boston, MA, USA). The crystal structure file of p65-NF-kB, TLR4, iNOS, and NADPH oxidase was obtained from the Protein Data Bank (http://www.rcsb.org/, accessed on 16 January 2023) (PDB: 1OY3, 3FXI, and 3E6T, 1HH4, respectively).

Non-polar hydrogen atoms were merged, and rotatable bonds were defined on the AutoDockTools® program. Flexible torsions, charges, and the grid size were assigned by AutoDock Tools [29], and the docking calculations were performed using AutoDock Vina [30]. The active site of target enzymes was based on an exhaustive search in the literature of studies which demonstrated the binding sites of the enzymes; then, based on these results, successive tests were carried out to locate the best active site of the enzymes. The binding pose with the lowest binding energy (highest binding affinity) was selected as a representative image to visualize in the Discovery Studio 2016 Client (Dassault Systèmes Biovia Corp®, Hudson, OH, USA) [31].

2.11. Statistical Analysis

The power analysis to determine the sample size was performed, as indicated by Lwanga [32], for analytical studies using $\alpha = 5\%$ and z $\alpha/2 = 1.96$, as used in health studies, accomplished using our previous study as a basis [11]. The statistical analysis procedures were conducted with software GraphPad Prism, version 9.0. The data normality were tested by the Kolmogorov–Smirnov test. The normal data were analyzed by ANOVA and the post hoc Newman–Keuls method. The Correlation Matrix analysis was carried out using the Person test. Data were expressed as means ± standard deviation (SD), using $p < 0.05$ as the level of significance.

3. Results

3.1. Yacon Composition

It was observed that yacon flour (in the dry basis) is a rich source of prebiotics, mainly FOS and inulin. Furthermore, we observed the presence of other fibers in its composition. The simple carbohydrates were the main macronutrient present, and we observed the presence of fructose, sucrose and glucose. Additionally, proteins and ash were identified; however, the amount of lipids was very small (Table 1).

3.2. Superoxide Anion and Nitric Oxide Release

It was observed that none of the groups, treated or not with yacon flour and with or without induced colon cancer, differed in the release of superoxide anion, either in the unstimulated (Figure 2A) or stimulated (Figure 2B) neutrophils with opsonized zymozan ($p > 0.05$).

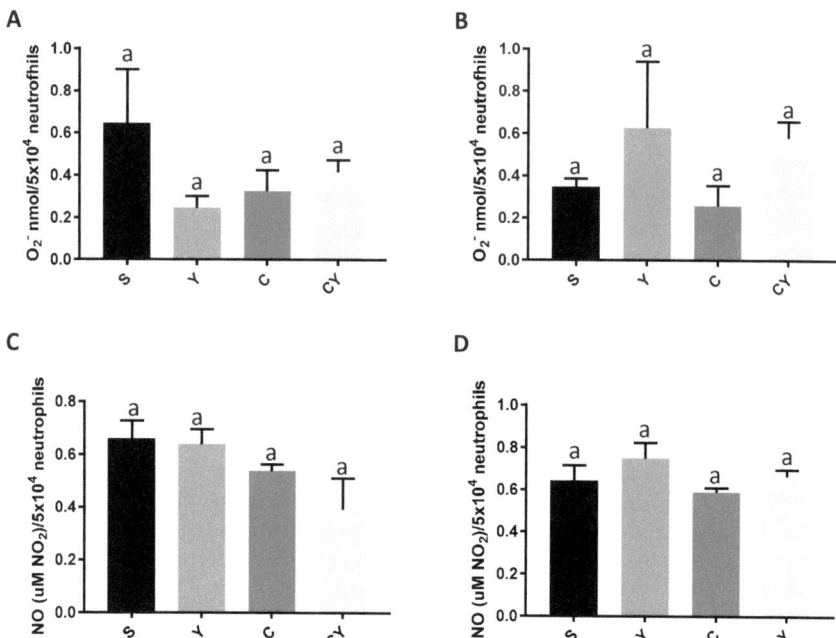

Figure 2. Superoxide anion and nitric oxide release by neutrophils from rats fed or not with yacon flour and induced or not to colorectal cancer. (**A**) Superoxide anion release by neutrophils not stimulated by opsonized zymozan; (**B**) superoxide anion release by neutrophils stimulated by opsonized zymozan; (**C**) nitric oxide release by neutrophils not stimulated by opsonized zymozan; (**D**) NO release by neutrophils stimulated by opsonized zymozan. Values are shown as means ± SD. Dates analyzed by one-way ANOVA and post hoc Newman–Keuls ($p < 0.05$). The lowercase letter "a" indicates that there is no difference between groups. Dates analyzed by absorbance. S = group without the induction of colon cancer and without yacon flour ($n = 10$); C = group with the induction of colon cancer and without yacon flour ($n = 10$); Y = group without the induction of colon cancer and with yacon flour ($n = 12$); CY = group with the induction of colon cancer and with yacon flour ($n = 12$). YF = yacon flour; CRC = colorectal cancer. O_2^-: superoxide anion; NO: nitric oxide.

Likewise, all groups showed similar nitric oxide secretions, regardless of whether they were stimulated by zimozan or not (Figure 2C,D) ($p > 0.05$).

3.3. Secretory IgA Production, Endotoxemia and Total Antioxidant Capacity

The Y group had the highest levels ($p < 0.05$) of sIgA, and the values were similar to the CY group, which also received yacon flour and had colorectal cancer induction. The C group had the lowest IgA secretion values ($p < 0.05$). The S group did not present statistically different values when compared to the Y, C, and CY groups (Figure 3A).

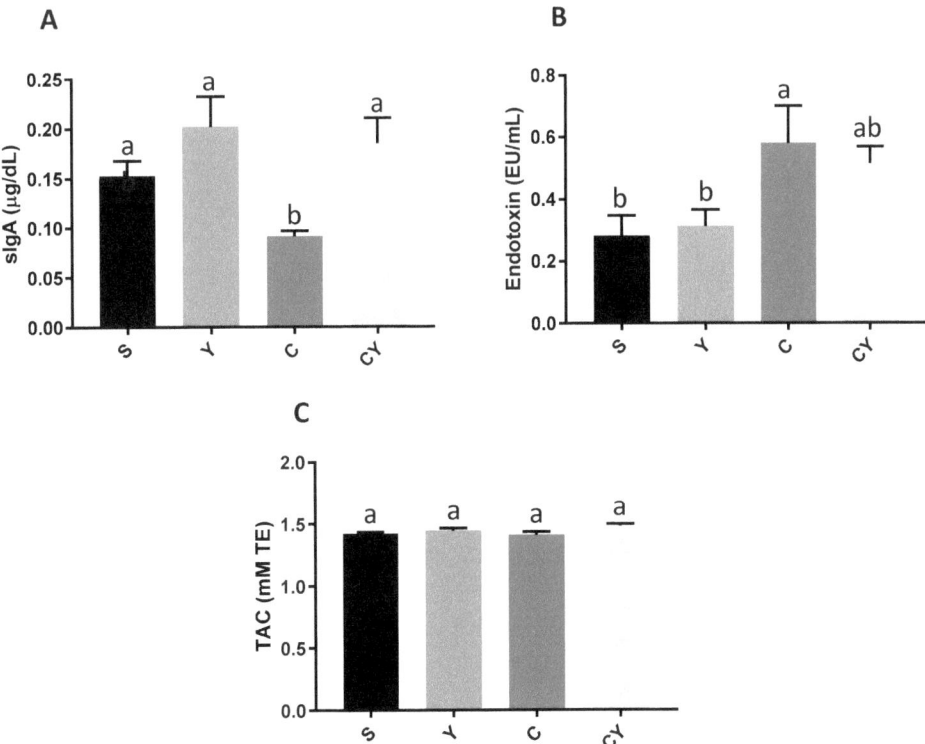

Figure 3. Immunologic and oxidative markers produced by rats fed or not with yacon flour and induced or not to colorectal cancer. (**A**) IgA release; (**B**) endotoxin levels; (**C**) TAC. Values shown as means ± SD. Dates are analyzed by one-way ANOVA and post hoc Newman–Keuls ($p < 0.05$). The different letters are the differences between groups. Dates analyzed by absorbance. S = group without induction of colon cancer and without yacon flour ($n = 10$); C = group with induction of colon cancer and without yacon flour ($n = 10$); Y = group without induction of colon cancer and with yacon flour ($n = 12$); CY = group with induction of colon cancer and with yacon flour ($n = 12$). YF = yacon flour; CRC = colorectal cancer. sIgA= secretory immunoglobulin A. TAC= total antioxidant capacity. mMTE= millimolar of Trolox equivalent. EU/mL: endotoxin unit/mL plasma.

Groups with induced colorectal cancer, the C and CY groups, showed the highest endotoxemia values ($p < 0.05$). However, the CY group had similar values to the S and Y groups, which had no induction of colorectal cancer. Furthermore, the S and Y groups showed similar and lower values of endotoxemia (Figure 3B).

In addition, all groups, regardless of treatment, had similar values for total plasma antioxidant capacity (Figure 3C).

3.4. Cytokines Release

The C group showed the highest plasma levels of pro-inflammatory cytokines TNFα (Figure 4A) and IL-12 (Figure 4B) ($p < 0.05$). The CY group had the lowest levels of those cytokines ($p < 0.05$) followed by the C group. The release of TNFα and IL-12 were similar between S, Y, and CY groups ($p > 0.05$) (Figure 4A,B).

However, the values of anti-inflammatory cytokine IL-10 were similar between S, Y and C groups. The CY group had the lowest plasma levels of this cytokine ($p < 0.05$) (Figure 4C).

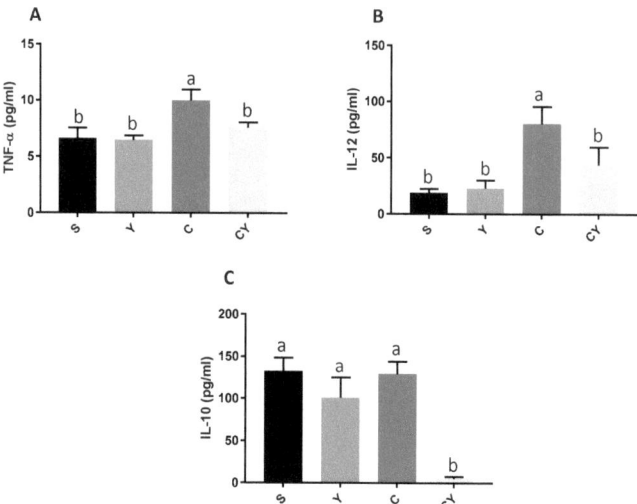

Figure 4. Plasmatic cytokine release by rats fed or not with yacon flour and induced or not to colorectal cancer. (**A**) TNF-α release; (**B**) IL-12 release; (**C**) IL-10 release. Values showed as means ± SD. Dates analyzed by one-way ANOVA and post hoc Newman–Keuls ($p < 0.05$). The different letters are the differences between groups. Dates analyzed by absorbance. S = group without induction of colon cancer and without yacon flour ($n = 10$); C = group with induction of colon cancer and without yacon flour ($n = 10$); Y = group without induction of colon cancer and with yacon flour ($n = 12$); CY = group with induction of colon cancer and with yacon flour ($n = 12$). TNF-α = tumoral necrosis factor alpha; IL-12 = interleukin-12; YF = yacon flour; CRC = colorectal cancer.

3.5. In Silico Analyses

Butyrate showed the highest interaction by lowest estimated free energy (EFE) with p65-NF-κB, iNOS, and NADPH oxidase (EFE of −3.4, −4.3, and −4.1, respectively), whereas acetate showed the lowest interaction with these markers. Propionate showed the highest interaction with TLR4 (EFE of −3.6) and butyrate showed the lowest interaction with TLR4 (EFE of −3.1) (Table 3 and Figure 5).

Table 3. Estimated free energy binding and chemical interactions among the main short-chain fatty acids from FOS fermentation and the catalytic site of the p65NF-κB, TLR4, iNOS, and NADPH oxidase.

	Acetate		Propionate		Butyrate	
	EFE	IAAR	EFE	IAAR	EFE	IAAR
p65 NF-KB	−2.9	GLU D: 302; GLY D: 279; THR D: 276	−3.2	GLU D: 302; GLY D: 279; PRO D: 301; THR D:276; ARD D: 275	−3.4	TRH D: 276; GLY D: 276; GLU D: 302; LEU D: 283
TLR4	−3.4	LYS B: 341; LYS B: 362; THR B: 319	−3.6	LYS B: 341; LYS B: 362; THR B: 319; TYR B: 292	−3.1	HIS B: 179; LYS B: 230
iNOS	−3.2	TYR B: 483; TRP B: 188; PHE B: 363	−3.9	TYR B: 483; TRP B: 188; PHE B: 363	−4.3	CYS B: 194; TRP B: 188; ILE B: 238; TYR B: 483; LEU B: 203; PHE B: 363

Table 3. Cont.

	Acetate		Propionate		Butyrate	
	EFE	IAAR	EFE	IAAR	EFE	IAAR
NADPH oxidase	−3.6	VAL B: 14; ALA B: 13; GLY B: 15; LYS B: 16; THR B: 17	−4	GLY B: 15; VAL B: 14; LYS B: 16; ALA B: 13; THR B: 17; CYS B: 18	−4.1	GLY B: 15; ALA B: 13; VAL B: 14; LYS B: 16; THR B: 17

EFE: Estimated free energy (kcal·mol^{-1}). IAAR: Interacting amino acid residues. Docking calculations were carried out using AutoDock Vina. Negative values mean spontaneous reaction. The most potent interaction between short-chain fatty acids and receptor is in bold.

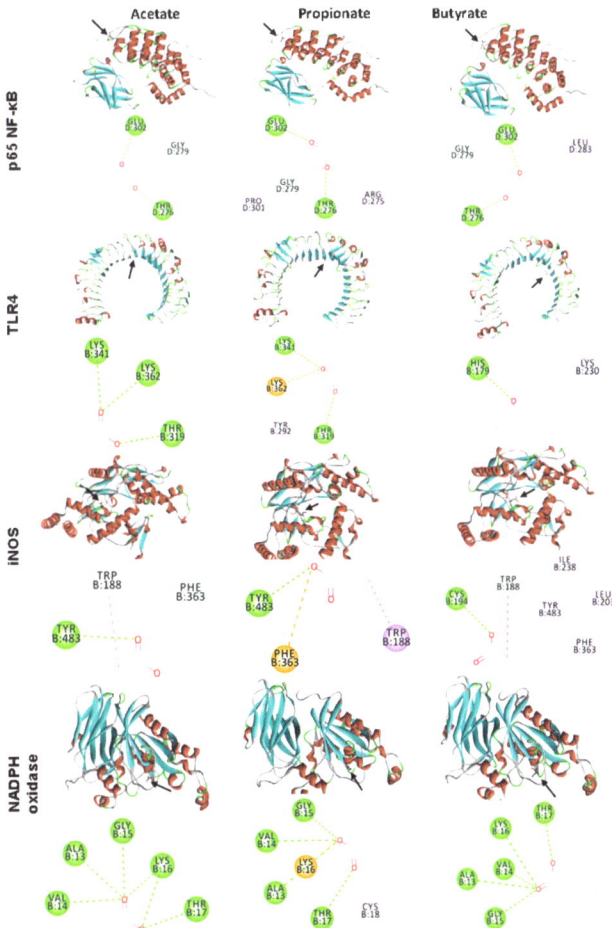

Figure 5. The in silico interaction of the main short-chain fatty acids generate by FOS fermentation after yacon consumption: acetate, propionate, and butyrate. Dates analyzed by AutoDock Vina® and visualized by Discovery Studio 2016 Client®. Color code indicates the residue interaction: heliotrope: Pi-sigma bond; lime green: conventional hydrogen bond; light green: carbon hydrogen bond; neon pink: Pi-Pi T-shaped bond; orange: Pi-cation bond. p65 NF-κB: nuclear factor kappa B. TLR4: Toll-like receptor 4. iNOS: inducible nitric oxide synthase. NADPH oxidase: nicotinamide adenine dinucleotide phosphate oxidase.

3.6. Correlation Analysis

It was observed that the urinary excretion of mannitol and lactulose had a positive correlation with each other ($p < 0.05$). In addition, both showed a positive correlation with fecal pH and IL-10. The mannitol had also a positive correlation with TNF and IL-12 ($p < 0.05$). On the other hand, these sugars showed an inverse correlation with the levels of propionate and butyrate in the feces ($p < 0.05$). The fecal pH showed an inverse correlation to the levels of propionate and IgA: the lower the pH, the higher the value observed of IgA and propionate in the feces. Conversely, the ACF values showed a significant inverse correlation only with acetate, and TAC had a significant positive correlation with butyrate in the feces ($p < 0.05$). Acetate also had an inverse correlation with serum LPS and a positive correlation with the anti-inflammatory cytokine IL-10 ($p < 0.05$). Propionate showed a positive correlation with sIgA and butyrate in the feces. The levels of the inflammatory cytokine IL-12 showed, in turn, a positive correlation ($p < 0.05$) with LPS and urinary mannitol (Figure 6).

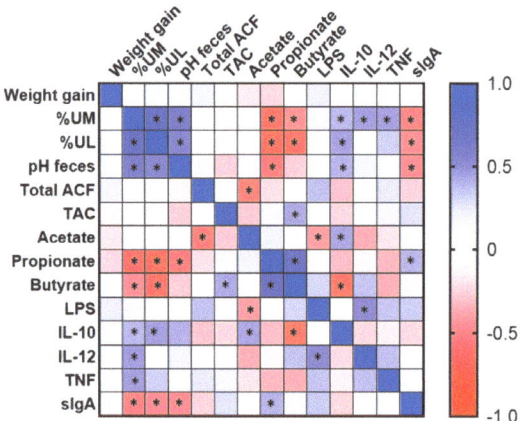

Figure 6. Heat map of the Pearson rank correlations between the biological outcomes of animals with induced colorectal cancer and fed with yacon flour for 8 weeks. * $p < 0.05$. %UM: percentage of urinary excretion of mannitol; %UL: percentage of urinary excretion of lactulose; total ACF: total aberrant crypt foci; TAC: total antioxidant capacity; LPS: lipopolysaccharide; IL: interleukin; TNF: tumor necrosis factor; sIgA: secretory immunoglobulin A.

4. Discussion

This study demonstrated that the yacon flour, as a source of FOS, was able to reduce inflammatory biomarkers in CRC-induced animals. Chronic inflammation can be modulated by some nutritional compounds, such as prebiotics. Prebiotics are non-digestible food components that modulate gut microbiota by stimulating the growth and/or activating the metabolism of probiotic bacteria, such as Lactobacillus and Bifidobacterium spp. [33].

Yacon (*Smallanthus sonchifolius*) flour is a rich source of prebiotics by providing 52.2% of FOS, 6.61% of inulin, and 10.68% of other fibers (Table 1). The FOS, as well as being associated with probiotics, can modulate the immune resistance [34] in addition to providing protective effects against early biomarkers and the development of tumors in the colon of rats [11,12,14]. Furthermore, FOS can be fermented by gut microbiota, generating SCFAs, mainly acetate, butyrate, and propionate, which are associated with health benefits, including anti-cancer effects [35]; this was shown in our results, whereby pH was inversely the production of acetate and inversely related with the ACF formation. The fermentation was confirmed since the pH was inversely correlated with propionate, i.e., the fermentation reduced the pH by the production of SCFAs, confirming our previous works [11,14]. Furthermore, the reduction in ACF, related with acetate, was also confirmed in our previous work [11]. ACFs are the first lesions detected microscopically in colorectal carcinogenesis;

they are true preneoplastic lesions, commonly used as an indicator of the early stages of the disease, and its reduction indicates a potential to suppress CRC [36].

The healthy gut microbiota has a key role in the induction of defense cell production, such as T cells and secretory immunoglobulin A (sIgA) [37]. In this study, the yacon flour improved the sIgA levels even in animals with CRC (CY group). This result may be due to microbiota modulation by prebiotic FOS, which stimulates the B lymphocyte to produce sIgA [37–39]; this was confirmed by the positive association between sIgA and propionate, which confirmed that the fermentation induced by yacon has the ability to induce sIgA. This immunoglobulin is predominant in secretions such as saliva, tears, colostrum, and feces; this immunoglobulin does not bind complement, and may act against microorganisms without triggering a progressive inflammatory process that damages the epithelium. In addition, sIgA acts by neutralizing toxins and pathogenic microorganisms, preventing them from binding or passing through the intestinal mucosa [40]. Other studies also observed an increase in sIgA levels after yacon ingestion in experimental studies [15,37,41] and human trials [16].

Furthermore, in the current study, the endotoxemia levels on CRC-induced animals treated with yacon flour (CY) were similar to those seen in healthy animals, which can contribute to the reduced inflammation process, as confirmed by the lower IL-12 and TNF-α levels, the major cytokines of the inflammation process [42], thus confirming our original hypothesis. These results are further supported by the verification that a higher excretion of mannitol is positively related to the values of inflammatory cytokines IL-12 and TNF by correlation analysis. Then, yacon consumption possibly reduced serum inflammation by reducing intestinal permeability, which reduces bacterial translocation (by reducing LPS release) and the induction of inflammatory cytokines.

Under normal conditions, the LPS in the intestinal lumen does not cause negative effects. However, some factors, such as dysbiosis, fat consumption, and obesity, may favor the transfer of LPS to the circulatory system, a process called endotoxemia [1,2]. Then, the intracellular signaling pathways and transcription factors such as NF-κB are activated in the plasma cells, such as neutrophils, macrophages, and lymphocytes, which release pro-inflammatory cytokines [43].

The low TNF-α levels observed can be associated with the suggested capacity of SCFAs to bind into NF-κB and TLR4, as proposed in the in silico analysis, which can reduce the activation of these biomarkers and, consequently, their associated pathways. Other studies observed a reduction in endotoxemia after xylo-oligosaccharide and inulin consumption by healthy patients [17] and by mice fed with a high-fat diet [44]. Nevertheless, the levels of anti-inflammatory IL-10 were not increased as expected, although acetate levels positively correlated with IL-10 levels. This result was probably due to the systemic evaluation instead of local IL-10 levels, as in the intestine, this cytokine is released by macrophages, dendritic cells, and epithelial cells [45,46]. A study with preschool children also did not find an increase in IL-10 levels associated with yacon flour intake, despite the increased levels of IL-4 [16].

We observed favorable interactions of the ligand-proteins in every in silico analysis, such as hydrogen bonding, the carbon–hydrogen bond, and Pi-sigma bond; they can contribute to lowering the system's free energy, especially the hydrogen bonds that play an essential role in protein–ligand binding [47,48]. Despite the observed supposed interaction between SCFAs and NADPH oxidase and iNOS by in silico analysis, we do not observe the results in oxidative stress between groups, independently of stimulus, in nitric oxide and superoxide levels. These results indicate that both cancer and yacon flour had no impact on these oxidative and inflammatory markers, the opposite of what we initially hypothesized for the study. Furthermore, a possible explanation of why cancer did not increase the oxidative stress is because the cancer was already present. This disease, to avoid cytotoxic signaling and to facilitate tumorigenic signaling, has a local mechanism in place that monitors ROS, such as signaling molecules that convey information about increases in oxidative stress to the nucleus in order to upregulate antioxidant genes [49].

High levels of ROS are associated with DNA damage, significant toxicity, cell apoptosis, endothelium dysfunction, among others, which have been implicated in many diseases, including cancer [50]. Healthy mice fed with FOS from yacon did not demonstrate any alteration on NO levels [51]. Another similar study which analyzed the effects of yacon flour on the prevention of CRC also found no changes in the antioxidant capacity of animals [14].

Those results were confirmed by the similarity of the TAC values between the groups, confirming that no oxidative stress was induced in the animals, regardless of the tested treatment. The organism had mechanisms to fight against ROS production, which include endogenous enzymes, like glutathione-peroxidase, superoxide dismutase, paraoxonase-1, catalase. In addition, yacon flour is a rich source of antioxidant compounds, such as phenolics, chlorogenic, caffeic, coumaric and protocatechuic acids [52], which can improve the oxidative stress; however, in this study, this effect was not observed. The TAC analyses provide more relevant biological information than individual components, once the cumulative effect of all antioxidants present in body fluids and plasma is considered [53].

The proposed effect of yacon flour in our study is that its consumption, as a rich source of FOS, increased fecal sIgA, improving the barrier that prevents pathogen bacteria from passing through the intestinal membrane, contributing to the reduction in endotoxemia. Such results directly contributed to the reduction in inflammatory cytokine secretion. These results may be related to the in silico interaction of the SCFAs produced by the fermentation of FOS with biomarkers of inflammation. However, despite the in silico effect of SCFAs on oxidative stress markers, none of the modifications to the antioxidant were observed in animals, which may have occurred due to the non-induction of oxidative stress by colorectal cancer. However, we emphasize that these connections between SCFAs and enzymes, demonstrated in the in silico analysis, are plausible to occur, but require caution in their interpretation, since in a physiological context, other factors can interfere in these connections and in the consequent actions of the enzymes [54]. The main limitation of this study was the lack of studies on the same topic, as it made it difficult to establish the exact dose of yacon flour, the treatment time and the main markers for assessing oxidative stress (Figure 7).

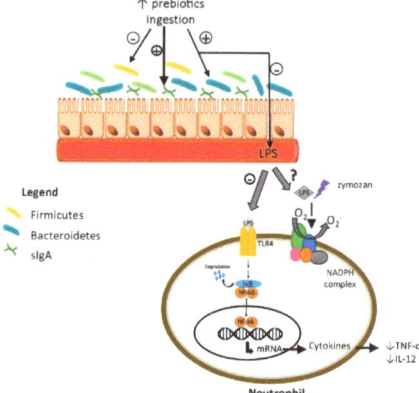

Figure 7. The proposal effect caused by the consumption of yacon flour as a FOS (prebiotic) source. The prebiotic ingestion stimulates the *Bacteroidetes* bacteria development instead of *Firmicutes* bacteria, which reduce the production and release of LPS to the blood circulation. Then, the binding of LPS on TLR4, and consequently the downstream pathway activation, is reduced on immune cells, like neutrophil, which reduces the cytokines' release and reduces the inflammation. LPS: lipopolysaccharide; O_2^-: superoxide anion; NADPH oxidase: nicotinamide adenine dinucleotide phosphate oxidase; sIgA: secretory immunoglobulin A. TLR4: Toll-like receptor 4; p65 NF-κB: nuclear factor kappa B; IκB: inhibitor of κB; TNF-α = tumoral necrosis factor alpha; IL-12 = interleukin-12.

5. Conclusions

We confirm our hypothesis that yacon flour improves the inflammation caused by colorectal cancer; however, we have not observed the effects on oxidative stress and endotoxemia. These results are innovative and highlight the effectiveness of yacon flour against inflammation in CRC-induced rats. Furthermore, this study could drive further studies to investigate the molecular mechanisms related to these systemic effects observed in CRC-induced rats, as well as clinical investigations.

Author Contributions: Conceptualization: M.G., N.M.B.C. and M.L.V.; methodology: M.G., N.M.B.C., M.d.G.V.T., M.D.C.I., D.F.d.O., A.G.V.C. and M.L.V.; software: M.G.; validation: N.M.B.C. and M.L.V.; formal analysis: M.G., N.M.B.C., M.D.C.I., D.F.d.O., A.G.V.C. and M.L.V.; investigation: M.G., N.M.B.C., M.d.G.V.T., M.D.C.I., D.F.d.O., A.G.V.C. and M.L.V.; resources: N.M.B.C., M.d.G.V.T., A.G.V.C. and M.L.V.; data curation: M.G., N.M.B.C. and M.L.V.; writing—original draft preparation: M.G., N.M.B.C. and M.L.V.; writing—review and editing: M.G., N.M.B.C., M.d.G.V.T., M.D.C.I., D.F.d.O., A.G.V.C. and M.L.V.; visualization: M.G., N.M.B.C. and M.L.V.; supervision: N.M.B.C. and M.L.V.; project administration: N.M.B.C. and M.L.V.; funding acquisition: N.M.B.C. and M.L.V. All authors have read and agreed to the published version of the manuscript.

Funding: Authors are grateful to the "Coordenação de Aperfeiçoamento de Pessoal de Nível Superior (CAPES)"—Brazil [Finance Code 001] for M.G.'s scholarship. This study was financed by "Fundação de Amparo à Pesquisa e Inovação do Espírito Santo (FAPES)"—Brazil [grant number 567/2018] and "Conselho Nacional de Desenvolvimento Científico e Tecnológico (CNPq)"—Brazil [grant number 486353/2013-3].

Institutional Review Board Statement: The experimental procedures with animals were performed in compliance with the ethical principles for animal experimentation, in accordance with Directive 86/609/EEC of 24 November 1986. The "Ethics Committee of Animals Use" of the Universidade Federal do Espírito Santo (No. 004/2014) approved the study.

Informed Consent Statement: Not applicable.

Data Availability Statement: Not applicable.

Acknowledgments: We acknowledge Eduardo Fornazier for lab assistance.

Conflicts of Interest: The authors have no conflict of interest.

References

1. Bardelcíková, A.; Šoltys, J.; Mojžiš, J. Oxidative Stress, Inflammation and Colorectal Cancer: An Overview. *Antioxidants* **2023**, *12*, 901. [CrossRef] [PubMed]
2. Katsaounou, K.; Nicolaou, E.; Vogazianos, P.; Brown, C.; Stavrou, M.; Teloni, S.; Hatzis, P.; Agapiou, A.; Fragkou, E.; Tsiaoussis, G.; et al. Colon Cancer: From Epidemiology to Prevention. *Metabolites* **2022**, *12*, 499. [CrossRef] [PubMed]
3. Sun, Y.H.; Li, J.; Shu, H.J.; Li, Z.L.; Qian, J.M. Serum Immunoinflammation-Related Protein Complexes Discriminate between Inflammatory Bowel Disease and Colorectal Cancer. *Clin. Transl. Oncol.* **2019**, *21*, 1680–1686. [CrossRef] [PubMed]
4. Nimptsch, K.; Aleksandrova, K.; Fedirko, V.; Jenab, M.; Gunter, M.J.; Siersema, P.D.; Wu, K.; Katzke, V.; Kaaks, R.; Panico, S.; et al. Pre-Diagnostic C-Reactive Protein Concentrations, CRP Genetic Variation and Mortality among Individuals with Colorectal Cancer in Western European Populations. *BMC Cancer* **2022**, *22*, 695. [CrossRef] [PubMed]
5. Dai, Z.; Zhang, J.; Wu, Q.; Chen, J.; Liu, J.; Wang, L.; Chen, C.; Xu, J.; Zhang, H.; Shi, C.; et al. The Role of Microbiota in the Development of Colorectal Cancer. *Int. J. Cancer* **2019**, *148*, 2032–2041. [CrossRef]
6. Li, Q.; von Ehrlich-Treuenstätt, V.; Schardey, J.; Wirth, U.; Zimmermann, P.; Andrassy, J.; Bazhin, A.V.; Werner, J.; Kühn, F. Gut Barrier Dysfunction and Bacterial Lipopolysaccharides in Colorectal Cancer. *J. Gastrointest. Surg.* **2023**, *ahead of print*. [CrossRef]
7. Lin, S.; Li, Y.; Zamyatnin, A.A.; Werner, J.; Bazhin, A.V. Reactive Oxygen Species and Colorectal Cancer. *J. Cell. Physiol.* **2018**, *233*, 5119–5132. [CrossRef]
8. De Almeida, C.V.; De Camargo, M.R.; Russo, E.; Amedei, A. Role of Diet and Gut Microbiota on Colorectal Cancer Immunomodulation. *World J. Gastroenterol.* **2019**, *25*, 151–162. [CrossRef]
9. Wang, F.; Ugai, T.; Haruki, K.; Wan, Y.; Akimoto, N.; Arima, K.; Zhong, R.; Twombly, T.S.; Wu, K.; Yin, K.; et al. Healthy and Unhealthy Plant-based Diets in Relation to the Incidence of Colorectal Cancer Overall and by Molecular Subtypes. *Clin. Transl. Med.* **2022**, *12*, e893. [CrossRef]
10. Nadai, L.D.; Fernando, L.; Moraes, D.S.; Cristina, B.; Dias, M.; Teixeira, D.O.; Calcagno, T.; Bruno, V.; Egídio, I.; Caroline, A.; et al. Yacon (*Smallanthus sonchifolius*)-Based Product Increases Fecal Short-Chain Fatty Acids and Enhances Regulatory T Cells by Downregulating RORγt in the Colon of BALB/c Mice. *J. Funct. Foods* **2019**, *55*, 333–342. [CrossRef]

11. Grancieri, M.; Costa, N.M.; Vaz Tostes, M.D.; de Oliveira, D.; Nunes, L.D.; Marcon, L.D.; Veridiano, T.; Viana, M. Yacon Flour (*Smallanthus sonchifolius*) Attenuates Intestinal Morbidity in Rats with Colon Cancer. *J. Funct. Foods* **2017**, *37*, 666–675. [CrossRef]
12. de Moura, N.A.; Caetano, B.F.R.; Sivieri, K.; Urbano, L.H.; Cabello, C.; Rodrigues, M.A.M.; Barbisan, L.F. Protective Effects of Yacon (*Smallanthus sonchifolius*) Intake on Experimental Colon Carcinogenesis. *Food Chem. Toxicol.* **2012**, *50*, 2902–2910. [CrossRef]
13. Martino, H.S.D.; Kolba, N.; Tako, E. Yacon (*Smallanthus sonchifolius*) Flour Soluble Extract Improve Intestinal Bacterial Populations, Brush Border Membrane Functionality and Morphology In Vivo (*Gallus Gallus*). *Food Res. Int.* **2020**, *137*, 109705. [CrossRef]
14. Verediano, T.A.; Viana, M.L.; das Graças Vaz Tostes, M.; de Oliveira, D.S.; de Carvalho Nunes, L.; Costa, N.M.B. Yacón (*Smallanthus sonchifolius*) Prevented Inflammation, Oxidative Stress, and Intestinal Alterations in an Animal Model of Colorectal Carcinogenesis. *J. Sci. Food Agric.* **2020**, *100*, 5442–5449. [CrossRef]
15. Grancieri, M.; Machado, P.A.; Oliveira, D.F.; Marcon, L.N.; Vaz Tostes, M.G.; Costa, N.M.B.; Ignacchiti, M.D.C.; Nunes, L.C.; Viana, M.L. Efeito Da Farinha de Yacon (*Smallanthus sonchifolius*) Na Resposta Imunológica Intestinal No Câncer Colorretal. *Braspen J.* **2016**, *31*, 335–339.
16. das Graças Vaz-Tostes, M.; Viana, M.L.; Grancieri, M.; dos Santos Luz, T.C.; de Paula, H.; Pedrosa, R.G.; Costa, N.M.B. Yacon Effects in Immune Response and Nutritional Status of Iron and Zinc in Preschool Children. *Nutrition* **2014**, *30*, 666–672. [CrossRef]
17. Machado, A.M.; da Silva, N.B.M.; de Freitas, R.M.P.; de Freitas, M.B.D.; Chaves, J.B.P.; Oliveira, L.L.; Martino, H.S.D.; Alfenas, R.d.C.G. Effects of Yacon Flour Associated with an Energy Restricted Diet on Intestinal Permeability, Fecal Short Chain Fatty Acids, Oxidative Stress and Inflammation Markers Levels in Adults with Obesity or Overweight: A Randomized, Double Blind, Placebo Controll. *Arch. Endocrinol. Metab.* **2020**, *64*, 597–607. [CrossRef]
18. Cocato, M.L.; Lobo, A.R.; Azevedo-Martins, A.K.; Mancini, J.; Sá, L.R.M.; Colli, C. Effects of a Moderate Iron Overload and Its Interaction with Yacon Flour, and/or Phytate, in the Diet on Liver Antioxidant Enzymes and Hepatocyte Apoptosis in Rats. *Food Chem.* **2019**, *285*, 171–179. [CrossRef]
19. AOAC. *Association of Official Analytical Chemistry Official Methods of Analysis*; AOAC: Gaithersburg, MD, USA, 2012; Volume 19.
20. Reeves, P.G.; Nielsen, F.H.; Fahey, G.C. AIN-93 Purified Diets for Laboratory Rodents: Final Report of the American Institute of Nutrition Ad Hoc Writing Commite on the Refomurlation of the AIN-76A Rodent Diet. *Am. Inst. Nutr.* **1993**, *123*, 1939–1951. [CrossRef]
21. Rodrigues, M.A.M.; Silva, L.A.G.; Salvadori, D.M.F.; De Camargo, J.L.V.; Montenegro, M.R. Aberrant Crypt Foci and Colon Cancer: Comparison between a Short- and Medium-Term Bioassay for Colon Carcinogenesis Using Dimethylhydrazine in Wistar Rats. *Braz. J. Med. Biol. Res.* **2002**, *35*, 351–355. [CrossRef]
22. Bird, J.K.; Raederstorff, D.; Weber, P.; Steinert, R.E. Cardiovascular and Antiobesity Effects of Resveratrol Mediated through the Gut Microbiota. *Adv. Nutr. Int. Rev. J.* **2017**, *8*, 839–849. [CrossRef]
23. Henson, P.M. The Immunologic Release of Constituents from Neutrophil Leukocytes. *J. Immunol.* **1971**, *107*, 1535–1546. [CrossRef] [PubMed]
24. Johnston, R.B.; Lehmeyer, J.E. Elaboration of Toxic Oxygen by Products by Neutrophils in a Model of Immune Complex Disease. *J. Clin. Investig.* **1976**, *57*, 836–841. [CrossRef] [PubMed]
25. Green, L.C.; Wagner, D.A.; Glogowski, J.; Skipper, P.L.; Wishnok, J.S.; Tannenbaum, S.R. Analysis of Nitrate, Nitrite, and [^{15}N] Nitrate in Biological Fluids. *Anal. Biochem.* **1982**, *126*, 131–138. [CrossRef] [PubMed]
26. Song, P.; Zhang, R.; Wang, X.; He, P.; Tan, L.; Ma, X. Dietary Grape-Seed Procyanidins Decreased Postweaning Diarrhea by Modulating Intestinal Permeability and Suppressing Oxidative Stress in Rats. *J. Agric. Food Chem.* **2011**, *59*, 6227–6232. [CrossRef]
27. Kotani, A.; Miyaguchi, Y.; Kohama, M.; Ohtsuka, T.; Shiratori, T.; Kusu, F. Determination of Short-Chain Fatty Acids in Rat and Human Feces by High-Performance Liquid Chromatography with Electrochemical Detection. *Anal. Sci.* **2009**, *25*, 1007–1011. [CrossRef]
28. de Sá, L.R.V.; de Oliveira, M.A.L.; Cammarota, M.C.; Matos, A.; Ferreira-Leitão, V.S. Simultaneous Analysis of Carbohydrates and Volatile Fatty Acids by HPLC for Monitoring Fermentative Biohydrogen Production. *Int. J. Hydrogen Energy* **2011**, *36*, 15177–15186. [CrossRef]
29. Morris, G.; Huey, R. AutoDock4 and AutoDockTools4: Automated Docking with Selective Receptor Flexibility. *J. Comput. Chem.* **2009**, *30*, 2785–2791. [CrossRef]
30. Trott, O.; Olson, A. AutoDock Vina: Improving the Speed and Accuracy of Docking with a New Scoring Function, Efficient Optimization and Multithreading. *J. Comput. Chem.* **2010**, *31*, 455–461. [CrossRef]
31. Grancieri, M.; Martino, H.S.D.; Gonzalez de Mejia, E. Digested Total Protein and Protein Fractions from Chia Seed (*Salvia Hispanica* L.) Had High Scavenging Capacity and Inhibited 5-LOX, COX-1-2, and INOS Enzymes. *Food Chem.* **2019**, *289*, 204–214. [CrossRef]
32. Lwanga, S.K.; Lemeshow, S.; World Health Organization. *Sample Size Determination in Health Studies: A Practical Manual*; World Health Organization: Geneva, Switzerland, 1991.
33. de Almeida Brasiel, P.G.; Luquetti, S.C.P.D.; Medeiros, J.D.; do Amaral Corrêa, J.O.; Machado, A.B.F.; Moreira, A.P.B.; Rocha, V.N.; de Souza, C.T.; Peluzio, M.d.C.G. Kefir Modulates Gut Microbiota and Reduces DMH-Associated Colorectal Cancer via Regulation of Intestinal Inflammation in Adulthood Offsprings Programmed by Neonatal Overfeeding. *Food Res. Int.* **2022**, *152*, 110708. [CrossRef]
34. Alatorre-Santamaría, S.; Cruz-Guerrero, A.; Guzmán-Rodríguez, F. Fructooligosaccharides (FOS). In *Handbook of Food Bioactive Ingredients*; Springer: Berlin/Heidelberg, Germany, 2022; p. 1.

35. Mahalak, K.K.; Firrman, J.; Narrowe, A.B.; Hu, W.; Jones, S.M.; Bittinger, K.; Moustafa, A.M.; Liu, L.S. Fructooligosaccharides (FOS) Differentially Modifies the in Vitro Gut Microbiota in an Age-Dependent Manner. *Front. Nutr.* **2023**, *9*, 1058910. [CrossRef]
36. Silva-Reis, R.; Castro-Ribeiro, C.; Gonçalves, M.; Ferreira, T.; Pires, M.J.; Iglesias-Aguirre, C.E.; Cortés-Martín, A.; Selma, M.V.; Espín, J.C.; Nascimento-Gonçalves, E.; et al. An Integrative Approach to Characterize the Early Phases of Dimethylhydrazine-Induced Colorectal Carcinogenesis in the Rat. *Biomedicines* **2022**, *10*, 409. [CrossRef]
37. Jangid, A.; Fukuda, S.; Kato, T.; Seki, M.; Suzuki, Y.; Taylor, T.D.; Ohno, H.; Prakash, T. Impact of Dietary Fructooligosaccharides (FOS) on Murine Gut Microbiota and Intestinal IgA Secretion. *3 Biotech* **2022**, *12*, 56. [CrossRef]
38. Matsumoto, K.; Ichimura, M.; Tsuneyama, K.; Moritoki, Y.; Tsunashima, H.; Omagari, K.; Hara, M.; Yasuda, I.; Miyakawa, H.; Kikuchi, K. Fructo-Oligosaccharides and Intestinal Barrier Function in a Methionine–Choline-Deficient Mouse Model of Nonalcoholic Steatohepatitis. *PLoS ONE* **2017**, *12*, e0175406. [CrossRef]
39. Xie, X.; He, Y.; Li, H.; Yu, D.; Na, L.; Sun, T.; Zhang, D.; Shi, X.; Xia, Y.; Jiang, T.; et al. Effects of Prebiotics on Immunologic Indicators and Intestinal Microbiota Structure in Perioperative Colorectal Cancer Patients. *Nutrition* **2019**, *61*, 132–142. [CrossRef]
40. Turula, H.; Wobus, C.E. The Role of the Polymeric Immunoglobulin Receptor and Secretory Immunoglobulins during Mucosal Infection and Immunity. *Viruses* **2018**, *10*, 237. [CrossRef]
41. Roche, L.D.; López, A.M.V.; Martínez-Sánchez, G. Procesos Moleculares Patogénicos de La Aterosclerosis y Alternativas Terapéuticas Para Su Control. *Rev. Cuba. Farm.* **2012**, *46*, 267–280.
42. Page, M.J.; Bester, J.; Pretorius, E. The Inflammatory Effects of TNF-α and Complement Component 3 on Coagulation. *Sci. Rep.* **2018**, *8*, 1812. [CrossRef]
43. Lazar, V.; Ditu, L.-M.; Pircalabioru, G.G.; Picu, A.; Petcu, L.; Cucu, N.; Chifiriuc, M.C. Gut Microbiota, Host Organism, and Diet Trialogue in Diabetes and Obesity. *Front. Nutr.* **2019**, *6*, 21. [CrossRef]
44. Cani, P.D.; Neyrinck, A.M.; Fava, F.; Knauf, C.; Burcelin, R.G.; Tuohy, K.M.; Gibson, G.R.; Delzenne, N.M. Selective Increases of Bifidobacteria in Gut Microflora Improve High-Fat-Diet-Induced Diabetes in Mice through a Mechanism Associated with Endotoxaemia. *Diabetologia* **2007**, *50*, 2374–2383. [CrossRef]
45. Bo Liu, D.; Tonkonogy, S.L.; Sartor, R.B. IL-10 Produced by Antigen Presenting Cells Inhibits Bacterial- Responsive TH1/TH17 Cells and Suppresses Colitis in Mice. *Gastroenterology* **2011**, *141*, 653–662. [CrossRef] [PubMed]
46. Krause, P.; Morris, V.; Greenbaum, J.A.; Park, Y.; Bjoerheden, U.; Mikulski, Z.; Muffley, T.; Shui, J.W.; Kim, G.; Cheroutre, H.; et al. IL-10-Producing Intestinal Macrophages Prevent Excessive Antibacterial Innate Immunity by Limiting IL-23 Synthesis. *Nat. Commun.* **2015**, *6*, 7055. [CrossRef] [PubMed]
47. Owoloye, A.J.; Ligali, F.C.; Enejoh, O.A.; Musa, A.Z.; Aina, O.; Idowu, E.T.; Oyebola, K.M. Molecular Docking, Simulation and Binding Free Energy Analysis of Small Molecules as Pf HT1 Inhibitors. *PLoS ONE* **2022**, *17*, e0268269. [CrossRef] [PubMed]
48. Du, X.; Li, Y.; Xia, Y.L.; Ai, S.M.; Liang, J.; Sang, P.; Ji, X.L.; Liu, S.Q. Insights into Protein–Ligand Interactions: Mechanisms, Models, and Methods. *Int. J. Mol. Sci.* **2016**, *17*, 144. [CrossRef]
49. Döppler, H.; Storz, P. Mitochondrial and Oxidative Stress- Mediated Activation of Protein Kinase D1 and Its Importance in Pancreatic Cancer. *Front. Oncol.* **2017**, *7*, 41. [CrossRef]
50. Khosravi, M.; Poursaleh, A.; Ghasempour, G.; Farhad, S.; Najafi, M. The Effects of Oxidative Stress on the Development of Atherosclerosis. *Biol. Chem.* **2019**, *400*, 711–732. [CrossRef]
51. Delgado, G.T.C.; Thomé, R.; Gabriel, D.L.; Tamashiro, W.M.S.C.; Pastore, G.M. Yacon (*Smallanthus sonchifolius*)-Derived Fructooligosaccharides Improves the Immune Parameters in the Mouse. *Nutr. Res.* **2012**, *32*, 884–892. [CrossRef]
52. Sousa, S.; Pinto, J.; Rodrigues, C.; Gião, M.; Pereira, C.; Tavaria, F.; Xavier Malcata, F.; Gomes, A.; Bertoldo Pacheco, M.T.; Pintado, M. Antioxidant Properties of Sterilized Yacon (*Smallanthus sonchifolius*) Tuber Flour. *Food Chem.* **2015**, *188*, 504–509. [CrossRef]
53. Kampa, M.; Nistikaki, A.; Tsaousis, V.; Maliaraki, N.; Notas, G.; Castanas, E. A New Automated Method for the Determination of the Total Antioxidant Capacity (TAC) of Human Plasma, Based on the Crocin Bleaching Assay. *BMC Clin. Pathol.* **2002**, *16*, 3. [CrossRef]
54. Viceconti, M.; Pappalardo, F.; Rodriguez, B.; Horner, M.; Bischoff, J.; Tshinanu, F.M. In silico trials: Verification, validation and uncertainty quantification of predictive models used in the regulatory evaluation of biomedical products. *Methods* **2021**, *185*, 120–127. [CrossRef]

Disclaimer/Publisher's Note: The statements, opinions and data contained in all publications are solely those of the individual author(s) and contributor(s) and not of MDPI and/or the editor(s). MDPI and/or the editor(s) disclaim responsibility for any injury to people or property resulting from any ideas, methods, instructions or products referred to in the content.

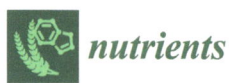

Article

Anti-Obesity Effects of *Pleurotus ferulae* Water Extract on 3T3-L1 Adipocytes and High-Fat-Diet-Induced Obese Mice

Seulmin Hong [1,2], Seonkyeong Park [1], Jangho Lee [1], Soohyun Park [1], Jaeho Park [1] and Yugeon Lee [1,*]

[1] Food Functionality Research Division, Korea Food Research Institute (KFRI), Wanju-gun, Jeonbuk-do 55365, Republic of Korea; h.seulmin@kfri.re.kr (S.H.); p.seonkyeong@kfri.re.kr (S.P.); jhlee@kfri.re.kr (J.L.); shpark0204@kfri.re.kr (S.P.); jaehopark@kfri.re.kr (J.P.)
[2] Department of Food Science and Technology, Chung-Ang University, Anseong, Gyeonggi-do 17546, Republic of Korea
* Correspondence: ugun2@kfri.re.kr; Tel.: +82-63-219-9585

Abstract: This study offers promising insights into the anti-obesity potential of *Pleurotus ferulae*, an edible mushroom valued in Asian cuisine for its nutritional benefits. A hot water extract of *P. ferulae* (PWE) administered to high-fat diet-induced obese mice over an 8-week period significantly reduced their body weight gain and fat accumulation. PWE not only improved the body weight metrics but also positively influenced the serum lipid profile of obese mice by lowering their total cholesterol and low-density lipoprotein cholesterol levels. In vitro studies using 3T3-L1 adipocytes showed that PWE inhibited adipocyte differentiation and lipid accumulation by downregulating key adipogenic transcription factors, particularly PPARγ and C/EBPα, as well as related lipogenic genes involved in fat synthesis and storage, such as Fabp4, Fasn, and Scd1. Chemical analysis revealed that PWE is rich in polysaccharides, which have been associated with various health benefits, including anti-obesity, anti-diabetic, and anti-cancer properties. These findings suggest that the bioactive compounds in PWE may serve as functional food components that could potentially be applied for the prevention and management of obesity and other metabolic disorders.

Keywords: *Pleurotus ferulae*; high-fat diet; obesity; adipogenesis; polysaccharides

Citation: Hong, S.; Park, S.; Lee, J.; Park, S.; Park, J.; Lee, Y. Anti-Obesity Effects of *Pleurotus ferulae* Water Extract on 3T3-L1 Adipocytes and High-Fat-Diet-Induced Obese Mice. *Nutrients* 2024, *16*, 4139. https://doi.org/10.3390/nu16234139

Academic Editor: Jacqueline Isaura Alvarez-Leite

Received: 12 November 2024
Revised: 27 November 2024
Accepted: 28 November 2024
Published: 29 November 2024

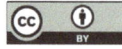

Copyright: © 2024 by the authors. Licensee MDPI, Basel, Switzerland. This article is an open access article distributed under the terms and conditions of the Creative Commons Attribution (CC BY) license (https://creativecommons.org/licenses/by/4.0/).

1. Introduction

Obesity is a prevalent metabolic disorder characterized by an increase in white adipose tissue mass, attributed to both adipocyte hypertrophy and hyperplasia [1]. Preadipocyte differentiation into mature adipocytes involves complex mechanisms regulated by key transcription factors, including peroxisome proliferator-activated receptor γ (PPARγ) and CCAAT/enhancer-binding protein (C/EBP) [2]. Both proteins play pivotal roles in the early stages of adipogenesis, with their cross-regulation being crucial for proper differentiation [3]. Specifically, PPARγ is considered indispensable for the formation of white adipocytes [4], considering its subsequent activation of genes related to free fatty acid uptake, intracellular transport, and lipid synthesis, including fatty acid-binding protein 4 (FABP4), fatty acid synthase (FASN), and ATP-citrate lyase (ACLY) [5]. Therefore, targeting lipogenic factors in adipose tissue and adipocytes could be an effective strategy for the prevention and management of obesity and its associated metabolic disorders.

Obesity is often associated with hyperlipidemia, a lipid disorder characterized by both quantitative and qualitative alterations in plasma lipoproteins [6]. The primary lipid abnormalities include elevated triglycerides, reduced high-density lipoprotein cholesterol levels, and elevated low-density lipoprotein cholesterol (LDL-C) levels [7]. Elevated serum triglycerides result from the increased production of hepatic very low-density lipoprotein particles and the impaired clearance of triglyceride-rich lipoproteins from the circulation [8]. Numerous studies have investigated the relationship between obesity and lipid profiles in animal models, focusing particularly on total cholesterol (TC) and LDL-C levels [9]. Notably, one study found that high-fat-diet (HFD)-induced obese mice showed significantly higher serum TC and LDL-C levels than mice on a normal diet [10,11]. Therefore, lipid profile alterations have been considered a critical factor in determining the anti-obesity effects of potential therapeutic options, including food components.

Dietary and medicinal mushrooms have been widely recognized for their extensive health benefits, which include immune system regulation and anti-viral, anti-diabetic, and anti-cancer effects [12]. Various species, such as *Lentinus*, *Auricularia*, *Hericium*, *Grifola*, *Flammulina*, *Tremella*, and *Pleurotus*, have demonstrated notable functional and nutritional properties [13]. Among these, *Pleurotus ferulae*, an edible mushroom prized for its culinary qualities, has been especially valued by consumers for its distinctive flavor and texture [14]. Beyond its culinary appeal, *P. ferulae* has shown promising medicinal properties, including anticancer activities [15]. However, research on its anti-obesity effects remains limited. The current study therefore sought to investigate the anti-obesity potential of *P. ferulae* using both an HFD-induced obese mouse model and a 3T3-L1 adipocyte cell line model.

2. Materials and Methods

2.1. Materials and Reagents

Dulbecco's Modified Eagle Medium (DMEM, #LM001-05), fetal bovine serum (FBS, #S001-01), and bovine calf serum (BCS, #S003-01) were purchased from Welgene (Gyeongsan, Republic of Korea). Penicillin–streptomycin solution (10,000 U/mL) was obtained from Gibco (Carlsbad, CA, USA). Dimethyl sulfoxide (DMSO, #276855), 3-isobutyl-1-methylxanthine (IBMX, #I5879), dexamethasone (DEX, #D1756), insulin (#I6634), Oil Red O (ORO, #O1516) solution, gallic acid (#G7384), D-(+)-glucose (#G7021), and quercetin (#Q4951) were obtained from Sigma-Aldrich (St. Louis, MO, USA). Antibodies against PPARγ (16643-1-AP, Proteintech, Chicago, IL, USA), ATP-citrate lyase (ACLY, #15421-1-AP, Proteintech, Chicago, IL, USA), and α/β-tubulin (#2148, Cell Signaling Technology, Danvers, MA, USA) were used for Western blotting.

2.2. P. ferulae Extract Preparation

P. ferulae was cultivated in Chilgok-gun (Gyeongsangbuk-do, Republic of Korea) and harvested in February 2020. After harvesting, the mushrooms were washed, dried, and crushed. To prepare the *P. ferulae* water extract (PWE), the sample was mixed with distilled water at a 1:20 (w/w) ratio. Extraction was performed twice using a reflux cooling method at 50 °C for 3 h. The resulting extract was then filtered, freeze-dried and stored at 20 °C until further use. For the *P. ferulae* ethanol extract (PEE), the dried sample was extracted with 70% ethanol (100 g/L) twice using a reflux cooling method for 3 h at 50 °C. This extract was then filtered, concentrated under reduced pressure, freeze-dried, and stored at 20 °C until further use.

2.3. Animal Experiment

Five-week-old male C57BL/6 mice were purchased from Orient Bio Inc. (Seongnam, Gyeonggi-do, Republic of Korea) and housed under controlled conditions at 22 ± 2 °C with 50 ± 5% humidity and a 12 h light/dark cycle. This study adhered to ethical guidelines for animal experimentation and was approved by the Institutional Animal Care and Use Committee of the Korea Food Research Institute (Approval No: KFRI-M-23007; approved on 4 December 2023). After a 1-week acclimation period, the mice were divided into the following groups: a normal diet control group (ND), an HFD control group, and an HFD group supplemented with PWE. The HFD provided 60% of kcal from fat (D12492, Research Diets, Inc., New Brunswick, NJ, USA). PWE was dissolved in drinking water and administered orally at a dose of 100 mg/kg of body weight. Weight changes in the mice were monitored through weekly body weight measurements for 8 weeks. The mice's body composition and fat mass were assessed using an InAlyzer (Medikors, Seoul, Republic of Korea). At the end of the feeding period, the mice were sacrificed for further analysis. Blood samples were collected, and serum was separated by centrifugation for lipid profiling analysis, conducted at OBEN Bio (Suwon, Republic of Korea) using a Beckman Coulter AU480 analyzer (Siemens, Germany).

2.4. Histological Analysis

Tissues were fixed with 3.7% paraformaldehyde (Biosesang, Yongin, Gyeonggi-do, Republic of Korea), embedded in paraffin wax, and sectioned sagittally to a thickness of 3 µm. Thereafter, the sections were stained with hematoxylin and eosin (H&E) to assess any morphological changes. Images of the stained adipose tissue were captured using a light microscope equipped with a camera (OBEN Bio). Image analysis was performed using ImageJ software (version 1.54d).

2.5. Cell Culture

Mouse 3T3-L1 preadipocytes were obtained from the American Type Culture Collection (Manassas, VA, USA) and maintained in high-glucose DMEM supplemented with 10% BCS and 1% penicillin–streptomycin solution at 37 °C in a 5% CO_2 atmosphere. For differentiation, confluent cells were incubated in DMEM containing 10% FBS and a differentiation mix (MDI) consisting of 10 µg/mL insulin, 0.5 mM of IBMX, and 1 µM of DEX for 2 days. Subsequently, the medium was replaced every other day with insulin-supplemented DMEM (10 µg/mL). During differentiation, the cells were treated with either DMSO (control) or PWE for 8 days.

2.6. Cell Viability Assay

Cell viability was evaluated using the MTT assay. Briefly, the cells were seeded into a 96-well plate at a density of 1×10^4 cells per well. After 2 days, the differentiation of the cells was induced using MDI-supplemented FBS-DMEM and they were treated with various concentrations of PWE for 8 days. Following treatment, MTT stock solution (5 mg/mL) was added to each well followed by incubation for 2 h. After subsequently removing the medium, the resulting formazan crystals were dissolved in DMSO. The absorbance was then measured at 570 nm using a microplate reader (Molecular Devices, Sunnyvale, CA, USA).

2.7. ORO Staining

Lipid droplet accumulation was determined using ORO staining. Briefly, differentiated cells were washed with Dulbecco's Phosphate-Buffered Saline and fixed with 3.7% paraformaldehyde (Biosesang) for 15 min. The cells were then washed with 60% isopropanol and subsequently stained with ORO solution for 20 min. Residual reagent was completely removed by washing the cells three times with distilled water, after which the stained cells were visualized using an Olympus IX73 light microscope (Olympus, Center Valley, PA, USA). To quantify lipid accumulation, the ORO stain was eluted using 100% isopropanol, and the absorbance was measured at 490 nm using a microplate reader (Molecular Devices).

2.8. Western Blot Analysis

Protein expression was confirmed using Western blotting. Briefly, the cells were lysed with RIPA buffer (#R0278, Cell Signaling Technology) containing phosphatase and protease inhibitor cocktails (Roche, Mannheim, Germany). Thereafter, the cell lysate was incubated on ice for 10 min and then centrifuged to collect the supernatant. The protein concentration was quantified using a BCA assay (iNtron Biotechnology, Inc., Seoul, Republic of Korea). Equal amounts of protein were mixed with 5× SDS-PAGE buffer (Biosesang), boiled at 95 °C for 5 min, and then cooled. Proteins were separated via SDS-PAGE and then transferred to polyvinylidene difluoride membranes (Bio-Rad, Hercules, CA, USA), which were then blocked with blocking buffer (#ML062-01, Welgene) for 1 h to prevent nonspecific binding. Subsequently, the membranes were incubated with primary antibodies at 4 °C for 12 h, followed by incubation with secondary antibodies at room temperature for 1 h.

Immunoblots were developed using Pierce ECL Western Blotting Substrate (Thermo Fisher Scientific, Sunnyvale, CA, USA), and densitometry analysis was conducted using ImageJ to quantify protein expression.

2.9. RNA Analysis

RNA expression was evaluated using real-time polymerase chain reaction (PCR). Total RNA was extracted using the RNeasy Mini Kit (Qiagen, Hilden, Germany), and complementary DNA (cDNA) was synthesized using the cDNA Reverse Transcription Kit (#FSQ-301, TOYOBO Co., Ltd., Osaka, Japan). Real-time PCR was performed using FastStart Universal SYBR Green (Roche Molecular Biochemicals), specific primers, and equal amounts of each cDNA sample. The primer sequences used for RT-PCR are listed in Table 1. The thermal cycling conditions were as follows: initial denaturation at 95 °C for 10 min, followed by 40 cycles of 95 °C for 15 s, 60 °C for 1 min, and a final step at 65 °C for 5 s. The relative expression of each gene was normalized to the expression level of RPLP0 and calculated using the ∆∆Ct method.

Table 1. Primer sequences used during RT-PCR analysis.

Origin	Gene	Direction	Sequence (5'-3')
Mouse	Acc	forward	TCTATTCGGGGTGACTTTC
		reverse	CTATCAGTCTGTCCAGCCC
	Fabp4	forward	GGGAACCTGGAAGCTTGTCT
		reverse	ACTCTCTGACCGGATGGTGA
	Fasn	forward	AGAAGCCATGTGGGGAAGATT
		forward	AGCAGGGACAGGACAAGACAA
	Gpat	forward	GTAGTTGAACTCCTCCGACA
		forward	ATCCACTACCACTGAGAGGA
	Scd1	forward	TTCTTGCGATACACTCTGGTGC
		reverse	CGGGATTGAATGTTCTTGTCGT
	Rplpo	forward	GTGCTGATGGGCAAGAAC
		reverse	AGGTCCTCCTTGGTGAAC

2.10. Total Phenolic Content

The total phenolic content was determined using the Folin–Ciocalteu method [16]. Briefly, 0.1 mL of the sample or standard (gallic acid) was mixed with 0.1 mL of Folin–Ciocalteu phenol reagent (#F9592, Sigma-Aldrich) and incubated for 5 min at room temperature. Subsequently, 1 mL of 7% Na_2CO_3 solution and 0.4 mL of distilled water were added, and the mixture was incubated for 2 h at room temperature in the dark. The absorbance of the resulting solution was measured at 760 nm using a microplate reader (Molecular Devices). The results were expressed as gallic acid equivalents per 1 mg of dry weight (μg GAE/mg of dried weight).

2.11. Total Flavonoid Content

The total flavonoid content was determined using a colorimetric method with slight modifications [17]. Briefly, 0.1 mL of the sample or standard (quercetin) was mixed with 1 mL of diethylene glycol (H26456, Sigma-Aldrich) and 0.1 mL of 1 N NaOH. The mixture was allowed to react at 30 °C for 1 h. Subsequently, the absorbance of the reaction product was measured at 420 nm using a microplate reader (Molecular Devices). The flavonoid content of the sample was expressed in quercetin equivalent units (μg QE/mg of dried weight).

2.12. Total Polysaccharide Content

The total polysaccharide content was determined using the phenol–sulfuric acid method [18]. Briefly, a 0.1 mL aliquot of a 5% phenol solution (#P4557, Sigma-Aldrich) was added to 0.1 mL of the sample or standard (glucose) and thoroughly mixed. Thereafter, 0.5 mL of sulfuric acid (#258105, Sigma-Aldrich) was added to the mixture, which was incubated at room temperature for 10 min. The absorbance of the resulting product was measured at 490 nm using a microplate reader (Molecular Devices). The polysaccharide content was expressed as glucose equivalent units (µg GE/mg of dried weight).

2.13. Statistical Analysis

All experiments were conducted in triplicate, with the results being presented as mean ± standard deviation (mean ± SD). Statistical significance was assessed using a one-way analysis of variance followed by Tukey's post hoc test for multiple comparisons or an unpaired two-tailed Student's *t*-test using Prism 8 software (GraphPad Software, San Diego, CA, USA). A *p* value of 0.05 indicated statistical significance.

3. Results

3.1. Effects of the PWE on Body Weight Changes in HFD-Induced Obese Mice

ORO staining analysis was conducted to compare the inhibitory effects of PWE and PEE on lipid accumulation. Our results showed that PWE had a stronger potential to inhibit lipid accumulation than PEE (Supplementary Figure S1). Based on these findings, an animal study was conducted to evaluate the effects of *P. ferulae* on obesity using its water extract (PWE). Mice were fed a HFD supplemented with PWE for 8 weeks while the changes in their body weight were monitored. The HFD group exhibited significantly greater body weight gain than the ND group, whereas the PWE group showed significantly lower body weight gain than the HFD group (Figure 1A). Specifically, after 8 weeks on the HFD, the HFD group had an average weight gain of 23.5 g, whereas the PWE group showed a weight reduction of 14.0 g (Figure 1B).

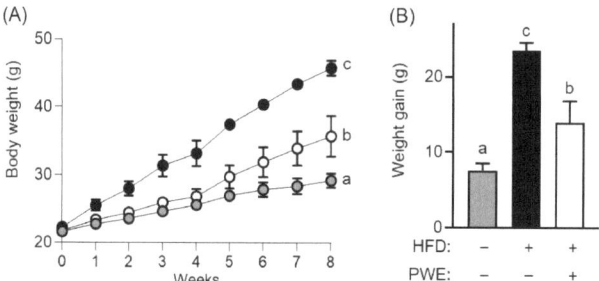

Figure 1. Anti-obesity effects of *Pleurotus ferulae* water extract (PWE) intake in high-fat-diet-induced obese mice. Alteration in body weight over 8 weeks (**A**) and weight gain after 8 weeks (**B**) in the high-fat-induced obese model with or without PWE intake. All results are expressed as mean ± standard deviation (SD) (*n* = 3). Different letters indicate significant differences (*p* < 0.05) determined via one-way analysis of variance followed by Tukey's post hoc test.

3.2. Effects of PWE on Body Fat Mass and Adipocyte Area in HFD-Induced Obese Mice

Consistent with the trend in body weight changes, the body fat mass measured using the InAlyzer was significantly greater in the HFD group (53.4%) than in the ND group (23%), with a lower increase observed in the PWE-supplemented group (46.5%) than in the HFD group (Figure 2A,B). Furthermore, PWE supplementation significantly reduced the tissue mass of adipose tissue (−23.9%) and liver (−41.8%) compared to the HFD group (Figure 2C,D). Additionally, H&E staining revealed that the adipocyte area in epididymal white adipose tissue was significantly larger in the HFD group (15,299.4 µm^2) than in the ND group (3287.9 µm^2). However, the PWE group (7560.9 µm^2) showed a significant reduction in adipocyte size despite receiving a HFD (Figure 2E,F). These findings suggest that PWE effectively suppressed HFD-induced weight gain and adipocyte hypertrophy.

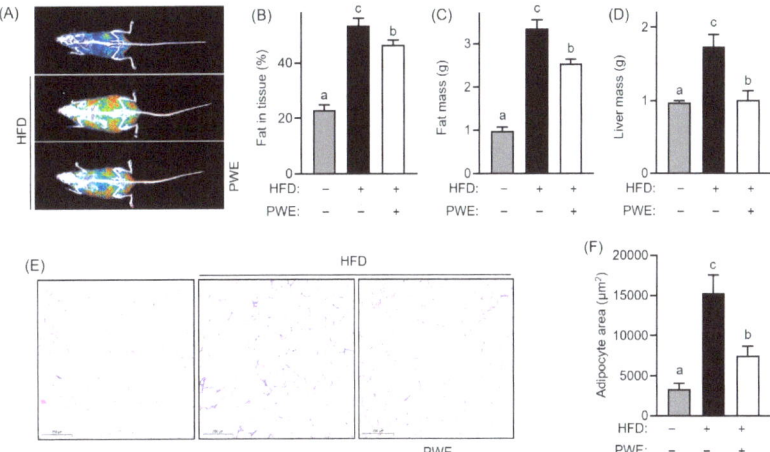

Figure 2. Effects of *Pleurotus ferulae* water extract (PWE) intake on tissue mass and morphological changes induced by a high fat diet. Alteration in body image (**A**), body fat content (**B**), fat mass (**C**), and liver mass (**D**). Hematoxylin and eosin (H&E) staining image (**E**) and adipocyte size (**F**) of epididymal white adipose tissue in a high-fat diet-induced obese model with or without PWE intake. All results are expressed as mean ± standard deviation (SD) (n = 3). Different letters indicate significant differences ($p < 0.05$) determined via one-way analysis of variance followed by Tukey's post hoc test.

3.3. Effects of PWE on Serum TC and LDL-C Levels in HFD-Induced Obese Mice

To further investigate the effects of PWE on lipid metabolism, the serum levels of TC and LDL-C were analyzed. Notably, both the TC and LDL-C levels were higher in the HFD group than in the ND group (Figure 3A,B). However, PWE treatment significantly reduced the TC and LDL-C levels in mice receiving the HFD. These results indicate that PWE intake effectively mitigated the lipid imbalances associated with HFD-induced obesity.

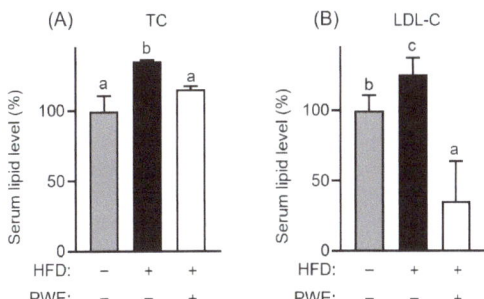

Figure 3. Effects of *Pleurotus ferulae* water extract (PWE) intake on lipid profiles following a high fat diet. Alterations in total serum cholesterol (**A**) and serum low-density lipoprotein cholesterol levels (**B**) in a high-fat-diet-induced obese model with or without PWE intake. All results are expressed as mean ± standard deviation (SD) (n = 3). Different letters indicate significant differences ($p < 0.05$) determined via one-way analysis of variance followed by Tukey's post hoc test.

3.4. Effects of PWE on Lipid Accumulation in 3T3-L1 Adipocytes

The 3T3-L1 preadipocyte differentiation model was utilized to investigate the effects of PWE on obesity at the cellular level. First, we conducted a cell viability assay using the MTT reagent. After the supplementation of PWE at various concentrations (0–200 µg/mL) during differentiation, no cytotoxicity was observed in the PWE-treated groups (Figure 4A).

Based on these results, treatment concentrations of 100 and 200 µg/mL were selected for further experiments. Subsequently, the inhibition of lipid accumulation was assessed using ORO staining (Figure 4B). More lipid droplets were observed in the differentiated group than in the control group. However, PWE treatment dose-dependently decreased lipid accumulation, with the group treated with 200 µg/mL of PWE showing an approximately 20% lower lipid accumulation than the DMSO-treated group (Figure 4C). These findings indicate that PWE effectively inhibited lipid accumulation during adipocyte differentiation without affecting cell viability.

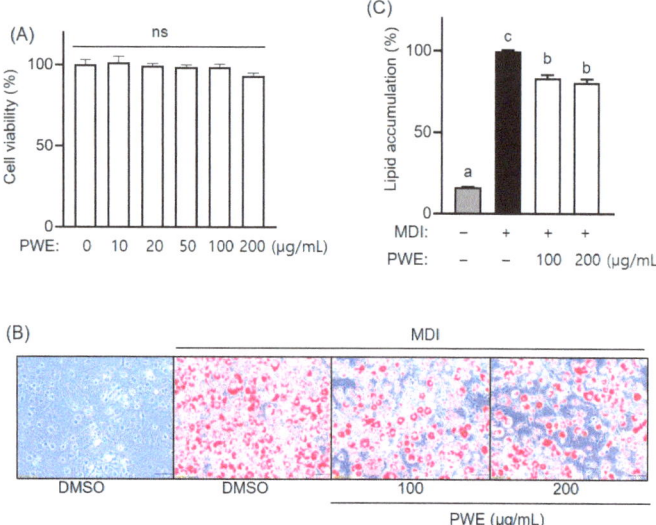

Figure 4. Effects of *Pleurotus ferulae* water extract (PWE) on cytotoxicity and lipid accumulation in 3T3-L1 cells. PWE cytotoxicity in 3T3-L1 adipocytes (**A**) was assessed using the MTT assay. Lipid droplet images were captured using microscopy (**B**), and lipid accumulation (**C**) after Oil Red O staining was measured in 3T3-L1 adipocytes with or without PWE treatment. All results are expressed as mean ± standard deviation (SD) (n = 3). Different letters indicate significant differences ($p < 0.05$) determined via one-way analysis of variance followed by Tukey's post hoc test. ns, not significant.

3.5. Effects of PWE on Lipid Metabolism-Related Factors in 3T3-L1 Adipocytes

To further assess the effects of PWE on lipid accumulation, the expression of the key proteins involved in adipogenesis and lipogenesis was analyzed. Our results showed that PPARγ, C/EBPα and ACLY expression significantly increased during adipocyte differentiation. However, differentiated adipocytes treated with PWE significantly reduced the expression levels of these proteins (Figure 5A,B). Additionally, the mRNA expression levels of genes essential for adipogenesis and lipogenesis, such as Acc, Fabp4, Fasn, Gpat, and Scd1, were upregulated during differentiation. However, PWE treatment decreased the expression levels of such genes (Figure 6). Collectively, these findings suggest that PWE effectively reduced lipid accumulation in adipocytes by suppressing the expression of genes associated with lipid metabolism during differentiation.

3.6. Analysis of the Major Bioactive Compounds in PWE

Finally, the total phenolics, flavonoids, and polysaccharides in PWE were quantified using colorimetric methods to identify the bioactive components in *P. ferulae*. Notably, phenolics and flavonoids were undetectable in the PWE; however, PWE contained a significant number of polysaccharides (662.2 µg GE/mg of dried weight; Table 2). In contrast, the PEE also lacked phenolics and flavonoids but contained lower polysaccharide levels than the PWE. This finding suggests that the high polysaccharide content in PWE may play a significant role in its potential effects on lipid accumulation and that polysaccharides are likely a key component in the health benefits of *P. ferulae*.

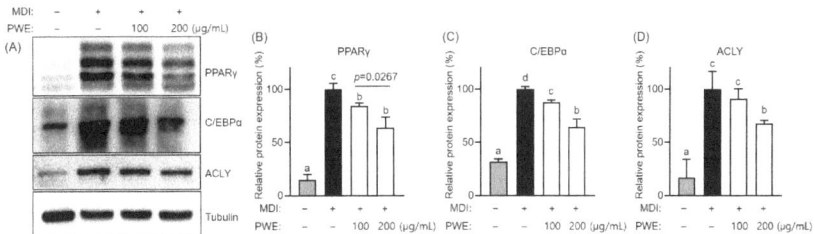

Figure 5. Effects of *Pleurotus ferulae* water extract (PWE) on adipogenesis-associated protein expression in 3T3-L1 adipocytes. Band images (**A**) and quantification of PPARγ (**B**), C/EBPα (**C**) and ACLY (**D**) by Western blot assay in 3T3-L1 adipocytes with or without PWE treatment. All results are expressed as mean ± standard deviation (SD) (n = 3). Different letters indicate significant differences ($p < 0.05$) determined via one-way analysis of variance followed by Tukey's post hoc test. Statistical significance (p value) was determined using the unpaired two-tailed Student's t-test.

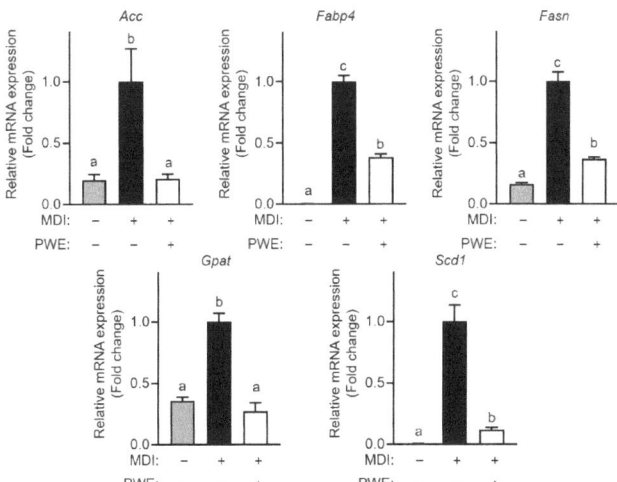

Figure 6. Effects of *Pleurotus ferulae* water extract (PWE) on adipogenesis-associated gene expression in 3T3-L1 adipocytes. qPCR analysis was conducted to quantify the mRNA expression of Acc, Fabp4, Fasn, Gpat, and Scd1 in 3T3-L1 adipocytes with or without PWE treatment. All results are expressed as mean ± standard deviation (SD) (n = 3). Different letters indicate significant differences ($p < 0.05$) determined via one-way analysis of variance followed by Tukey's post hoc test.

Table 2. Total phenolic acid content, total flavonoid content, and total polysaccharide content of *Pleurotus ferulae* water extract (PWE) or *Pleurotus ferulae* ethanol extract (PEE).

	PWE	PEE
Total phenolic content (μg GAE)/mg dried weight)	Not detected	Not detected
Total flavonoid content (μg QE)/mg dried weight)	Not detected	Not detected
Total polysaccharide content (μg GE)/mg dried weight)	662.17 ± 8.78	549.59 ± 3.89

GAE; gallic acid equivalents, QE; quercetin equivalents, GE; glucose equivalents.

4. Discussion

Obesity is characterized by an increase in body weight due to excessive fat accumulation [19]. This condition not only affects physical appearance but also significantly contributes to the development of metabolic diseases, such as diabetes and cardiovascular diseases [20]. These metabolic disturbances have been closely associated with insulin resistance and chronic inflammation, which together disrupt lipid homeostasis [21]. Consequently, this vicious cycle has been considered a major risk factor for numerous health issues, underscoring the need for strategies that effectively address and manage excessive fat accumulation and its systemic effects.

Adipose tissue, an insulin-sensitive peripheral organ, plays a critical role in maintaining energy homeostasis by secreting various hormones [22]. Adipogenesis involves a complex transcriptional cascade wherein transcription factors, such as PPARγ, are sequentially activated at the molecular level [23]. Additionally, PPARγ works synergistically with C/EBPα to support the synthesis and transport of free fatty acids (FFAs), processes that are vital for lipid metabolism and the proper functioning of adipose tissue in energy regulation [24]. However, under conditions of obesity, these transcription factors, PPARγ and C/EBPα, not only enhance insulin-mediated glucose uptake but also contribute to increased FFA production. Therefore, targeting these transcriptional pathways in differentiating adipocytes represents a promising therapeutic strategy for addressing obesity [25]. Our findings revealed that PWE treatment significantly reduced the protein expression levels of PPARγ and C/EBPα in differentiated 3T3-L1 cells, a widely used model for studying adipocyte differentiation. Additionally, PWE suppressed the insulin-induced activation of lipogenic genes, lipid transport, and lipid droplet formation. These findings suggest that PWE exerts anti-adipogenic and anti-lipogenic effects by modulating the key transcription factors involved in insulin-stimulated adipocyte differentiation. Furthermore, an 8-week administration of PWE in high-fat-diet-induced obese mice resulted in significant reductions in body weight, fat mass, and serum levels of TC and LDL-C.

Recent studies have highlighted the anti-obesity potential of various edible mushrooms, attributing their effects to bioactive compounds [26,27]. For example, the phenolic-rich fractions of *Melanoleuca stridula*, *Chlorophyllum agaricoides*, and *Tricholoma populinum* showed higher radical-scavenging activity than their organic solvent extracts [28,29]. Moreover, a phenolic-rich extract of *Pleurotus eryngii* was reported to exert anti-inflammatory activity by inhibiting NF-κB signaling-mediated inflammation pathways [30]. Fiber intake from *Agaricus bisporus* mushrooms significantly reduced serum cholesterol and LDL levels by upregulating LDL receptor expression [31]. The administration of Yamabushitake mushroom (*Hericium erinaceus*) in HFD-induced obese mice significantly decreased their body weight gain and fat weight by modulating the expression of lipid metabolic genes, including PPARα [32]. Another study found that the consumption of a HFD supplemented with alkaloid mushrooms from *Lentinus edodes* reduced HFD-induced increases in serum triglyceride and LDL levels [33]. Additionally, *P. ostreatus* has been shown to suppress lipid synthesis by modulating the gut microbiota, thereby improving lipid and glucose metabolism in HFD-supplemented mouse models [34]. Overall, these findings suggest that supplementation with *P. ferulae*, which is rich in polysaccharides, could be a promising strategy for alleviating obesity and its associated metabolic dysregulation. However, further research is needed to fully understand the specific molecular pathways through which *P. ferulae* reduces lipid accumulation in mature adipocytes and in vivo models.

Although phenolic acids and flavonoids have been considered the most common bioactive components in mushroom species, other functional compounds, including sterols, terpenoids, and polysaccharides, have also been found in mushrooms [35,36]. Polysaccharides, in particular, have garnered significant attention for their anticancer and immunomodulatory activities [37]. Furthermore, polysaccharides have been shown to alter gut microbiota composition, support the growth of beneficial bacteria, and reduce fat accumulation in obese mice, thereby promoting weight reduction [38]. Evidence also shows that they are capable of reducing oxidative stress and improving lipid profiles in diabetic mice by lowering triglyceride and TC levels [39]. Furthermore, recent clinical trials have suggested that polysaccharides can act as prebiotics, positively influencing the composition of the human gut microbiota [40]. Several polysaccharides with lipid-lowering effects, including glucans, heteroglycans, fucoidan, ulvan A, ulvan B, gentiobiose, and agaropectin, have been identified [41]. In addition, pectic-type polysaccharides such as rhamnogalacturonan-I (RG-I) and homogalacturonan (HG) have demonstrated potential in addressing metabolic disorders, including insulin resistance, inflammation, and diet-induced obesity [42]. Interestingly, the lipid-lowering activity of polysaccharides appears to be closely linked to their monosaccharide composition. For example, $(1\rightarrow3,1\rightarrow4)$-$\beta$-D-glucan and arabinoxylan can inhibit the reabsorption of bile acids in the large intestine, promoting bile salt excretion [43]. This process stimulates the use of plasma cholesterol for bile synthesis, effectively reducing blood TC and LDL-C levels. Additionally, polysaccharides with higher molecular weights tend to form more viscous gels, which increase the viscosity within the gastrointestinal tract [44]. This property restricts the diffusion of lipids and lipases, thereby slowing the lipolytic process and reducing blood lipid levels. Accordingly, exploring the polysaccharide components in PWE with lipid-lowering effects could provide valuable insights and significant therapeutic opportunities for managing metabolic disorders.

Consequently, polysaccharides from natural sources have been attracting considerable attention owing to their potential to improve various metabolic disorders, including obesity. In the current study, we confirmed that PWE was rich in polysaccharides, suggesting that its anti-obesity effects may be attributed to these compounds. However, further analysis is necessary to identify the individual active components and clarify their mechanisms of action. Conducting liquid chromatography–mass spectrometry analysis to isolate and characterize the polysaccharides present in PWE is essential. Such efforts could spearhead the application of mushroom polysaccharides in the functional food industry and support the development of targeted functional ingredients for obesity prevention and management.

5. Conclusions

Our findings suggest that *P. ferulae* effectively alleviated HFD-induced obesity and its associated metabolic disturbances. Using both animal and cellular models, we demonstrated that PWE supplementation significantly reduced body weight, fat mass, and the serum levels of TC and LDL-C in HFD-induced obese mice. Furthermore, PWE supplementation decreased lipid accumulation and adipocyte hypertrophy in white adipose tissue. In 3T3-L1 adipocytes, PWE inhibited lipid accumulation, reduced lipid droplet formation, and suppressed the expression of key adipogenic and lipogenic transcription factors, including PPARγ and C/EBPα. A further compound analysis of PWE revealed high levels of polysaccharides, which have been previously shown to exhibit anti-obesity, antioxidant, anti-inflammatory, and metabolic regulatory properties. Given the observed effects in our study, polysaccharides appear to be promising active components that account for the beneficial impact of PWE on lipid metabolism and adipocyte regulation. The influence of PWE on both systemic lipid regulation and cellular lipid metabolism presents a promising pathway for developing functional food ingredients targeting obesity and metabolic health.

Supplementary Materials: The following supporting information can be downloaded at: https://www.mdpi.com/article/10.3390/nu16234139/s1, Figure S1: Effects of *Pleurotus ferulae* water extract (PWE) or Pleurotus ferulae ethanol extract (PEE) on lipid accumulation in 3T3-L1 cells.

Author Contributions: Conceptualization, J.P. and Y.L.; writing—original draft. S.H.; methodology, S.H., S.P. (Soohyun Park) and Y.L.; data curation, S.H., S.P. (Seonkyeong Park) and J.L.; formal analysis, S.H., J.L., S.P. (Seonkyeong Park) and S.P. (Soohyun Park); funding acquisition, J.P.; supervision, Y.L.; writing—review and editing, Y.L. All authors have read and agreed to the published version of the manuscript.

Funding: This work was supported by the Main Research Program (E0210400 and E0210601) of the Korea Food Research Institute and funded by the Ministry of Science, ICT, and Future Planning. The authors thank members of the Personalized Diet Research Group for their support, collegiality, and critical review of the manuscript.

Institutional Review Board Statement: This study adhered to ethical guidelines for animal experimentation and was approved by the Institutional Animal Care and Use Committee of the Korea Food Research Institute (Approval No: KFRI-M-23007; approved on 4 December 2023).

Informed Consent Statement: Not applicable.

Data Availability Statement: The data presented in this study are available upon request from the corresponding author.

Conflicts of Interest: The authors declare no conflicts of interest.

References

1. Longo, M.; Zatterale, F.; Naderi, J.; Parrillo, L.; Formisano, P.; Raciti, G.A.; Beguinot, F.; Miele, C. Adipose Tissue Dysfunction as Determinant of Obesity-Associated Metabolic Complications. *Int. J. Mol. Sci.* **2019**, *20*, 2358. [CrossRef] [PubMed]
2. Guo, L.; Li, X.; Tang, Q.-Q. Transcriptional regulation of adipocyte differentiation: A central role for CCAAT/enhancer-binding protein (C/EBP) β. *J. Biol. Chem.* **2015**, *290*, 755–761. [CrossRef] [PubMed]
3. Zuo, Y.; Qiang, L.; Farmer, S.R. Activation of CCAAT/enhancer-binding protein (C/EBP) α expression by C/EBPβ during adipogenesis requires a peroxisome proliferator-activated receptor-γ-associated repression of HDAC1 at the C/ebpα gene promoter. *J. Biol. Chem.* **2006**, *281*, 7960–7967. [CrossRef] [PubMed]
4. Audano, M.; Pedretti, S.; Caruso, D.; Crestani, M.; De Fabiani, E.; Mitro, N. Regulatory mechanisms of the early phase of white adipocyte differentiation: An overview. *Cell Mol. Life Sci.* **2022**, *79*, 139. [CrossRef]
5. Pettinelli, P.; Videla, L.A. Up-regulation of PPAR-γ mRNA expression in the liver of obese patients: An additional reinforcing lipogenic mechanism to SREBP-1c induction. *J. Clin. Endocrinol. Metab.* **2011**, *96*, 1424–1430. [CrossRef]
6. Vekic, J.; Zeljkovic, A.; Stefanovic, A.; Jelic-Ivanovic, Z.; Spasojevic-Kalimanovska, V. Obesity and dyslipidemia. *Metabolism* **2019**, *92*, 71–81. [CrossRef]
7. Giudetti, A.M. Editorial: Lipid metabolism in obesity. *Front. Physiol.* **2023**, *14*, 1268288. [CrossRef]
8. Vekic, J.; Stefanovic, A.; Zeljkovic, A. Obesity and Dyslipidemia: A Review of Current Evidence. *Curr. Obes. Rep.* **2023**, *12*, 207–222. [CrossRef]
9. Stadler, J.T.; Marsche, G. Obesity-related changes in high-density lipoprotein metabolism and function. *Int. J. Mol. Sci.* **2020**, *21*, 8985. [CrossRef]
10. Zhou, M.; Huang, J.; Zhou, J.; Zhi, C.; Bai, Y.; Che, Q.; Cao, H.; Guo, J.; Su, Z. Anti-Obesity Effect and Mechanism of Chitooligosaccharides Were Revealed Based on Lipidomics in Diet-Induced Obese Mice. *Molecules* **2023**, *28*, 5595. [CrossRef]
11. Li, J.; Wu, H.; Liu, Y.; Yang, L. High fat diet induced obesity model using four strains of mice: Kunming, C57BL/6, BALB/c and ICR. *Exp. Anim.* **2020**, *69*, 326–335. [CrossRef] [PubMed]
12. Sumaira, S.; Muhammad, S.; Muhammad, M.; Sumia, A.; Ayoub, R. Wild Mushrooms: A Potential Source of Nutritional and Antioxidant Attributes with Acceptable Toxicity. *Prev. Nutr. Food Sci.* **2017**, *22*, 124–130.
13. Ganesan, K.; Xu, B. Anti-Obesity Effects of Medicinal and Edible Mushrooms. *Molecules* **2018**, *23*, 2880. [CrossRef] [PubMed]
14. Cirlincione, F.; Gargano, M.L.; Venturella, G.; Mirabile, G. Conservation Strategies of the Culinary-Medicinal Mushroom *Pleurotus nebrodensis* (Basidiomycota, Fungi). In Proceedings of the 2nd International Electronic Conference on Diversity (IECD 2022)—New Insights into the Biodiversity of Plants, Animals and Microbes, Online, 15–31 March 2022.
15. Wang, W.; Chen, K.; Liu, Q.; Johnston, N.; Ma, Z.; Zhang, F.; Zheng, X. Suppression of tumor growth by Pleurotus ferulae ethanol extract through induction of cell apoptosis, and inhibition of cell proliferation and migration. *PLoS ONE* **2014**, *9*, e102673. [CrossRef] [PubMed]
16. Gutfinger, T. Polyphenols in olive oils. *J. Am. Oil Chem. Soc.* **1981**, *58*, 966–968. [CrossRef]
17. Moreno, M.I.N.; Isla, M.I.; Sampietro, A.R.; Vattuone, M.A. Comparison of the free radical-scavenging activity of propolis from several regions of Argentina. *J. Ethnopharmacol.* **2000**, *71*, 109–114. [CrossRef]
18. DuBois, M.; Gilles, K.A.; Hamilton, J.K.; Rebers, P.t.; Smith, F. Colorimetric method for determination of sugars and related substances. *Anal. Chem.* **1956**, *28*, 350–356. [CrossRef]
19. Björntorp, P. Metabolic implications of body fat distribution. *Diabetes Care* **1991**, *14*, 1132–1143. [CrossRef]
20. Sarma, S.; Sockalingam, S.; Dash, S. Obesity as a multisystem disease: Trends in obesity rates and obesity-related complications. *Diabetes Obes. Metab.* **2021**, *23* (Suppl. S1), 3–16. [CrossRef]
21. Gasmi, A.; Noor, S.; Menzel, A.; Pivina, L.; Bjørklund, G. Obesity and insulin resistance: Associations with chronic inflammation, genetic and epigenetic factors. *Curr. Med. Chem.* **2021**, *28*, 800–826. [CrossRef]
22. Hwang, I.; Kim, J.B. Two faces of white adipose tissue with heterogeneous adipogenic progenitors. *Diabetes Metab. J.* **2019**, *43*, 752–762. [CrossRef] [PubMed]

23. Ambele, M.A.; Dhanraj, P.; Giles, R.; Pepper, M.S. Adipogenesis: A complex interplay of multiple molecular determinants and pathways. *Int. J. Mol. Sci.* **2020**, *21*, 4283. [CrossRef] [PubMed]
24. Oger, F.; Dubois-Chevalier, J.; Gheeraert, C.; Avner, S.; Durand, E.; Froguel, P.; Salbert, G.; Staels, B.; Lefebvre, P.; Eeckhoute, J. Peroxisome proliferator-activated receptor γ regulates genes involved in insulin/insulin-like growth factor signaling and lipid metabolism during adipogenesis through functionally distinct enhancer classes. *J. Biol. Chem.* **2014**, *289*, 708–722. [CrossRef] [PubMed]
25. Kopchick, J.J.; Berryman, D.E.; Puri, V.; Lee, K.Y.; Jorgensen, J.O. The effects of growth hormone on adipose tissue: Old observations, new mechanisms. *Nat. Rev. Endocrinol.* **2020**, *16*, 135–146. [CrossRef] [PubMed]
26. Mustafa, F.; Chopra, H.; Baig, A.A.; Avula, S.K.; Kumari, S.; Mohanta, T.K.; Saravanan, M.; Mishra, A.K.; Sharma, N.; Mohanta, Y.K. Edible Mushrooms as Novel Myco-Therapeutics: Effects on Lipid Level, Obesity and BMI. *J. Fungi* **2022**, *8*, 211. [CrossRef]
27. Abdelshafy, A.M.; Belwal, T.; Liang, Z.; Wang, L.; Li, D.; Luo, Z.; Li, L. A comprehensive review on phenolic compounds from edible mushrooms: Occurrence, biological activity, application and future prospective. *Crit. Rev. Food Sci. Nutr.* **2022**, *62*, 6204–6224. [CrossRef]
28. Bahadori, M.B.; Sarikurkcu, C.; Yalcin, O.U.; Cengiz, M.; Gungor, H. Metal concentration, phenolics profiling, and antioxidant activity of two wild edible Melanoleuca mushrooms (*M. cognata* and *M. stridula*). *Microchem. J.* **2019**, *150*, 104172. [CrossRef]
29. Sezgin, S.; Dalar, A.; Uzun, Y. Determination of antioxidant activities and chemical composition of sequential fractions of five edible mushrooms from Turkey. *J. Food Sci. Technol.* **2020**, *57*, 1866–1876. [CrossRef]
30. Hu, Q.; Yuan, B.; Xiao, H.; Zhao, L.; Wu, X.; Rakariyatham, K.; Zhong, L.; Han, Y.; Kimatu, B.M.; Yang, W. Polyphenols-rich extract from Pleurotus eryngii with growth inhibitory of HCT116 colon cancer cells and anti-inflammatory function in RAW264.7 cells. *Food Funct.* **2018**, *9*, 1601–1611. [CrossRef]
31. Fukushima, M.; Nakano, M.; Morii, Y.; Ohashi, T.; Fujiwara, Y.; Sonoyama, K. Hepatic LDL Receptor mRNA in Rats Is Increased by Dietary Mushroom (*Agaricus bisporus*) Fiber and Sugar Beet Fiber. *J. Nutr.* **2000**, *130*, 2151–2156. [CrossRef]
32. Hiwatashi, K.; Kosaka, Y.; Suzuki, N.; Hata, K.; Mukaiyama, T.; Sakamoto, K.; Shirakawa, H.; Komai, M. Yamabushitake mushroom (*Hericium erinaceus*) improved lipid metabolism in mice fed a high-fat diet. *Biosci. Biotechnol. Biochem.* **2010**, *74*, 1447–1451. [CrossRef] [PubMed]
33. Yang, H.; Hwang, I.; Kim, S.; Hong, E.J.; Jeung, E.B. Lentinus edodes promotes fat removal in hypercholesterolemic mice. *Exp. Ther. Med.* **2013**, *6*, 1409–1413. [CrossRef] [PubMed]
34. Hu, Y.; Xu, J.; Sheng, Y.; Liu, J.; Li, H.; Guo, M.; Xu, W.; Luo, Y.; Huang, K.; He, X. Pleurotus Ostreatus Ameliorates Obesity by Modulating the Gut Microbiota in Obese Mice Induced by High-Fat Diet. *Nutrients* **2022**, *14*, 1868. [CrossRef] [PubMed]
35. Łysakowska, P.; Sobota, A.; Wirkijowska, A. Medicinal Mushrooms: Their Bioactive Components, Nutritional Value and Application in Functional Food Production—A Review. *Molecules* **2023**, *28*, 5393. [CrossRef] [PubMed]
36. Kumar, K.; Mehra, R.; Guiné, R.P.; Lima, M.J.; Kumar, N.; Kaushik, R.; Ahmed, N.; Yadav, A.N.; Kumar, H. Edible mushrooms: A comprehensive review on bioactive compounds with health benefits and processing aspects. *Foods* **2021**, *10*, 2996. [CrossRef] [PubMed]
37. Kiddane, A.T.; Kim, G.-D. Anticancer and immunomodulatory effects of polysaccharides. *Nutr. Cancer* **2021**, *73*, 2219–2231. [CrossRef]
38. Chang, C.J.; Lin, C.S.; Lu, C.C.; Martel, J.; Ko, Y.F.; Ojcius, D.M.; Tseng, S.F.; Wu, T.R.; Chen, Y.Y.; Young, J.D.; et al. Ganoderma lucidum reduces obesity in mice by modulating the composition of the gut microbiota. *Nat. Commun.* **2015**, *6*, 7489. [CrossRef]
39. Huang, H.-Y.; Korivi, M.; Chaing, Y.-Y.; Chien, T.-Y.; Tsai, Y.-C. Pleurotus tuber-regium polysaccharides attenuate hyperglycemia and oxidative stress in experimental diabetic rats. *Evid.-Based Complement. Altern. Med.* **2012**, *2012*, 856381. [CrossRef]
40. Ho Do, M.; Seo, Y.S.; Park, H.-Y. Polysaccharides: Bowel health and gut microbiota. *Crit. Rev. Food Sci. Nutr.* **2021**, *61*, 1212–1224. [CrossRef] [PubMed]
41. Tang, C.; Wang, Y.; Chen, D.; Zhang, M.; Xu, J.; Xu, C.; Liu, J.; Kan, J.; Jin, C. Natural polysaccharides protect against diet-induced obesity by improving lipid metabolism and regulating the immune system. *Food Res. Int.* **2023**, 113192. [CrossRef]
42. Lee, H.-B.; Kim, Y.-S.; Park, H.-Y. Pectic polysaccharides: Targeting gut microbiota in obesity and intestinal health. *Carbohydr. Polym.* **2022**, *287*, 119363. [CrossRef]
43. Gunness, P.; Flanagan, B.M.; Gidley, M.J. Molecular interactions between cereal soluble dietary fibre polymers and a model bile salt deduced from 13C NMR titration. *J. Cereal Sci.* **2010**, *52*, 444–449. [CrossRef]
44. Espinal-Ruiz, M.; Restrepo-Sánchez, L.-P.; Narváez-Cuenca, C.-E.; McClements, D.J. Impact of pectin properties on lipid digestion under simulated gastrointestinal conditions: Comparison of citrus and banana passion fruit (*Passiflora tripartita* var. *mollissima*) pectins. *Food Hydrocoll.* **2016**, *52*, 329–342. [CrossRef]

Disclaimer/Publisher's Note: The statements, opinions and data contained in all publications are solely those of the individual author(s) and contributor(s) and not of MDPI and/or the editor(s). MDPI and/or the editor(s) disclaim responsibility for any injury to people or property resulting from any ideas, methods, instructions or products referred to in the content.

MDPI AG
Grosspeteranlage 5
4052 Basel
Switzerland
Tel.: +41 61 683 77 34

Nutrients Editorial Office
E-mail: nutrients@mdpi.com
www.mdpi.com/journal/nutrients

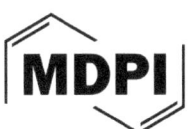

Disclaimer/Publisher's Note: The title and front matter of this reprint are at the discretion of the Guest Editor. The publisher is not responsible for their content or any associated concerns. The statements, opinions and data contained in all individual articles are solely those of the individual Editor and contributors and not of MDPI. MDPI disclaims responsibility for any injury to people or property resulting from any ideas, methods, instructions or products referred to in the content.

www.ingramcontent.com/pod-product-compliance
Lightning Source LLC
LaVergne TN
LVHW072334090526
838202LV00019B/2420